Nursing Care of Older People with Diabetes

Edited by Trisha Dunning
AM, RN, MEd, PhD, CDE, FRCNA

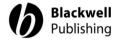

Blackwell
Publishing

Editorial offices:
Blackwell Publishing Ltd, 9600 Garsington Road, Oxford OX4 2DQ, UK
    Tel: +44 (0)1865 776868
Blackwell Publishing Inc., 350 Main Street, Malden, MA 02148–5020, USA
    Tel: +1 781 388 8250
Blackwell Publishing Asia Pty Ltd, 550 Swanston Street, Carlton, Victoria 3053, Australia
    Tel: +61 (0)3 8359 1011

First published 2005 by Blackwell Publishing Ltd

ISBN-10: 1-4051-2364-8
ISBN-13: 978-1-4051-2364-8

Library of Congress Cataloging-in-Publication Data
Nursing care of older people with diabetes/edited by Trisha Dunning.
        p. ; cm.
    Includes bibliographical references and index.
    ISBN-13: 978-1-4051-2364-8 (pbk. : alk. paper)
    ISBN-10: 1-4051-2364-8 (pbk. : alk. paper)
    1. Diabetes in old age–Nursing.
    [DNLM: 1. Diabetes Mellitus–nursing–Aged.   2. Diabetes Complications–Aged.   WY
155 N9736 2005] I. Dunning, Trisha. II. Title.
    RC660.75.N87 2005
    618.97′6462—dc22
    2004028171

A catalogue record for this title is available from the British Library

Set in 10/12pt Souvenir
by Graphicraft Limited, Hong Kong
Printed and bound in India
by Replika Press Pvt Ltd, Kundli

The publisher's policy is to use permanent paper from mills that operate a sustainable forestry policy, and which has been manufactured from pulp processed using acid-free and elementary chlorine-free practices. Furthermore, the publisher ensures that the text paper and cover board used have met acceptable environmental accreditation standards.

For further information on Blackwell Publishing, visit our website:
www.blackwellnursing.com

Contents

Author profiles

Trisha Dunning AM, RN, MEd, PhD, CDE, FRCNA
Department of Endocrinology and Diabetes
St. Vincent's Hospital
Victoria, Australia
Professor Trisha Dunning is Director of Endocrinology and Diabetes Nursing Research at St. Vincent's Hospital and the University of Melbourne. She has been a diabetes educator for 20 years and is passionate about holistic nursing care. Trisha is the author of several books for people with diabetes and many books and papers for health professionals. She is an active researcher with a focus on people's beliefs and attitudes and how they affect professional care and self-care. Trisha is a very active worker on a great many Australian and international diabetes committees.

Angus Forbes BSc, MSc, PhD, RGN, RHV, DNCert, CPT
Primary Care Section
Florence Nightingale School of Nursing and Midwifery
King's College London
London, United Kingdom
Dr Angus Forbes is Research Fellow at King's College London, School of Nursing and Midwifery. Angus has a clinical background in community nursing and primary health care, having worked as a district nurse, health visitor and community practice teacher. Angus' academic background is in health services research, particularly in chronic disease management, including work examining diabetes care for older people. Angus conducts diabetes courses for nurses and other professionals and he is still actively providing diabetes care.

Susan Hunt
Independent Practitioner
Victoria, Australia
Susan Hunt is currently working in independent practice while she completes her PhD thesis entitled *Quality Use of Medicines in Residential Aged Care.* She has extensive experience working with older people in the community, rehabilitation and residential settings, specialising in quality use of medicines, continence promotion and care of people with dementia. Susan has authored a number of books, papers and educational materials for health professionals. She has been highly active in medicine policy development since the late 1980s and is currently a director of the National Prescribing Service in Australia.

Michelle Robins BN, CDE, M. Health Sc (Health Education and Health Promotion), Grad Cert Nursing (Gerontology), Grad Cert Health Sc (Wound Management)

Logan Beaudesert Health Service
Queensland, Australia

Michelle has been a Diabetes Educator since 1993, working in a variety of hospital and community settings. In 1998 she worked at Melbourne Extended and Rehabilitation Service, which included transition services, amputee and neurological rehabilitation, dementia assessment in low and high aged care settings. This experience enabled Michelle to identify and appreciate the differences and complexities of managing older people with diabetes and fuelled a desire to communicate with and mentor other health professionals about diabetes care in older people. Currently Michelle is the Integrated Team Leader at Logan Beaudesert Health Service. Although this district covers a wide area and population, it also has a large number of retirement villages. Michelle is chair of the Queensland Branch of the Australian Diabetes Educators Association and was a steering committee member for the development of the *Guidelines for the Management and Care of Diabetes in the Elderly.*

List of Figures

List of Tables

Foreword

Most health professionals and an increasing number of people within the community are recognising that Type 2 Diabetes Mellitus is one of our most common disabling medical disorders that is associated with a significant health, social, and economic burden. We know that in some northern European countries, for example, diabetes may be present in nearly 1 in 3 subjects above the age of 70 and older people with diabetes constitute the largest proportion of acute hospitalisations for diabetes. Hospital care is, of course, extremely expensive care and whilst equity of access to investigation and to specialist care must be present in our aging population at the same time, there are many advantages to focusing diabetes care within the community and keeping older people closer to home. Whilst in many cases, diabetes care may be relatively straightforward for patients in their 60s and early 70s but, with advancing age and with increasing levels of medical comorbidities, diabetes care for frail elderly people can take on a very complex nature with many challenges. This book, edited by Trisha Dunning, has taken on one of these important challenges and in my view, has produced a text which is a delight to read.

First of all, this book is incredibly comprehensive and should be able to deal with the majority of problems encountered in older people and as such will not only be first line reading for nurses and other non-medical health professionals, but I think will also be informative for many physicians delivering diabetes care for this often vulnerable group of subjects. I was particularly impressed with the layout of the book which starts off with a very useful introduction to diabetes and older people and then follows with a discussion of assessment processes and developing care systems. The important emphasis on nutrition and on maintaining mobility is vitally important to such a text. And the later emphasis on promoting quality of life and optimising mental health is spot on! Of course, quite naturally, many of these areas apply equally to much younger patients, especially those who may have had a serious vascular episode in their early 40s or 50s. In essence, part of their diabetes care will revolve around a model of disability and part around a model of therapeutic intervention. The importance of recognising and treating hypoglycaemia is well illustrated in this book and the section on education and communication is particularly pertinent. Later chapters dealing with rehabilitation, mental health, medication, and sexuality are well organised in this marvellous textbook. I was particularly intrigued with the section on complementary therapies.

I have always been a strong advocate for nurses specialising in the management of older people with diabetes and this textbook is one of a few resources that are available that provide a unique insight into the complexity of care in older people and also bring with this some of the joy that is experienced in managing patients with this disorder.

Professor Alan J. Sinclair MSc MD FRCP (Edin) FRCP (Lond)
Professor of Medicine (Geriatrics) and Consultant Diabetologist

Preface

Older people have a special place in my heart, especially now, as I join their ranks.

I spent a great deal of my early childhood being cared for by my grandmother, great aunt and great grandmother – active country women who loved the land and animals and who were problem solvers. Grandma had wonderful sayings that influenced the person I became, such as 'a whistling woman is good to neither God nor man'. Needless to say, I can't whistle!

Many of the first people I cared for as a trainee nurse were old and demented. I was taught holistic nursing practice by the Government Medical Officer in the country hospital where I trained. My love of poetry and writing was fostered by another elderly doctor, who also taught me how they could be used in nursing and self-care. Although none of these people had diabetes, they showed the contribution older people make to health care and society in general. Diabetes was relatively uncommon. My first encounter with a person with diabetes was a school friend who developed gestational diabetes, which was devastating and frightening for all concerned.

For the last few years I have been receiving phone calls from nursing colleagues seeking advice about how to manage diabetes in older people. I have watched them struggle with staff shortages and the undervalued status of aged care nursing. I watched outstanding leaders and advocates of nursing older people, including Sally Garrett and Rhonda Nay, promote aged care nursing.

My fellow authors are experts in their own right and have made a significant contribution to aged care nursing through their writings, teachings and examples. Angus has conducted research into improving care systems for older people. Michelle is well recognised in the Australian diabetes scene for her contribution to diabetes care in general and particularly to wound care in elderly people with diabetes. Susan Hunt was involved at the inception of the Quality Use of Medicines programme in Australia and has made a significant contribution to the care of older people.

Diabetes presents particular challenges to aged care nurses regardless of whether the person is self-caring and living in the community, requires considerable assistance in the community or lives in residential aged care facilities. Diabetes is a serious and increasing global health problem associated with life-threatening conditions and is the commonest cause of blindness in people over 60, the most common cause of lower limb amputation and the second commonest reason for commencing renal dialysis. The prevalence of diabetes in people over 65 is currently 16.8% in Australia and somewhere between 8% and 10% in the UK. Managing diabetes in older people presents many difficulties due to the 'silent' nature of the disease and its complications, and the impact of other disease processes and intercurrent illness on metabolic control. Managing medicines for older people with diabetes is a complex issue and the potential for adverse medicine events increases with the need for multiple medicines, memory impairment and reduced physical capacity. Ideal metabolic targets have been defined for people with diabetes, including older people, but are accompanied by the risk of hypoglycaemia and hypotension.

Falls risk is increased in older people generally. Diabetes significantly increases the falls risk over and above the general risk factors through hypo- and hyperglycaemia and the effect of diabetes complications. Recently, the increased rates of depression and dementia associated with diabetes have been recognised. Nutritional factors are becoming increasingly important as the role of micronutrients in reducing morbidity and mortality becomes clearer.

At present there is little specific information available about the nursing management of older people with diabetes. Diabetes *is* different in older people and specific nursing considerations may not be apparent from most current nursing texts. The aims of the book are to address the apparent deficiency by:

- Developing a comprehensive nursing text that addresses the specific nursing management of older people with diabetes. It adopts a staged approach to aged care and addresses the elderly living in the community and hostel care, but the focus is on nursing care in residential aged care facilities.
- By using research evidence, where possible, to support the care suggested.

This book is a companion to *Care of People with Diabetes* (2003, Blackwell Publishing) and expands the nursing management of older people suggested in that book. Certainly a holistic approach to care is essential. We began to decide on the content for the book in 2003. In that year the logo for World Diabetes Day, 14 November, was the yin yang symbol, now an almost universal symbol of balance.

Trisha Dunning

Acknowledgements

My sincere thanks go to Blackwell Publishing, especially Beth Knight and Lisa Whittington for embracing the proposal for this book and seeing it through to the completed product.

Thank you also to our copy editor, Holly Regan-Jones, for checking our grammar, structure and style and ensuring the book meets the house style.

Especial thanks to Susan and Angus for their contributions and particularly Michelle, for her constant emails, early morning phone calls, ideas and unstinting support.

I am indebted to Jane Ford for typing a great deal of the manuscript, especially for her ability to decipher the additional inserts.

The people who deserve special acknowledgement are my family and especially the 'wind beneath my wings' or should I say taxi driver – my husband John.

Terms used in the book

Aged care nursing
Aged care nursing refers to nursing older people and encompasses nursing older people in a diverse range of settings including hospital, the community and residential aged care homes/facilities. Other terms are 'geriatric nursing' and 'gerontological nursing'.

Aged care facilities
The term 'aged care facilities' refers to care facilities that specifically cater for older people. In Australia they may be low-level care, where the individual is largely self-caring and independent, or high-level care, where nursing care and supervision are required. Sometimes low- and high-level care facilities are located together. Other terms are 'old people's homes', 'special accommodation', 'hostel and aged care' and 'residential aged care'.

Dedication

This book is dedicated to all elderly people with diabetes and the relatives and nurses who care for them. We hope this book will make the path a little easier for both.

Other books of interest

Care of People with Diabetes
Second edition
T. Dunning
ISBN-10: 1-4051-0111-3
ISBN-13: 978-14051-0111-0

Handbook of Diabetes
Third edition
G. Williams and J.C. Pickup
ISBN-10: 1-4051-2052-5
ISBN-13: 978-14051-2052-4

Slide Atlas of Diabetes (CD-ROM)
J.C. Pickup and G. Williams
ISBN-10: 1-4051-2618-3
ISBN-13: 978-14051-2618-2

Practical Manual of Diabetic Footcare
M.E. Edmonds, A.V.M. Foster and
L.J. Sanders
ISBN-10: 1-4051-0715-4
ISBN-13: 978-14051-0715-0

Managing the Diabetic Foot
Second edition
M.E. Edmonds and A.V.M. Foster
ISBN-10: 1-4051-2970-0
ISBN-13: 978-14051-2970-1

Diabetes and its Management
Sixth edition
P.J. Watkins, S.L. Howell, S.A. Amiel
and E. Turner
ISBN-10: 1-4051-0725-1
ISBN-13: 978-14051-0725-9

Diabetes Management: Step by Step
M.H. Drucquer and P.G. McNally
ISBN-10: 0632-04848-4
ISBN-13: 978-0632-04848-9

Nursing in Care Homes
Second edition
L. Nazarko
ISBN-10: 0632-05226-0
ISBN-13: 978-0632-05226-4

Chapter 1
Introduction to Diabetes in Older People

Trisha Dunning

Key points

- Diabetes is an increasing global health problem.
- Increasing age is associated with insulin resistance that predisposes older people to diabetes.
- Type 1 diabetes can present for the first time in older people and people with Type 1 diabetes now survive longer with modern management.
- The onset of diabetes in older people can be insidious with non-specific symptoms and is often overlooked.
- Addressing the metabolic abnormalities associated with hyperglycaemia improves physical and mental functioning and quality of life.

1.1 Diabetes mellitus

Normal glucose homeostasis is dependent on several simultaneously operating variables: hormones, food intake, nutritional status, tissue sensitivity to insulin and physical activity. Table 1.1 outlines normal glucose metabolism.

Diabetes mellitus, usually known as diabetes, is a metabolic disorder in which carbohydrate, protein and fat metabolism is disturbed due to insulin resistance (Type 2 diabetes), or insulin deficiency/absence (Type 1 diabetes). Both these states lead to elevated blood glucose and glycosuria. When insulin is deficient or absent, glucose cannot be utilised for energy and accumulates in the blood. Fat stores and, in the longer term, protein are mobilised as substrates for gluconeogenesis in the liver. However, insulin is needed for the complete metabolism of fats. In the absence of insulin (Type 1 diabetes), ketone bodies accumulate and predispose the individual to ketoacidosis. Insulin deficiency in Type 2 diabetes predisposes the person to hyperosmolar states (see Chapter 4). Protein breakdown contributes to the hyperglycaemia, since the new glucose cannot enter the cells without insulin. In addition, fat breakdown leads to weight loss, and protein breakdown to loss of muscle mass and delayed wound healing. These can be significant problems in older people who are already predisposed to skin trauma and who are often malnourished.

Table 1.1 Normal glucose metabolism is a complex process depending on a balance between glucose uptake and glucose utilisation, production and storage. A constant supply of glucose is necessary for optimal mental functioning.

Ready fuel	Fuel stores	
Circulating blood glucose	Hepatic glycogen stores	
After food	Between meals	Longer term
• Glucose enters bloodstream and stimulates the pancreas to secrete insulin (glucose-mediated insulin production).	• Other hormones, e.g. adrenaline, cortisol and growth hormone, release glucose stores from the liver and muscle.	• In the longer term glucose is manufactured in the liver from fat and protein stores (gluconeogenesis and glycogenolysis). These are known as fuel substrates.
• Insulin attaches to receptor sites on the cell membranes.	• Insulin is required for the new glucose to enter the cells.	• Insulin is needed for the new glucose to enter the cells.
• Initiates a cascade of intracellular events that allows glucose to enter the cells.		
• Used for immediate energy or stored.		

The diagnosis of diabetes depends on finding persistently elevated blood glucose levels. The currently accepted diagnostic criteria are shown in Table 1.2. Recently, the World Health Organization and the International Diabetes Federation launched a new initiative, Diabetes Action Now, that aims to stimulate support for appropriate diabetes screening, prevention and management measures to achieve global awareness of diabetes and its complications.

1.2 Classification of diabetes

The American Diabetes Association (ADA) and the World Health Organization (WHO) revised the classification of diabetes in 1997. As part of the revised classification the terms insulin dependent diabetes mellitus (IDDM) and non-insulin dependent diabetes mellitus (NIDDM) were replaced with Type 1 and Type 2 diabetes respectively (Expert Committee on the Diagnosis and Classification of Diabetes Mellitus 1997). The new classification consists of:

(1) Type 1 diabetes, which has two forms:
   - immune-mediated diabetes mellitus as a result of autoimmune destruction of the pancreatic beta cells
   - idiopathic diabetes mellitus, which refers to forms of the disease that have no known aetiologies.

Table 1.2 Diagnostic criteria for diabetes mellitus based on Coleman *et al.* 1999. Fasting plasma glucose is preferred for diagnosis, however, in certain circumstances random plasma glucose or oral glucose tolerance tests are needed to make the diagnosis. In this table venous plasma glucose values are shown. Glucose in capillary blood is about 10–15% higher than venous blood.

Stage	Fasting plasma glucose	Random plasma glucose	Oral glucose tolerance test (OGTT)
Normal	<5.5 mmol/L	<5.5 mmol/L	2 hour plasma glucose <7.8 mmol/L
Impaired glucose tolerance is possible. Diabetes cannot be excluded. Repeat the test. If the repeat test is abnormal, do an OGTT.	5.5–6.9 mmol/L	5.5–11 mmol/L	Impaired glucose tolerance – 2 hour plasma glucose ≥7.8 and <11.1 mmol/L
Diabetes present.	≥7.0 mmol/L	≥11.1 mmol/L and symptoms	2 hour plasma glucose >11.1 mmol/L

(2) Type 2 diabetes mellitus, in which relative insulin deficiency and insulin resistance occur. The majority of older people have Type 2 diabetes and more than 20% of people diagnosed with diabetes already have retinopathy and macrovascular disease (National Health and Medical Research Council 1992).

(3) Impaired glucose homeostasis, which is an intermediate metabolic stage between normal glucose homeostasis and diabetes. It carries a significant risk of cardiovascular disease and is divided into two forms:
   - impaired fasting glucose (IFG) where the fasting plasma glucose is higher than normal but lower than the diagnostic criteria.
   - impaired glucose tolerance (IGT) where the plasma glucose is higher than normal and lower than the diagnostic criteria after a 75-gram glucose tolerance test.

   There is a considerable overlap between IFG and IGT but these are not synonymous or mutually exclusive states and people in this category can be considered to have impaired glucose regulation (WHO 1999).

(4) Gestational diabetes mellitus (GDM), which occurs during pregnancy and then usually resolves. However, women who develop GDM are at risk of Type 2 diabetes, which may first manifest in older age.

(5) Other specific types include diabetes caused by other identifiable disease processes such as:
   - genetic defects of beta cell function such as maturity onset diabetes of the young (MODY)
   - genetic defects of insulin action
   - diseases of the exocrine pancreas that affect beta cell function, such as cancer and pancreatitis
   - endocrine disorders such as Cushing's disease and acromegaly

- drug- or chemical-induced diabetes, which may be a more common contributing factor in older age than previously recognised with increasing drug treatment of comorbidities and depression where medicines such as glucocorticoids and olanzapine induce hyperglycaemia.

1.2.1   Older people at high risk of diabetes

Understanding the different diabetes states can help nurses plan health care and appropriately allocate resources, identify individuals at risk of diabetes and institute appropriate screening programmes in aged care environments so that early management can be instituted and coexisting morbidity reduced. In particular, people who should be monitored regularly in the community and care facilities:

- Are older, especially if they have IFG or IGT and become unwell.
- Have a family history of diabetes.
- Come from high-risk ethnic groups such as people from the Indian subcontinent, China and Aboriginal and Torres Strait Islander peoples.
- Had gestational diabetes when they were young.
- Have known complications of diabetes such as renal and cardiovascular disease, hypertension, dyslipidaemia.
- Are overweight and inactive.
- Are commenced on diabetogenic drugs such as glucocorticoids, thiazide and diuretics, beta blockers and some antipsychotic drugs such as olanzapine.

1.2.2   Prevalence of diabetes

The prevalence of diabetes in all ages and both sexes has slowly increased globally, with a steep rise occurring since the 1960s. The overall global prevalence in 2004 was 2.8% with a projected rise to 4.4% in 2030 (Wild *et al.* 2004). Some of the increase is due to the lower normal range for blood glucose set out in the diagnostic criteria determined in 1999, greater awareness of the condition, knowledge of the pathogenesis of complications, better screening processes and improved diagnostic methods (Sinclair & Finucane 1995). Perhaps the most significant factor is the enhanced survival rate due to modern treatment methods, which means people live longer and diabetes and other diseases are more effectively managed. Age is one of the most important factors that accounts for the increasing prevalence of diabetes in most societies and the majority of people with diabetes are aged over 65 years, with prevalence rates up to 40% (Popplewell *et al.* 1997; Dunstan *et al.* 2001).

However, the sex ratio for diabetes varies widely between countries; for example, in Africa and the Americas there is a male dominance whereas in the Pacific countries, females predominate (King & Rewers 1993). Migrant populations are particularly at risk of developing diabetes, which may be associated with changes in lifestyle. In addition, population subgroups, including those who live in institutional care, have a high prevalence of diabetes. Therefore, the recommendation for regular screening to detect diabetes early is justified.

Often diet and inactivity associated with residential care and comorbidities make it difficult for people to eat an appropriate diet and remain active. Diabetes occurs in up to 18% of older people and a further 11% have IGT. One in four older people in residential aged care facilities has diabetes.

The high prevalence of diabetes alone represents significant direct health costs spent on screening and diagnosis, preventive education and managing the disease and its short- and long-term complications. Indirect costs include pain, suffering and effects on the individual's physical and psychological being that profoundly affect their quality of life.

1.3 Normal ageing and the development of diabetes

1.3.1 Classification of older people

Ageing is not a disease but it does involve a gradual decline in physiological function that results in a reduced ability to respond to stress. Older people are a diverse group which can be divided chronologically into the:

- Young old 65–74 years.
- Middle old 75–79 years.
- Old, over 80 years.

However, the characteristics of ageing are very individual – that is, people age at individual rates and their specific organs age at different rates. The term 'old' is used loosely to describe anyone over 65 years, based on an arbitrary figure set in Germany 100 years ago, which largely related to when people retired from paid work. Retirement age is changing: some people retire earlier and some work until they are well past 65. Perhaps a more useful classification might be active old age, old age and advanced old age, where the criteria are concerned with quality of life, independence and state of mind (Hammond & Jilek 2003).

Some people have a positive outlook on life and are able to maintain vitality and energy until well into old age. These people have an inbuilt coping style and resilience that enable them to cope with their changing physical status, which is a normal part of ageing. Some older people are better at compensating for ageing decline than others. Much of the way people cope depends on their inherent personality, resilience and locus of control.

Physical decline occurs when the body can no longer adapt to the changes, especially when illness or trauma occurs. The focus often then becomes coping with the consequences of the illness – frailty, weakness, pain and, in the case of diabetes, the unremitting quest for blood glucose control and a great deal of self-care. Older people often focus on survival. People with a positive mental outlook live longer and are usually more fulfilled (Levy *et al.* 2002). Health problems increase with advancing age, fatigue, stress, anxiety and depression are common and older people often have financial constraints. However, older age can be a period of growth and fulfilment.

Older people are often also divided into two basic groups. The first group, the majority, are self-caring and live at home. The second much smaller group live in residential aged care facilities. Regardless of where the person lives and their age and functional status, their diabetes must be adequately managed within their physical, social and psychological context and their family and carers adequately supported to reduce the effects of diabetes and its complications on these parameters. However, the management is often complex and difficult (see Chapter 2). The major normal age-related changes occurring in each body system are shown in Table 1.3.

Table 1.3 Major normal age-related changes according to the body systems, the consequences of the changes and some suggested management strategies.

Body system changes	Consequences	Management strategies
Integumentary system Thin wrinkled skin Dry skin Heat intolerance More prominent bone structure Prominent veins and capillaries Reduced secretion of natural oils Reduced perspiration	Trauma, pressure areas, burns and bruises occur more easily.	Wear protective clothing, bed coverings. Heat to appropriate ambient temperatures. Bath or shower less frequently to maintain natural skin oils. Use non-soap options free from harsh chemicals. Use emollient creams if skin is particularly dry.
Respiratory system Increased residual lung volume and vital capacity that leads to lower gaseous exchange Reduced cough reflex These factors are complicated by osteoporosis and kyphosis that limit chest expansion	Easy fatiguability. Breathlessness. Increased risk of URTI and pneumonia. Impaired tissue oxygenation and nourishment, therefore delayed wound healing. Difficulty coughing up secretions and increased potential for prolonged pneumonia. Sleep apnoea. Reduced activity levels. Confusion. Falls during acute episodes.	Encourage regular activity and deep breathing exercises. Avoid smoking. Ensure fluid intake is adequate. Avoid exposure to airborne infections in care facilities by using appropriate infection control practices. Regular, yearly influenza vaccinations and other vaccinations as indicated.
Cardiovascular system	Reduced cardiac output. Heart valves become thicker and stiffer due to calcium deposits. Reduced increase in heart rate and stroke volume in response to stress (e.g. CCF, cancer, PVD and MI) and slower recovery rate when the stress subsides. Dysrrhythmias. Increased blood pressure, especially systolic due to primary hypertension and diabetes. Fatiguability. Intermittent claudication. Falls risk.	Encourage regular physical activity. Stop smoking. Encourage low-fat, high-fibre, low-salt diet and weight control. Consider antioxidant supplements. Education to recognise urgency of need to seek medical advice and appropriate symptoms since MI is often silent in people with diabetes. Stress management. Regular health checks, e.g. blood pressure, glucose and lipids and general health status. Regular medication reviews. Preventive vaccines.

Musculoskeletal system

Loss of bone density, increasing the risk of osteoporosis and stress fractures.
Reduced muscle strength and mass.
Reduced height.
Joint degeneration and increased stiffness, making activity and fine motor skills more difficult.
Pain.
Falls and trauma risk.
Pressure ulcer risk

Regular physical activity, especially weight bearing and tai chi.
High-calcium, well-balanced diet.
Calcium and vitamin D supplements.
Modify the environment to reduce falls risk.
Manage pain.
Provide options to encourage the person to continue self-care activities.

Gastrointestinal system

Reduced salivation, dry mouth.
Dysphagia, which increases the risk of aspiration and the need for enteral feeding.
Reduced oesophageal and gut motility.
Reduced pepsin and hydrochloric acid production in the stomach, which affects digestion and absorption of iron, calcium and vitamin D, which in turn increase the risk of anaemia and osteoporosis.
Increased tendency to heartburn, indigestion, flatulence and constipation.
Reduced number of taste receptors, which affects appetite and enjoyment of food.
Mouth and dental changes that mean the dentures may not fit correctly, predisposing the individual to mouth ulcers.

Regular mouth and dental care.
Small frequent meals. Supplements such as vitamins and calcium.
Sit up after meals.
High-fibre, low-fat diet, with adequate fluids.
Note foods that cause problems and avoid.
Consider possibility of coeliac disease.
Regular toileting and gentle aperients if necessary.
Avoid strenuous activity after food.
Antacids if necessary.

Nervous system

Reduced number of brain cells.
Slower reaction to stimuli.
Confusion during illness and in unfamiliar environments.
Reduced cerebral circulation which affects balance and can precipitate falls, fainting, postural hypotension and TIAs.
Reduced amount of sleep needed.

Plan education appropriately.
Provide sensory stimulation.
Encourage regular exercise.
Encourage individual to change position slowly (lying to sitting to standing), bend from the knees rather than bending over and/or rise slowly after bending over.

Table 1.3 *(cont'd)*

Body system changes	Consequences	Management strategies
	Takes longer to absorb and remember information. Neuropathies that increase falls and pressure area risk. Reduced thirst sensation and consequent risk of dehydration, especially in hot weather.	Stay awake in the daytime. Investigate confusion. Manage sleep apnoea and investigate for associated diseases such as cardiovascular if present. Treat illnesses quickly and adequately. Remind individual to drink during hot weather. Appropriate foot care including footwear.
Genitourinary system		
Men: Benign prostatic hyperplasia and cancer.	Urinary retention and/or frequency. Incomplete bladder emptying. Nocturia. Falls risk.	Ready access to toilet facilities. Wear easy-to-remove clothing. Pelvic floor exercises. Drink adequate fluids, including before and after investigative procedures involving the urinary tract and radiocontrast media.
Women: Relaxed perineal muscles and detrusor and urethral dysfunction.	Urge and stress incontinence.	Avoid constipation, appropriate high-fibre diet and aperients if necessary. Avoid substances that irritate the bladder such as caffeine, carbonated drinks, alcohol and artificial sweeteners.
Both: Nephron loss with reduced filtration rate and reabsorption. Slower correction of acid–base balance.	Changed drug metabolism and elimination. Increased risk of metabolic abnormalities. Falls risk.	Monitor fluid balance and hydration status, especially in hot weather. Regular medication review.
Reproductive system		
	Men: Reduced size of the penis and testes. Delayed erections and orgasm. Slower arousal. Women: Reduced vaginal elasticity and secretions leading to vaginal dryness, painful intercourse and vaginal trauma during sexual activity and medical procedures. Slower sexual responses.	Careful sex history and appropriate sensitive examination. Sex education, including how to give and receive pleasure. Management of erectile dysfunction in men. Appropriate vaginal lubrication during sexual activity and medical examinations. Providing privacy and confidentiality in care facilities and keeping couples together. Regular pap smears and mammograms. Avoid ageist attitudes.

The senses: vision, hearing, taste and smell	*Vision*: reduced ability to focus on near objects. Glare intolerance. Difficulty adjusting to changes in light intensity. Poor night vision, which affects night driving. Reduced ability to distinguish colours, especially blue and green, which affects education and reading. *Hearing*: more difficult to hear high-pitched sounds. Inappropriate responses during conversation. Leans forward to hear. Boredom, confusion, social isolation. Reduced quality of life and depression. *Taste and smell*: both reduced, which affects food enjoyment and appetite.	Use appropriate education material. Wear glasses or hearing aid. Regular eye checks and change of glasses prescription when necessary. Regular assessment of suitability to drive. Modify lighting to avoid glare yet provide adequate lighting for reading and safety. Regular hearing assessment. Reduce noise. Look at the person when speaking to them, speak slowly and clearly and use non-verbal cues. Consider whether poor intake is due to reduced vision. Check ability to shop and prepare food at home.
Psychosocial and cognitive changes Although not strictly a system, psychological health and quality of life are affected by ageing and affect all the physical systems.	Brain changes that lead to reduced ability to learn and process information. Reduced short-term memory (5–30 seconds), recent memory (one hour to several days). Slower to acquire, register, retain and retrieve information. Easy distraction. Coping and resilience may be reduced. Confusion. Behavioural problems. Falls risk Depression, self-care deficits.	Life care plans. Regular cognitive and mental health assessments performed at optimal times in suitable environments. Appropriate management of sensory deficits. Provide cues to memory. Community social support systems.

References

Ebersole, P. & Hess, P. (1998) *Toward Healthy Aging: Human Needs and Nursing Response*, 5th edn. Mosby, St Louis.
Leuckenotte, A. (1996) Gerontologic assessment. In: *Gerontologic Nursing* (ed. A. Leuckenotte). Mosby, St Louis.
Whitehead, C. & Finucane, P. (1995) Is it just my age doctor? Separating normality from pathology in old age. *Modern Medicine of Australia*, **163**, 94–101.

1.3.2   The normal ageing process

Intrinsic ageing (within the individual) is genetically determined and is essentially common to everybody. Extrinsic ageing results from factors external to the individual such as illness, pollution, excess sun exposure and smoking. These factors cause changes in physical appearance and in physical and mental functioning. At a cellular level the ability to maintain homeostasis and cellular regeneration diminishes with age. The major normal age-related changes are shown in Table 1.3 according to the body system they affect. Particular problems encountered in older people due to the effects of diabetes are shown in Table 1.4. The net effect of these age-related and diabetes changes for acute and residential care is:

- Increased risk of comorbidities and diabetes complications that predispose the person to infection and functional decline.
- Frequent assessment is necessary to detect changes early.
- Encouraging ambulation, activity, deep breathing and sometimes medicines is necessary to reduce the risk of respiratory infections and venous thrombosis.
- Assistance may be required with activities of daily living on a temporary or permanent basis.
- The assessment carried out in acute settings may not reflect functional status or cognitive ability once the acute problem resolves.
- Environmental issues such as noise, light and frequent disturbance can affect an older person's adjustment to new situations.
- Controlling blood glucose levels reduces hospital morbidity and mortality rates (Krinsley 2004).

Practice point

People may have been given information about what to do when they become sick and may know what to do but be too unwell or incapacitated to undertake necessary self-care. Sometimes the best advice to give an older community-dwelling person is to call a relative or their doctor.

As people age pharmacological intervention becomes more likely to maintain homeostasis and manage abnormalities. Polypharmacy is likely in older people with diabetes due to the long-term complications, normal ageing process and comorbidities. All of these factors increase the possibility that the person will require:

- Assessment in the emergency department.
- Admission to hospital.
- Community services to maintain them in the community.
- Assistance from family or carers.
- Admission to residential aged care.
- Multidisciplinary, co-ordinated assessment and management.

1.3.3   Pharmacology and ageing

There is no doubt that medicines improve health and wellbeing. However, the normal ageing process affects the pharmacodynamics and pharmacokinetics of most drugs

Table 1.4 Particular problems encountered in older people with diabetes and the resultant risks associated with the problem. Many of these problems are accompanied by significant pain and disability. Adapted with permission from Dunning 2003.

Problem	Associated risk
Hyperglycaemia leading to short-term complications: • polyuria and polydipsia leading to dehydration, electrolyte imbalance and changed fuel substrate use for energy • dry skin and mucous membranes • constipation • postural hypotension • impaired cognition.	Incontinence. Infections including urinary tract infections. Delayed wound healing. Thrombosis. Lethargy and reduced activity. Sleep disturbances. Hyperosmolar states. Ketoacidosis. Impaired cognition. Reduced mood and depression. Compromised self-care. Falls and trauma. Chronic long-term complications if not corrected.
Inadequate food intake, absorption, utilisation.	Nutritional deficiencies. Impaired immune response, which increases the risk of infection, delayed wound healing and other morbidities and mortality. Reduced plasma albumin that can alter drug transport. Hypoglycaemia. Lethargy. Falls.
Cerebral insufficiency and increased prevalence of vascular dementia and Alzheimer's disease.	TIAs and stroke. Non-recognition of hypoglycaemia TIAs mistaken for hypoglycaemia. Impaired cognition and compromised self-care. Education difficulties. Safety issues, e.g. when driving. Falls and trauma risk.
Cardiac insufficiency.	Cardiac dysrhythmias and cardiomyopathy. Myocardial infarction. Confusion. Reduced peripheral circulation and poor tissue perfusion increasing the risk of foot and leg ulcers and pressure ulcers. Peripheral oedema. Altered drug distribution, which affects medicine choices. Intermittent claudication and reduced exercise capacity. Falls and trauma.
Neuropathy: • peripheral • autonomic • other isolated neuropathies such as Bell's palsy.	Peripheral: • unstable gait • non-recognition of trauma • foot ulcers • pressure ulcers • burns • falls and trauma • pain

Table 1.4 (*cont'd*)

Problem	Associated risk
	• sleep disturbances • reduced quality of life. Autonomic: • postural hypotension • non-recognition of hypoglycaemia • silent myocardial infarction • silent urinary tract infections • incontinence • gastroparesis, leading to delayed food absorption, inadequate nutrition, bloating, food fermenting in the stomach and bacterial overgrowth and delayed drug absorption • erratic blood glucose pattern • erectile dysfunction in men • pain • depression and compromised self-care • falls and trauma. Isolated neuropathies may lead to feeding difficulties, reduced mobility, muscle wasting and body image problems depending on the nerves involved. Increased risk of enteral feeding.
Renal disease.	Reduced urine output. Increased risk of urinary tract infections. Reduced drug clearance and increased risk of toxicity. Increased hypoglycaemia risk. Risk of lactic acidosis with metformin. Oedema. Skin itch and potential infection. Falls and trauma. Nausea and changed appetite that lead to nutritional deficiencies. Increased likelihood of needing dialysis.
Increased tissue glycosylation.	Carpal tunnel syndrome, Dupuytren's contracture. Joint stiffness. Self-care deficits including managing medicines. Potential need for surgery. Stiffening blood vessel walls leading to hypertension.
Visual impairment.	Self-care deficits including managing medicines and blood glucose testing. Compromised diabetes care increasing the possibility of hyper- or hypoglycaemia. Education difficulties. Social isolation – failure to keep appointments, reduced activity. Loss of independence, e.g. ability to drive safely and read. Depression. Falls and trauma.

Table 1.4 (*cont'd*)

Problem	Associated risk
Skin atrophy.	Pressure ulcers. Skin tears. Foot pathology.
Mental health, including cognitive impairment, depression and dementia.	Communication difficulties. Inappropriate eating. Self-care deficits. Social isolation. Education difficulties. Possibility of being prescribed diabetogenic drugs. Stress on family and carers.

and adjustments or changes to the dose or dose interval may be necessary (see Chapters 2 and 9), as well as adjustments for specific reasons such as surgery, investigative procedures and enteral feeding (see Chapter 7). Some specific pharmacological issues to consider are shown in Table 1.5.

1.3.4   Metabolic changes associated with ageing

Research into the pathophysiology of diabetes in older people is a relatively new occurrence (Sinclair & Finucane 1995). The genetic make-up of the individual is an important contributing factor to the development of diabetes and is exacerbated by the factors outlined in Section 1.2.1. In addition, glucose metabolism changes with increasing age. Glucose-induced insulin release and glucose-mediated glucose disposal change and contribute to glucose intolerance (Iozzo *et al.* 1999). Importantly, the degree of the reduction in insulin secretion is more apparent to an oral glucose load than to intravenous glucose. The relevance of this issue to clinical care is unknown but it may be relevant to diagnostic and hypoglycaemic management procedures.

The most important pathophysiologic mechanism underlying glucose intolerance in older people is insulin resistance, especially tissue resistance to insulin-mediated glucose disposal (Ferrannini 1996). Specifically, the person may produce sufficient quantities of insulin but the tissues do not respond to insulin and glucose does not readily enter the cells. Under usual circumstances, the individual shows few effects of insulin resistance. However, stress states further increase the degree of insulin resistance and metabolic decompensation can occur and require treatment. It is not clear whether age-related insulin resistance is part of the normal ageing process or is a result of lifestyle changes that occur with increasing age, especially in care facilities. Both factors probably play a part.

Regardless of the underlying mechanism, the outcome is that older people are often diagnosed when they become ill and less able to cope with the diagnosis or the self-care tasks required. Regular screening can identify people with glucose intolerance and allow lifestyle modification and management strategies to be implemented early. Checking for existing diabetes complications is an important aspect of

Table 1.5 Relative and absolute contraindications to exercise in older people with diabetes. Supervision may be needed if the person is cognitively impaired or has visual deficits.

Issue	Possible consequences
Polypharmacy	Drug–drug and drug–food interactions that increase the risk of emergency presentations and hospital admission. Confusion and compliance difficulties may mean medicines are less effective but conversely, non-compliance may actually reduce some potential adverse effects.
Nutritional intake	Reduced appetite is often present, sometimes as a consequence of drugs. Conversely, some oral hypoglycaemic agents stimulate appetite and contribute to weight gain. Nausea and vomiting or bloating may mean drugs are not absorbed. Presence of gastrointestinal comorbidities and use of medicines that delay or increase absorption of medicines or nutrients, e.g.: • antacids reduce Vitamin B_{12} absorption • antibiotics and phenytoin reduce absorption of folic acid • steroids, thiazide diuretics and some antipsychotic agents cause hyperglycaemia. Hyperglycaemia, protein malnutrition and weight loss lead to reduced serum proteins and body water that leads to reduced drug binding sites and therefore more circulating free drug. Weight gain and increased deposition of body fat lead to increased drug storage and delayed elimination and therefore unpredictable action profile. High-fibre diet may increase gut transit time and reduce drug absorption.
Renal status	Accuracy of creatine clearance as a measure of renal function. Compromised renal function leads to reduced drug metabolism and clearance, which influences the choice of medicines. Risk of kidney damage with some drugs, complementary therapies and investigative procedures.
Reduced cardiac output and reduced peripheral blood flow	Delayed drug transport to target tissues, therefore delayed action. Increased tissue levels of drugs and longer duration of action. Need to consider dose form and dose interval.
Reduced gastric acid	Changed metabolism and absorption of some drugs.
Reduced saliva production	Difficulty swallowing some tablets and capsules, especially if they are large. Difficulty distinguishing dry mouth caused by hyperglycaemia from dry mouth as a side effect of drugs. Increased risk of tooth enamel damage by some drugs.

screening programmes, since more than 20% of newly diagnosed older people already have complications (National Health and Medical Research Council 1992).

Lean and obese middle-aged people have elevated fasting glucose production and reduced insulin release and insulin resistance. In contrast, lean and obese older people have normal fasting hepatic glucose production. Lean older people have impaired insulin secretion but minimal insulin resistance, which has implications for management. Obese older people usually have intact glucose-induced insulin secretion (often hyperinsulinaemia) but marked insulin resistance. An important finding is that insulin-enhanced blood flow is reduced in older obese insulin-resistant people (Meneilly & Elliott 1999). Insulin-mediated vasodilation is believed to be responsible for 30% of normal glucose disposal, yet hyperinsulinaemia is associated with vasoconstriction. The reason for the vasodilatory action of insulin has not yet been specifically identified but normalising insulin levels as well as blood glucose may increase the delivery of both insulin and glucose to the tissues.

It is increasingly being recognised that autoimmune factors and beta cell destruction play a role in the pathogenesis of diabetes in a subset of older people with diabetes. These people often have high levels of islet cell and GAD antibodies, which are markers of autoimmune beta cell destruction. The presence of these antibodies predicts the need for insulin. Some experts suggest that GAD antibody testing should be routine practice since a large proportion of lean older people with diabetes have islet cell and GAD antibodies (Zimmet 1999). Others believe the clinical significance of these antibodies in older people, and whether they predict the need for insulin or a role for therapies that modify the autoimmune destruction of the pancreas, is not clear cut (Sinclair & Finucane 1995).

However, it is important to consider the underlying metabolic abnormality when deciding on treatment options. For example, lean older people have profoundly impaired glucose-induced insulin secretion and therefore insulin is the treatment of choice. Obese people require treatments that enhance insulin-mediated glucose disposal (reduce insulin resistance) such as metformin (see Chapter 2).

Glucose can also stimulate its own uptake in the absence of insulin. This is known as glucose-mediated glucose disposal and occurs under fasting conditions and in the central nervous system, where 70% of the glucose uptake occurs by this mechanism. This phenomenon is known as glucose effectiveness. In healthy older people glucose effectiveness is impaired during fasting but is normal under hypoglycaemic conditions. Older people with diabetes have even greater impairment of glucose effectiveness. The cause of these abnormalities is currently unknown and may become increasingly important in the future.

A significant factor for diabetes management in older people is the changes in the counterregulatory hormone response, especially glucagon and growth hormone, to hypoglycaemia in normal older people and to an even greater extent in people with diabetes. As a consequence, the autonomic hypoglycaemic warning signs may not be recognised (see Chapter 4). In addition, older people have significantly impaired psychomotor performance during hypoglycaemia that prevents them from appropriately treating the hypoglycaemia, even if they have been appropriately educated about hypoglycaemia.

Practice point

Preventing short-term metabolic abnormalities and long-term diabetes complications is a priority given the current life expectancy and the high costs associated with managing complications.

1.3.5   Environmental factors and older people

Lifestyle factors affect whether or not genetically susceptible people develop diabetes when they grow older. Diabetes is more likely to develop in older people who:

- Have diets high in simple sugar and saturated fat that lead to obesity, hyperglycaemia and hyperlipidaemia. Such diets are often deficient in important vitamins and trace elements due to the production of free radicals that contribute to tissue damage. Antioxidant foods that contain Vitamin C and E improve insulin action and blood glucose levels. Supplements of zinc and magnesium also improve glucose metabolism (Paolisso *et al.* 1994).
- Are obese, especially if they have truncal obesity.
- Are inactive.
- Consume excess alcohol, which predisposes the person to intercurrent illnesses and malnutrition.

Socio-economic factors may also be a contributing factor, for example for people with lower incomes (Gullitural *et al.* 2003).

1.3.6   Effects of medicines

Many older people have coexisting diseases and intercurrent illnesses that require medicines. The disease itself can predispose the person to glucose abnormalities, for example thyroid disease and infection. In addition, many of the medicines commonly prescribed to manage pre-existing conditions and intercurrent illness induce insulin resistance, for example thiazide diuretics, glucocorticoids and some antipsychotic drugs such as olanzapine, which may not be solely due to weight gain (Proietto 2004). The diagnosis of diabetes associated with olanzapine occurs within six months of commencing treatment in 73% of cases. Weight should be monitored and a healthy lifestyle encouraged. Although diabetes appears to be a risk associated with olanzapine, the drug is more effective and better tolerated than many other antipsychotics and the risks and benefits need to be carefully considered. The hyperglycaemia usually resolves when the drug is withdrawn.

Regular physical activity appears to improve tissue response to insulin. However, some medicines such as ACE inhibitors improve insulin sensitivity in older people with diabetes and hypertension (Paolisso *et al.* 1992). Therefore, medicines that enhance blood flow may play a valuable role in blood glucose control. Of 100 unplanned emergency admissions of older people to hospital, only 21% were for acute reasons. Early intervention could have prevented the admission and a planned elective admission would have been more appropriate in 18% of admissions. It is not clear what proportion of these people had diabetes. The factors affecting physical and mental status of and service utilisation by older people are shown in Figure 1.1.

1.4   Diagnosing diabetes in older people

Early detection to reduce morbidity and mortality and maintain independence and quality of life is mandatory. Containing health costs is essential. Early diagnosis

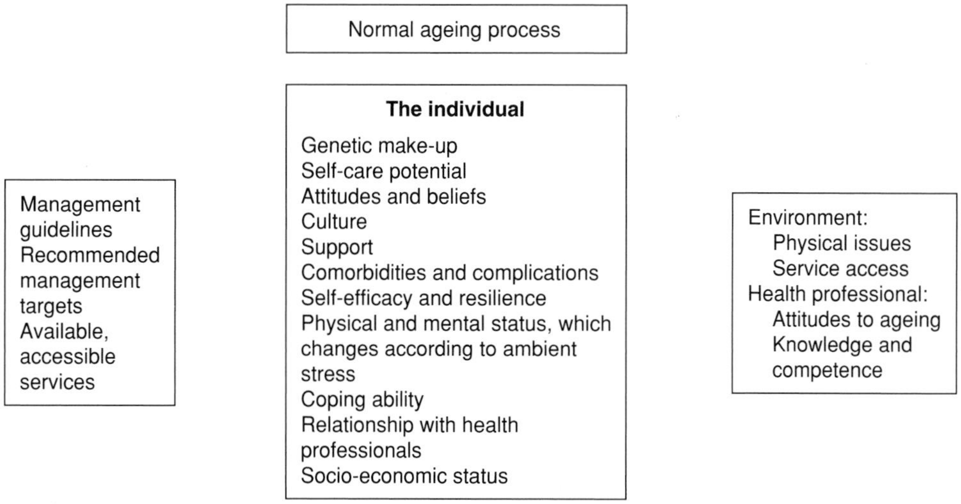

```
┌─────────────────────────────────┐
│      Normal ageing process      │
└─────────────────────────────────┘
```

The individual

Genetic make-up
Self-care potential
Attitudes and beliefs
Culture
Support
Comorbidities and complications
Self-efficacy and resilience
Physical and mental status, which
changes according to ambient
stress
Coping ability
Relationship with health
professionals
Socio-economic status

Management
guidelines
Recommended
management
targets
Available,
accessible
services

Environment:
  Physical issues
  Service access
Health professional:
  Attitudes to ageing
  Knowledge and
  competence

Figure 1.1 Multifactorial factors affecting the physical and mental status of, and service utilisation by, older people with diabetes. The interrelated and continuing nature of these factors means that a holistic, collaborative approach with clear communication between all service providers to set appropriate management targets and maintain quality of life, is essential.

requires a high degree of suspicion and regular screening since many older people with established diabetes are asymptomatic (Sinclair & Finucane 1995). The classic signs and symptoms of diabetes and the possible clinical features of diabetes in older people are shown in Table 1.6. However, many older people only exhibit non-specific symptoms that are mistaken for 'normal ageing'. Even the classic symptoms outlined in Table 1.6 may not be present. Some possible reasons for presenting to a health professional are also shown in Table 1.6.

The prevalence of diabetes, diagnosed and undiagnosed, after 80 years could be as high as 80%. Appropriate treatment reduces the morbidity and allows appropriate palliative care. The oral glucose tolerance test (OGTT) should not be performed in older people who:

- Already have a diabetes diagnosis because it could result in hyperglycaemia and increase the risk of hyperglycaemic short-term consequences.
- Have a fasting blood glucose >7 mmol/L, especially if symptoms are present.
- Who are acutely unwell or undergoing surgical procedures likely to cause metabolic stress, where false-positive results could be obtained. Screening should be undertaken after the person recovers. The hyperglycaemia should be managed in these circumstances.
- Are chronically malnourished, because the person may have limited reserves to respond to the stress of the glucose load.
- Are confined to bed for three or more days.

Table 1.6 The classic signs and symptoms of diabetes and the clinical features that are more likely to be present in older people. These features are often attributed to another cause or 'old age'. When present, they have a significant effect on quality of life.

Classic symptoms of diabetes	Clinical features of diabetes in older people	Consequences, possible reason for presentation to a health professional
Polyuria Polydipsia Polyphagia Lethargy Weight loss Hyperglycaemia Glycosuria	Osmotic diuresis.	Incontinence, dehydration. Nocturia and sleep disturbance. Impaired cognition. Risk of falls.
	Visual changes.	Impaired activities of daily living, including driving and reading. Risk of falls.
	Red blood cell deformity. Platelet adhesiveness.	Intermittent claudication, stroke, myocardial infarction, gangrene. Risk of falls.
	Recurrent infections. Poor wound healing.	Increased risk of hospitalisation. Hyperglycaemia, DKA or HONK.
	Non-specific complaints.	
	Mental changes. Depression.	Reduced self-care, memory changes. Increased risk of intercurrent illness.
	Reduced pain tolerance. Painful shoulder and other pain syndromes.	Reduced quality of life. Depression.
	Impaired recovery from a major illness.	Rehabilitation. Inability to cope. Palliative care
	Hyperosmolar non-ketotic states (see Chapter 4). Ketoacidosis (see Chapter 4).	Dehydration, seizures, thrombosis. Falls. Death.

Practice points

(1) Presentation of diabetes is atypical in older people.
(2) Diabetes can be present without any symptoms in older people or the symptoms can be mistaken for normal ageing.
(3) These factors mean the diagnosis is often delayed or made when significant morbidity is already established.
(4) Diabetes often coexists with and complicates other disease processes.

Table 1.6 illustrates the clinical features of hyperglycaemia in older people. The presence of one or more of these features should prompt the nurse to suspect diabetes, regardless of whether they are working in the community, an outpatient department or in acute or residential aged care. Managing the underlying metabolic abnormality significantly improves the outcome. Capillary blood glucose tests are not adequate to detect diabetes and venous blood samples are recommended.

1.4.1 Prevention and screening

All people over 65 years of age should be regularly screened for diabetes. Screening aims to identify people likely to have diabetes and can be accomplished by measuring the random venous plasma glucose level but fasting samples or OGTTs have a greater predictive value. They do, however, put added stress on the individual. The diagnostic values are shown in Table 1.2. Two diagnostic test results on two separate days are required unless there are definite symptoms of diabetes present.

When diabetes is not diagnosed, a repeat screen should be undertaken in 12 months or if any of the clinical features occur. The procedure for the OGTT is clearly described in a number of texts such as Sinclair & Finucane (1995) and Dunning (2003). It should be noted that the usefulness of the OGTT in older people is disputed by experts because approximately 75% of people diagnosed with IGT never develop diabetes (Sinclair & Finucane 1995) and many diagnosed using an OGTT never develop fasting hyperglycaemia or symptoms of diabetes. The diagnosis of diabetes can be socially, psychologically and financially devastating for older people and health professionals must be very sure of the diagnosis before informing the individual or their family. Conversely, it is important that people realise that there is no such thing as 'mild diabetes', especially in older people.

1.5 Nursing responsibilities

'The specialised knowledge and support required in providing care for complex, ill and elderly patients is growing in a manner that is unlikely to be addressed in the currently prevailing model of general practice.'

(Ferguson 2004)

The same sentiment could apply to other areas of practice, especially outside residential aged care facilities. The need to improve health services for older people was recognised in the UK with the development of practice guidelines (British Diabetes Association 1999) and the standards of care for aged care homes for older people (Department of Health 2001). Standards for residential aged care facilities have been in place in Australia for a number of years (Australian Quality Council 1998) and were recently revised following government reforms in aged care. Guidelines for the management of diabetes in older people were launched in 2003. However, these guidelines are concerned with defining evidence-based metabolic targets and do not address frail older people, residential care or nursing care (see Chapter 2). Guidelines for people over 80 are not well defined (Croxon 2002). Research to define safe management targets for this group is needed that takes account of cognitive deficits, falls risk, functional status, available support and quality of life.

1.5.1 Prevention and detection

(1) Be aware of the risk factors for diabetes in older people.
(2) Use nursing encounters to promote a healthy lifestyle to older people and inform at-risk individuals about the need to have regular checks for diabetes.
(3) Include diabetes risk factor screening in nursing history and assessments when caring for older people.
(4) Monitor the outcomes of medicines prescribed for older people, especially those likely to cause hyperglycaemia.
(5) Consider whether the person is using complementary therapies and over-the-counter medicines, some of which may contribute to hyperglycaemia.

1.5.2 Management

The aims of management are to:

- Set an appropriate blood glucose range to achieve freedom from the symptoms of hyperglycaemia and avoid hypoglycaemia.
- Limit the impact of coexisting diseases and intercurrent illness.
- Maintain adequate nutrition.
- Maintain functional status and quality of life.

(1) Prepare the individual appropriately for any diagnostic investigations such as fasting glucose and lipids and OGTT.
(2) Deliver care according to the presenting diagnosis, considering the special requirements of diabetes set out in Chapter 2.
(3) Be aware that diabetes impacts on the key clinical issues seen in residential aged care facilities:
    - impaired mobility and manual dexterity
    - falls and the consequent trauma
    - urinary incontinence
    - constipation and faecal incontinence
    - polypharmacy
    - cognitive impairment
    - depression
    - behavioural problems and dementia
    - pain
    - infections
    - skin integrity and wound healing.
(4) Co-ordinate care and ensure referrals are made in a timely manner to specialists or community services when appropriate.

References

Australian Quality Council (1998) *Accreditation Standards for Aged Care*. AQC, Canberra.
British Diabetes Association (1999) *Guidelines for Practice for Residents with Diabetes in Care Homes*. Diabetes UK, London.
Coleman, P., Thomas, D., Zimmet, P., Welborn, T., Garcia-Webb, P. & Moore, N. (1999) New classification and criteria for diagnosis of diabetes mellitus. Position statement from

Australian Diabetes Society, New Zealand Society for the Study of Diabetes, Royal College of Pathologists of Australasia and Australasian Association of Clinical Biochemists. *Medical Journal of Australia*, **170**(8), 375–8.

Croxon, S. (2002) Diabetes in the elderly: problems of care and service provision. *Diabetic Medicine*, **19** (suppl 4), 66–72.

Department of Health (2001) *Care Homes for Older People: National Minimal Standards of Care*. Standards Act 2000. HMSO, London.

Dunning, T. (2003) *Care of People with Diabetes. A Manual of Nursing Practice*. Blackwell Publishing, Oxford.

Dunstan, D., Zimmet, P. & Welborn, T. (2001) *Diabetes and Associated Disorders in Australia. The Accelerating Epidemic. The Australian Diabetes, Obesity and Lifestyle Study (AusDiab)*. International Diabetes Institute, Melbourne.

Expert Committee on the Diagnosis and Classification of Diabetes Mellitus (1997) Report of the Expert Committee on the Diagnosis and Classification of Diabetes Mellitus. *Diabetes Care*, **20**, 1183–97.

Ferguson, H. (2004) GPs need support in aged care. *Medical Observer*, 16 January, 8.

Ferrannini, E. (1996) European Group for the Study of Insulin Resistance. Insulin action and age. *Diabetes*, **45**, 949.

Gullitural, M., Mahahir, D. & Roke, B. (2003) Diabetes-related inequities in health status and financial barriers to health care access in a population based study. *Diabetic Medicine*, **21**, 45–51.

Hammond, G. & Jilek, R. (2003) *Caring for the Aged*. Media 21 Publishing, Sydney, Australia.

Iozzo, P., Beck-Neilsen, J., Loakso, M., Smith, U., Yki-Jarvinen, H. & Ferrannini, E. (1999) Independent influence of age on basal insulin secretion in non-diabetic humans. European Group for the Study of Insulin Resistance. *Journal of Clinical Endocrinology and Metabolism*, **84**, 863–8.

King, H. & Rewers, M. (1993) Global estimates for prevalence of diabetes mellitus and impaired glucose tolerance in adults. WHO Ad Hoc Diabetes Reporting Group. *Diabetes Care*, **16**(1), 157–77.

Krinsley, J. (2004) Effect of an intensive glucose management protocol on the mortality of critically ill adult patients. *Mayo Clinic Proceedings*, **79**(8), 992–1000.

Levy, B., Slade, M., Kunkel, S. & Kasl, S. (2002) Longevity increased by positive self-perceptions of ageing. *Journal of Personality and Social Psychology*, **83**(2), 261–70.

Meneilly, G. & Elliott, T. (1999) Metabolic alterations in middle-aged and elderly obese patients with Type 2 diabetes. *Diabetes Care*, **22**, 112–18.

National Health and Medical Research Council Series on Diabetes (1992) *Diabetes in Older People*. Australian Government Publishing Service, Canberra.

Paolisso, G., Gambardella, A., Verza, M., D'Amora, A., Sgambato, S. & Varrichio, M. (1992) ACE-inhibition improves insulin sensitivity in age insulin resistant hypertensive patients. *Journal of Human Hypertension*, **6**, 175–9.

Paolisso, G., D'Amora, A., Balbi, V., Volpe, C., Galzerano, D. & Giugliano, D. (1994) Plasma Vitamin C affects glucose homeostasis in healthy subjects in non-insulin dependent diabetes. *American Journal of Physiology*, 266, E261–8.

Popplewell, P., Burston, R. & Lowther, B. (1997) *Diabetes in Older People. Report of the Health Care Expert Committee Panel on Diabetes*. National Health and Medical Research Council, Canberra.

Proietto, J. (2004) Diabetes and antipsychotic drugs. *Australian Prescriber*, **27**(5), 118–19.

Sinclair, A. & Finucane, P. (1995) *Diabetes in Old Age*. John Wiley, Chichester.

Wild, S., Roglic, G., Green, A., Sicree, R. & King, H. (2004) Global prevalence of diabetes. *Diabetes Care*, **27**(5), 1047–53.

World Health Organization (WHO) (1999) *Report of a WHO Consultation. Part 1: Diagnosis and Classification of Diabetes Mellitus*. WHO, Geneva.

Zimmet, P. (1999) Diabetes epidemiology as a tool to trigger diabetes research and care. *Diabetologia*, **42**, 499–518.

Chapter 2
Managing Diabetes in Older People

Trisha Dunning

Key points

- Effective diabetes management in older people requires a holistic, proactive, risk management approach.
- A physical, psychological, social and environmental assessment is necessary to ensure management strategies are appropriate for the individual.
- Independent self-care should be encouraged within the individual's capabilities.
- Metabolic targets should be set that meet the recommended guidelines, but care must be taken to ensure the person is not placed at risk of adverse events such as hypoglycaemia, hyperglycaemia or falls when targets are set.

2.1 Introduction

Chronic disease management initiatives are becoming an important focus of health service providers. The needs of older people are slowly being addressed. At the very least, older people with diabetes should receive a minimal standard of care to prevent acute and chronic complications, regardless of where they live. Annual recall systems can facilitate appropriate screening and follow-up care. Standard care involves:

- Access to a general practitioner to ensure appropriate preventive health care, disease management, early intervention or referral and diabetes-specific care delivered according to available evidence.
- Basing therapeutic decisions on functional level and desirable metabolic control rather than age.
- The therapeutic relationship between the individual and care providers and between care providers and carers.
- Appropriate communication and documentation.

The discovery of insulin in 1922 and sulphonylureas in the 1950s, the development of blood glucose self-monitoring techniques in 1978 and the HbA_{1c} assay are four of the greatest advancements in diabetes care in the twentieth century. Such advances are continuing in the twenty-first century and include more accurate blood glucose monitoring techniques, new oral hypoglycaemic agents and insulin analogues, which hold great benefits for managing diabetes in older people.

The Australian Diabetes Educators Association (ADEA) developed a set of guidelines for managing diabetes in older people (ADEA 2003) to address a worldwide lack of specific guidelines for this vulnerable group of people. The ADEA guidelines specifically address older people but are primarily concerned with documenting evidence-based methods for screening for diabetes, metabolic targets (blood glucose and lipids), complication screening (blood pressure targets, renal function, eye examination and cognitive function) and nutrition in older people with diabetes. The guidelines apply to healthy older people and do not address nursing care.

According to the American Geriatric Society, controlling blood pressure and lipids is essential. These recommendations include screening for depression, polypharmacy, falls risk, incontinence, pain and memory deficits in addition to diabetes complications. HbA_{1c} should be individualised but recommended targets are <7% or 8% in frail older people (Brown *et al.* 2003). The National Service Framework for Diabetes Standards (Department of Health 2001) in the UK does not specifically cover older people. However, it does state that all adults with diabetes should receive high-quality care throughout their lifetime.

The most comprehensive set of guidelines was developed by the European Diabetes Working Party for Older People (2004). These guidelines are evidence based and apply to people 70 years and over with Type 2 diabetes. They cover important issues such as the ethical and moral aspects of caring for older people, depression and quality of life, education, screening and prevention, as well as metabolic targets. Unlike most guidelines, they address management in residential aged care.

Managing diabetes in older people is a complex undertaking. Although the majority of older people are able to manage their own health care, as they grow older they often have age-related changes such as reduced levels of independence, impaired dexterity and mobility, inadequate social support and financial constraints that reduce their self-care capacity. These changes make accessing health services difficult and they are compounded by the presence of diabetes. Controlling hyperglycaemia is just as important in older people as it is in any other age group, to reduce the short- and long-term consequences of hyperglycaemia and the consequent effects on wellbeing and quality of life, even if multiple medicines are required. People managed with diet alone have more complications and are monitored less frequently (Reuters 2004).

Practice points

(1) Vision can become blurred when glycaemic control improves. This phenomenon is not sight threatening but is does interfere with self-care and can be very frightening.

(2) Rapid improvement in glycaemic control can lead to hypoglycaemic symptoms even when the blood glucose level is not in the hypoglycaemic range (so-called relative hypoglycaemia).

(3) Haemodynamic changes that occur when blood glucose levels are improved quickly may predispose the individual to bleeding, especially if they are on anticoagulant medications or complementary medicines or subject to trauma.

New models of care are being developed, for example in Nottingham, UK, where an integrative service was developed to ensure equity of diabetes care for older people (Peck 2003). In the Nottingham model, a working relationship was established between the relevant care providers to standardise patient care and facilitate older people to meet in a support group and have a say in their care. Another strategy is currently under way in Melbourne, Australia, where an experienced diabetes educator provides a consultant service from a tertiary acute care hospital to a residential aged care facility. The role of the diabetes educator is to assess the diabetic and complication status of people with diabetes living in the facility and liaise with the nursing staff, allied health and visiting doctors to develop care plans as well as providing education for residents and staff and emergency advice as required.

2.2   Assessment and nursing diagnosis

A careful assessment of the physical, psychological, spiritual and social issues likely to affect self-care, nursing management and, where relevant, discharge planning is essential. In addition, these parameters need to be revised on a regular basis to account for age- and disease-related changes. Assessing the older person with diabetes is basically the same as any other nursing assessment and there are many examples available (see Chapter 3). One such proforma, developed specifically for diabetes, could be used for older people, provided cognitive function and assessment of activities of daily living, conducted in the person's usual environment, were included (Dunning 2003).

In particular, it is important to identify the degree of disability present at any given time to predict the amount of assistance needed and estimate the likelihood of adverse events such as hypoglycaemia, pressure ulcers, urinary tract infections and falls, which may have a further financial impact on the individual and the health system. Assessing disability involves four key questions that help decide appropriate management (see Table 2.1). In addition, constructing a combination geomap and ecomap can provide a great deal of information about the relationships in an individual's social network and help identify appropriate support people (see Figure 2.1).

Practice points

(1)   The individual's physical, psychological, spiritual and social circumstances are rarely fixed.
(2)   Regular reassessment is advisable, especially in the frail older group.
(3)   Regular assessments should be viewed as proactive, preventive measures that can help predict future care requirements.

It is also useful to consult the person's home blood glucose testing record, which often incorporates a list of their current medicines and relevant lifestyle issues. Water-resistant pages have added benefits. However, some older people find the print in commercial record books too small and record their results in an exercise book. Paper-based patient-held records are still popular with many people despite modern meter technology that includes a memory capacity and the capacity to download directly onto computers (Davis 2003).

Table 2.1 Four key questions to consider when assessing disability in older people with diabetes and the implications of the responses. Repeat measures may be needed, especially in acute settings where factors can change rapidly. In community settings such assessments should be part of the standard diabetes complication screening process.

Questions	Implications
(1) What activities are limited and to what degree?	A precise description of the disability is important in order to plan appropriate medical and nursing care and evaluate outcomes.
(2) Which disease processes are causing the disability?	Attributing disability to 'old age' is not an appropriate diagnosis. Common causes of disability include arthritis, cardiovascular disease, respiratory disease, stroke and visual impairment. One or more of these comorbidities often coexist with diabetes. Polypharmacy is likely. In some cases the medicine of choice for some comorbidities increases blood glucose levels.
(3) What is the person's mental state? Various assessment tools are used to assess mental status but their limitations need to be considered.	Evidence of memory loss, disorientation, confused behaviour and personality change may indicate diseases of the brain, dementia states or metabolic changes such as high or low blood glucose levels that impair mental processing. Consideration should also be given to the presence of anxiety, depression and the individual's general mental approach to life (positive or pessimistic) and hearing deficits.
(4) What is the person's social situation? See Figure 2.1.	Disability implies dependence on others. It is important to identify the services and people likely to be able to support the individual if they do require help. In addition, it is important to ensure the person who takes on the care is supported and their personal health and wellbeing considered to prevent stress, sleep disturbance and ill health in the carer, especially if they are also elderly.

The precise management, services required and division of responsibility depend on the individual health professionals involved in providing care and on local guidelines and services. As previously stated, there are two categories of older people:

● Those who are independent, self-caring and mobile, living in the community.
● Those who require assistance, either in low-level care where they are still mobile or living in high-level residential care facilities. It is important to realise that older people in hospital or living in residential aged care facilities do not represent the majority of individuals living in the community (Australian Institute of Health and Welfare (AIHW) 2002).

It is important to differentiate between the physical activities of daily living (PADL), which include essential basic daily activities such as bathing and dressing, and

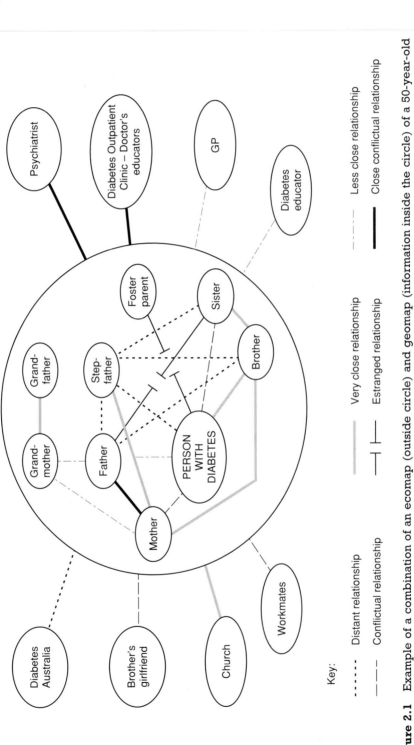

Figure 2.1 Example of a combination of an ecomap (outside circle) and geomap (information inside the circle) of a 50-year-old woman with Type 2 diabetes and a history of childhood molestation. It shows a great deal of conflict within and outside the family and identifies where her support base is. Reproduced with permission from Dunning 2003.

Key:

· · · · · · · Distant relationship   ———— Very close relationship   - - - - - - Less close relationship

— — — Conflictual relationship   -·-·-·- Estranged relationship   ▬▬▬ Close conflictual relationship

instrumental activities of daily living (IADL), which are more complex and necessary to live independently in society (Koch & Garratt 2001). The assessment of IADL must be based on activities pertinent to the individual and take account of their physical surroundings, culture and interests.

2.3   Principles of managing diabetes in older people

Successful management of diabetes in older people requires a preventive model of health care (see Figure 2.2 and Chapter 3).

2.3.1   Management aims

The aim of diabetes management in older people is to maintain their quality of life and independence, keep them free from unpleasant symptoms of hypo- or hyperglycaemia and manage complications and comorbidities quickly by adopting proactive, preventive, risk management models of care that acknowledge the role of the individual in their care and the significant contribution of their carers. Effective management requires a team approach where consistency and good communication are key features.

Specific aims include:

● Detecting and managing IGT.
● Maintaining an acceptable weight and adequate nutrition.
● Maintaining physical activity and other ADLs within the individual's capabilities for as long as possible.

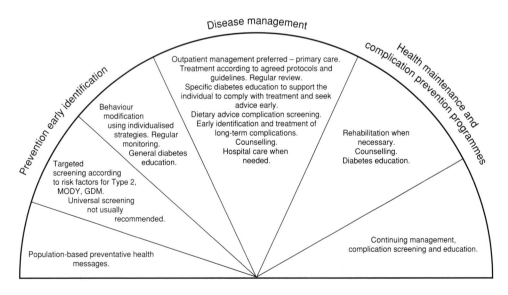

Figure 2.2   Example of a screening and preventive model of health care that can be used to plan the management of older people with diabetes. Adapted with permission from Dunning 2003.

- Achieving an acceptable blood glucose and lipid profile using lifestyle measures initially and medicines if indicated, according to the Quality Use of Medicines (see Chapter 9).
- Preventing complications of diabetes (short and long term).
- Limiting the effects of intercurrent illness.
- Maintaining psychological wellbeing and quality of life.
- Managing risks such as falls.

2.3.2 Managing older people with impaired glucose tolerance

The person should be informed that they have an increased chance of developing diabetes and macrovascular complications and the health professional should ensure regular screening checks occur.

General management issues include:

- Appropriate dietary modification to manage weight and ensure adequate nutrition.
- Exercise within the individual's capabilities and safety levels.
- Medication review to assess the need to continue current medicines, especially diabetogenic agents.
- Regular general health checks to manage hypertension, dyslipidaemia and other cardiovascular risk factors.
- Managing intercurrent illness risk to reduce the likelihood of stress-induced hyperglycaemia, for example pneumonia and influenza vaccinations.

2.3.3 Managing older people with established diabetes

Aims of management

The strategies necessary for managing IGT also apply to managing established diabetes. In addition, the following aims apply:

- Preventing hypo- and hyperglycaemia.
- Screening for, preventing and managing diabetic complications, when present.
- Managing coexisting illnesses to reduce metabolic stress and improve functional ability and quality of life.
- Helping the person develop and maintain a positive attitude and preventing depression, which compromises self-care and metabolic control.
- Maintaining a safe environment to limit adverse events such as infections and falls.

A number of factors affect diabetes management in older people and these are shown in Table 2.2. In addition, the following factors need to be considered.

- Age, although age alone may not give an accurate picture of an individual's ability to cope with self-care tasks and activities of daily living. The functional level may be a more reliable indicator.
- Current diabetes status, blood glucose and lipid levels and complication status, including the presence of liver and kidney disease, which may affect drug choice.
- Presence and severity of comorbidities.
- Mental and physical capacity to manage self-care tasks such as nutrition, blood glucose testing and medications and the choice of suitable education methods.

Table 2.2 Factors that can affect diabetes management and blood glucose control in older people. Adapted with permission from Dunning 2003.

Factors	Consequences
Health professionals	Attitudes and beliefs about diabetes. Ageist attitudes. Inadequate knowledge about nutrition and diabetes and its management. Personal treatment preferences.
Altered senses	Diminished vision and smell. Altered taste. Decreased proprioception.
Food issues	Food preferences and eating patterns. Purchasing, preparing and consuming food. Understanding of nutritional requirements. Poor appetite and early satiety. Gastrointestinal problems, including autonomic neuropathy. Effect of medicines on food absorption.
Concurrent diseases and their symptoms	Tremor, arthritis, poor dentition, gastrointestinal abnormalities, altered thirst sensation, altered renal and hepatic function, infection (acute or chronic).
Mobility and dexterity	Reduced ability to exercise and perform self-care tasks.
Drugs	Alcohol, medication such as corticosteroids, interactions and adverse effects, self-prescribed medications and complementary therapies.
Malabsorption	Due to diabetes medications, disease processes, drug interactions, diabetes complications and comorbidities.
Psychological issues	Bereavement, depression, loss, cognitive deficits. Acceptance of diabetes. Beliefs about and attitudes towards diabetes. Past experience with diabetes.
Social factors	Social isolation. Living alone or in care facilities. Family expectations and relationships. Hobbies and interests.
Financial status	Ability to purchase recommended foods, monitoring equipment, attending for diabetes complication screening and other health services.

- Nutritional status. Inadequate nutrition predisposes the person to hypoglycaemia, falls, reduced immunity, delayed wound healing and infections. These aspects need to be considered when planning the type and content of full meals, enteral feeds and vitaminised diets, as well as the requirements to limit fat, sugar, salt and alcohol.
- Sensory changes that will impact on diabetes education such as sight, hearing, cognitive ability. A suitable environment, appropriate timing and duration of the

session and the type of education aids used all need to be carefully considered (see Chapter 4). Where appropriate, patients should have their glasses and hearing aid with them during diabetes education sessions (Rosenstock 2001; Esler *et al.* 2002).

- Available social support.
- Life expectancy.

Recommended management targets

It is difficult to identify specific quality research on which to base management recommendations but a range of guidelines, position statements and journal articles are available. Generally accepted metabolic and complication screening targets are shown in Table 2.3. In Australia the National Diabetes Information Audit and Benchmarking

Table 2.3   Management targets for older people based on the ADEA *Guidelines for the Management and Care of Diabetes in the Elderly* 2003. It should be noted that these targets were determined for healthy people over age 65 and may not apply to older people living in residential aged care facilities. Specific management targets should be determined based on individual needs.

Management targets	Frequency of assessment
Blood glucose control HbA$_{1c}$ <7% Blood glucose pattern 4–8 mmol/L	Self-capillary blood glucose monitoring at least daily. Measure HbA$_{1c}$ twice a year if control is adequate and four times a year if control is inadequate. Hypoglycaemia should be avoided and higher HbA$_{1c}$ may be appropriate.
Blood lipids Cholesterol <4 mmol/L LDL <2.5 mmol/L Triglycerides <2.0 mmol/L	Measured annually if within the target range. Measured every 3–6 months if outside the range.
Blood pressure <140/90 mmHg	Measured every three months in people with hypertension. Measured every six months in normotensive people.
Maintain renal function and detect early decline	Microalbumin measured annually but 3–6 monthly if microalbuminuria is detected. Serum creatinine annually. Regular medication review.
Preserve vision	Eye examination at diagnosis to determine presence of retinopathy. If no retinopathy, screen in two years. If retinopathy is present, screen yearly. More frequent examinations may be needed. Screen for macular degeneration. Assess adequacy of glasses prescription.
Prevent foot pathology	Determine risk factors for foot ulceration. Self-foot checks regularly. Assess both feet annually if no risk factors of pathology present. Assess at least 3–6 monthly if at risk.
Reduce mental cognitive impairment associated with diabetes.	A range of measures can be used such as the MiniMental State Examination (MMSE) and the Brief Case Find for Depression (BCD).

Project (ANDIAB) data collection proforma can be used to document some of the assessment outcomes to help establish a national profile of older people with diabetes. The audit can be completed electronically.

Specific diabetes management

Managing metabolic abnormalities in older people usually consists of adopting a stepwise approach and using non-pharmacological measures where possible. These steps consist of:

(1) Dietary modification and exercise.
(2) Oral agents such as biguanides and sulphonylureas.
(3) Insulin.

Practice point

'The barriers to good control are often in the minds of physicians rather than the capacity of the elderly person with diabetes.'

(Halter 2001)

2.4 Nutritional aspects of caring for older people with diabetes

It is important to take a broad approach to nutritional management in older people with diabetes rather than just the usual focus on reducing fat and sugar. In addition to reducing fat to <1% of total energy intake and sugar to <25 g/day, older people need to be encouraged to:

- Eat a variety of nutritious foods in at least three meals every day.
- Eat plenty of cereals, wholegrain bread and pasta, especially those with a low Glycemic Index™, which should be 50–60% of total intake.
- Have adequate protein intake, consisting of at least 15% of the total intake.
- Eat plenty of fruit and vegetables to reduce the risk of cardiovascular disease and degenerative diseases and supply essential vitamins and minerals, such as calcium.
- Have an adequate fluid intake, including water (about 1500 mL per day) to reduce the likelihood of dehydration, especially in hot weather, unless fluid restriction is indicated.
- Drink alcohol in moderation. Because of the reduced muscle mass, the volume in which alcohol is distributed is smaller and therefore the concentration of circulating alcohol is higher, putting the person at risk of cognitive impairment, hypoglycaemia and falls. However, moderate consumption of alcohol might have health benefits.
- Use low-salt food and only add small amounts of salt to food to help prevent hypertension. (National Health and Medical Research Council 1999)

The nutritional plan for an older person must be revised on a regular basis because requirements change due to ageing and the presence of concomitant disease. An exercise or 'keep active' plan must also be considered. The nutritional status of older people generally is affected by a number of factors such as financial constraints, oral health, limited mobility and vision, inadequate knowledge and social factors such as living alone, ability to shop and prepare meals, living in residential aged care facilities or having home-delivered meals where personal choice is limited. Recent research suggests that older people with Type 2 diabetes, mean age 78, have healthier nutrition profiles than older non-diabetics, resulting in a lower body mass index (BMI) and alcohol intake and a higher intake of Vitamins C and E, higher HDL and lower LDL (Bates *et al.* 2004).

Practice points

(1) Many older people are malnourished even though they appear overweight. Malnutrition is common, occurring in 15% of homebound community dwellers, 35–65% of hospitalised people and 50% of residential aged care residents (Szoryi 2004).
(2) There are limited data about the nutritional needs of very old people.
(3) People over the age of 70 have special nutritional needs (Drewnowski & Warren-Mears 2001), especially if they have diabetes.
(4) Enteral feeding is required in the absence of a swallowing reflex.

2.4.1   Incidence and consequences of malnutrition

Older people with and without diabetes are at risk of malnutrition and the risk increases with increasing age (Department of Health 1992). The risk might be further increased in people with uncontrolled diabetes. Malnutrition is associated with increased morbidity and mortality, infections and poor wound healing (Baines & Roberts 2001), increased health service utilisation and length of stay in hospital (Szoryi 2004). The effects of malnutrition on physical status are shown in Table 2.4. In addition, some medications can impair the absorption of essential vitamins and minerals, for example metformin (see section 2.6.2). Low levels of these nutrients reduce immunity. Iron, zinc and Vitamin C deficiencies are relatively common in older people and there is some evidence that people with diabetes have higher deficiency rates of these nutrients than non-diabetics.

Factors that affect nutritional requirements

Many factors can affect nutritional requirements. These include:

● Usual eating pattern.
● Ability to feed themselves.
● Usual activity level.
● Metabolic rate and body composition.
● The weather pattern; people often eat less in hot weather.
● Psychological status.
● Medications being used including complementary and over-the-counter medicines such as vitamin and mineral supplements.
● Current physical status such as the presence of fever, wounds, active diabetic complications (renal and cardiovascular disease). Extra protein may be needed to

Table 2.4 Effects of malnutrition on the physical status of older people with diabetes. The weight loss may be due to undiagnosed or inadequately controlled diabetes or other comorbidities and the effects of medicines on appetite and taste and the gastrointestinal tract.

Malnutrition and associated effects	Consequences
Reduced immunity	• Increased rate of infection. • Slowed wound healing. • Reduced production of IgA, which protects mucosal surfaces. Therefore, opportunistic infections such as thrush, urinary tract and chest infections occur, especially if hypoglycaemia occurs frequently. • Limited phagocyte ability to ingest bacteria, which is also a factor in poor blood glucose control; therefore infections are likely to be more severe. • Limited immunoresponse to immunisation so prophylactic vaccinations such as FluVax are less effective.
Loss of respiratory muscle mass	• Increased risk of chest infections. • Poor respiratory function, which might increase the risk of lactic acidosis in the presence of biguanide. • Reduced ability to cough and expectorate.
Constipation	• Poor appetite, which exacerbates the poor nutritional status and weight loss. • Urinary retention and increased risk of urinary tract infection and incontinence. • Malabsorption. • Falls.
Limited glucose stores and glucose substrates	• Reduced ability to mount an effective response to hypoglycaemia. • Increased falls risk.
Reduced mobility	• Reduced appetite, which contributes to malnutrition and weight loss. It may be difficult to distinguish weight loss and lethargy associated with malnutrition from hyperglycaemic symptoms. • Loss of muscle mass and weakness. • Increased falls risk.
Exhaustion and weakness	• Poor mobility. • Poor appetite and difficulty eating. • Reduced mood. • Increased falls risk.
Changes in cognitive function	• Diminished cognitive performance. • Feeding dificuties. • Reduced sense of wellbeing. • Increased falls risk.

promote wound healing and replace protein loss, for example through a fistula or venous leg ulcer. Extra fluid may be required in hyperglycaemic states or during vomiting but fluid may need to be restricted if renal failure is present.

● Current blood glucose pattern.

Further malnourishment can occur in hospital (McWhirter & Pennington 1994); for example, cook/chill systems reduce Vitamin C content by between 45% and 76%. The incidence of malnutrition in residential care facilities is estimated to be at least 36% (Friedman & Kalant 1998) and possibly up to 43% (Visvanathan *et al.* 2004). Concomitant factors that increase the risk of malnutrition in older people with diabetes include:

● Psychiatric disorders, including depression (see Chapter 8).
● Parkinson's disease.
● Chronic obstructive pulmonary disease.
● Those with chewing and swallowing difficulties.
● Polypharmacy, which is common in diabetes.
● Dental problems.
● Disabled house-bound individuals.
● People with cancer or HIV/AIDS.

In addition, many older people have limited exposure to sunlight and therefore lack Vitamin D and often also calcium, which increases the risk of osteoporosis and fractures. Dietary fluctuations, especially in the intake of Vitamin K-rich vegetables, may make it difficult to maintain a stable International Normalisation Ratio (INR) in people on anticoagulant therapy. Increased intake of these foods leads to reduced INR. Conversely, when the diet is low in Vitamin K the INR increases (Ishida & Kawai 2004). Maintaining a stable Vitamin K intake appears to be important.

A number of factors can help maintain optimal nutrition and it is important to elicit what these are for the individual and acknowledge and enhance them when planning care. Callan and Wells (2003) interviewed community-dwelling people over 80 years who indicated that the top four aids to nutritional health were:

● Family and friends.
● Microwave ovens.
● Transportation.
● Proximity to a grocery store.

It should be noted the people surveyed were well motivated and well educated and may not be representative of other older community-dwelling people.

2.4.2 Assessing nutritional status

A full nutritional assessment may be difficult for many nurses to undertake and referral to a dietitian is recommended. Nurses can effectively use some simple screening tools to help identify people at risk of poor nutrition. Such assessments should include a physical assessment and dietary history. Nurses can identify actual or potential nutritional deficiencies and therefore gauge the urgency of the need to refer to a dietitian for a complete assessment and appropriate dietary advice. Dietary assessment and referral to a dietitian is essential for older people requiring enteral feeds (see section 2.4.13).

A number of screening tools have been designed to assess nutritional status and these include:

- Nutrition Screening Initiative.
- Subjective Global Assessment (SGA). This tool determines whether restricted nutrient assimilation has occurred because of inadequate food intake or is a consequence of a medical condition. There is good correlation between the SGA and biochemical and anthropometric measures of nutrition status.
- Australian Nutrition Screening Initiative is a checklist developed to raise awareness of the importance of nutrition and identify older people at risk of malnutrition. This is an appropriate screening tool for nurses to use to identify people who need further detailed assessment by a dietitian.
- Nutritional Screening Initiative checklist.
- Hydration Assessment checklist, which is an in-depth tool designed to detect hydration problems in older people. Adequate hydration is essential to support cell and organ health, electrolyte balance, medication absorption and distribution, and kidney and bladder function (Zembrzuski 1997).
- Mini Nutritional Assessment (MNA) (Nestlé Nutrition Services), which detects actual and potential malnourishment and is validated for people over 65. It examines anthropometrics, general issues and diet and incorporates the consumer's subjective perspective (Reilly 1996). The MNA may predict mortality in older people (Persson *et al.* 2002).

Practice point

Obese older people may be malnourished. Biochemical assessments include plasma proteins, but the concentration can be influenced by non-nutritional factors such as liver disease, some cancers, sepsis and inflammatory bowel disease. Low serum albumin is an indication of chronic protein deficiency but because albumin has a long half-life (~20 days) it is not an accurate indicator of short-term protein deficiency (Baines & Roberts 2001). Blood tests are also available to test for specific deficiencies such as zinc and vitamins.

Tiredness, fatigue and obesity may indicate inadequate protein intake, which can be calculated by comparing the blood urea nitrogen (BUN) with the serum creatinine. If the creatinine is low, protein intake is low. If both the creatinine and BUN are low, it is possible that a state of tissue catabolism, such as that associated with hyperglycaemia, exists.

2.4.3 Measuring nutritional status

Serial weights are a simple anthropometric measure. Serial weights are most useful if the person is weighed on the same scales, wearing approximately the same clothing. They may be the simplest, most practical measure to use for older people. Changes in weight, especially a 10% change over six months, usually represent changed nutritional status, but oedema should be excluded.

Body mass index (BMI), or Quetelet's Index, is usually used as a measure of body fat but can be unreliable in some cultural groups and muscular people and the defined ranges differ between health-care organisations. BMI is calculated according to the following formula:

Weight in kilograms (kg) divided by height in metres squared (m^2)

The following BMI levels indicate nutritional status.

BMI <18.5 kg/m^2 – significant malnutrition risk.
BMI <19 kg/m^2 – underweight.
BMI 20–25 kg/m^2 – acceptable.
BMI >25 kg/m^2 – overweight.

BMI can also be confounded by changes in hydration, oedema and ascites. Weight loss can be masked by oedema. Osteoporotic changes can lead to vertebral collapse and undercalculation of height.

Skinfold thickness, measured using callipers, is also an indication of body fat. Other anthropometric measures include:

- Mid-arm circumference (MAC) that can provide useful information about nutritional status provided serial measurements are taken. MAC measurements are useful for people who are too frail to stand to be weighed.
- Waist–hip ratio, which reflects abdominal adiposity, which is a particular risk factor for impaired glucose and diabetes. This is frequently the preferred method.

Dual energy X-ray absorptiometry (DEXA), which measures total body fat, and bioelectrical impedance, conduction or resistance, which measures the percentage of fat, are sometimes used, especially for research purposes.

2.4.4 Effect of medicines on nutritional status

Medicines can affect nutritional status by reducing the appetite or altering taste or smell and food appreciation. Some medicines such as antipsychotics, sulphonylureas and glucocorticoids lead to weight gain. Others, such as anticholinergic drugs, lead to dry mouth and difficulty swallowing.

Some medicines impair absorption of vitamins and minerals; for example, antacids reduce iron absorption whereas Vitamin C enhances the absorption of iron. There is increasing evidence that people with diabetic renal disease are at earlier risk of renal-associated anaemia, but the exact mechanism and role of nutrition in this process are not known.

Phenytoin, which is sometimes used to relieve painful diabetic peripheral neuropathy and seizures, reduces absorption of Vitamin D and folic acid. Conversely, food can modify the absorption of some drugs, which explains why the timing of medication doses in relation to food is important, especially in percutaneous endoscopic gastrostomy (PEG) and enteral feeding regimens.

2.4.5 Obesity

Obesity is common in people with Type 2 diabetes and has reached epidemic proportions in many parts of the world. Measuring obesity can be difficult and controversial (see section 2.4.3). Immobility, some drugs and high-fat, high-sugar and high-alcohol diets contribute to obesity in older people. Obesity occurs if the energy consumed outweighs the energy expended. Recently, obesity has been recognised as a disease in its own right (Marks 2000). Forty to sixty per cent of obesity is inherited through an obesity gene expressed in adipose tissue. Leptin, which appears to modulate the appetite and the metabolic rate, was discovered recently but its exact role is yet to be defined. Most obese people are leptin deficient. Likewise, a substance called resistin, found in adipocytes, leads to insulin resistance and increased abdominal fat deposition (truncal obesity) and may have a role in the pathogenesis of Type 2 diabetes (McTernan *et al.* 2002).

People with truncal obesity are at greatest risk of obesity-related disease such as diabetes, dyslipidaemia and fatty liver. Obesity is a chronic condition and long-term management goals and a great deal of support are required to achieve weight loss. Losing weight is very difficult for some older people with limited mobility. The focus in these people may be to improve functional ability and strength training, rather than weight loss. Reducing fat and sugar intake and increasing activity within the individual's capacity are the basis of any weight loss programme. In some circumstances very low-calorie diets such as Modifast™ and Optifast™ might be considered but need to be balanced against the need for adequate nutrition and long-term expectations.

Reviewing the need for medicines that contribute to weight gain is important. Glucocortoids are commonly used. These drugs are very similar to human glucocortoid hormones that are linked to human evolution. They motivate people to eat when food is available and support the capacity to store energy through abdominal fat deposition, a readily available fuel substrate for the liver, in times of necessity. Using drugs such as lipase inhibitors (orlistat) or serotonin reuptake inhibitors such as sibutamide could be considered. If Xenical is used, providing a low-fat diet is essential.

2.4.6 Measures to maintain adequate nutrition

Nurses caring for older people with diabetes in acute or residential care settings can introduce some general measures to maintain adequate nutrition and manage blood glucose levels. These include:

- Identifying the individual's food preferences and eating habits.
- Providing snacks, especially for cognitively impaired people and those unable to feed themselves.
- Encouraging and assisting older people to eat independently by providing appropriate aids such as plates with deep rims and non-slip surfaces and ensuring the food is placed where the person can see and reach it.
- Observing uneaten food to estimate intake and the types of foods that are consistently left so that alternatives can be offered.
- Providing supplements if the appetite is poor or a meal is declined, especially if the person is using oral hypoglycaemic agents (OHAs) or insulin.
- Organise meal times to reduce interruption and ensure staff are available to assist people to eat if necessary. Ensure meals are not rushed and are associated with pleasure. Present the meal attractively.
- Ensure medicines are given before or after meals as appropriate. Examples of drugs whose absorption can be modified by food are shown in Table 2.5. Although oral

Table 2.5 Drugs whose absorption can be modified by food. Reproduced with permission from Dunning 2003.

Reduced absorption	Delayed absorption	Increased absorption
Aspirin	Aspirin	Diazepam
Cephalexin	Cefaclor	Dicoumarol
Erythromycin	Cephalexin	Erythromycin
Penicillin V and G	Cimetidine	Hydrochlorothiazide
Phenacetin	Digoxin	Metoprolol
Tetracycline	Indoprofen	Nitrofurantoin
Theophylline	Metronidazole	Propranolol

hypoglycaemic agents and insulin are usually given before meals, it may be safer to give them after the meal to people who have a poor appetite, do not consume adequate carbohydrate during the meal or eat erratically, to reduce the risk of hypoglycaemia.

● Undertaking or participating in regular nutrition assessments.

2.4.7 Role of dietary supplements

Older people who do not consume adequate nutrients may benefit from supplements. Referral to a dietitian is recommended. In some cases deficiencies may be due to poor food absorption generally, or poor absorption of specific nutrients. A medication review may be warranted to ensure food–drug interactions are not occurring. In addition, prolonged or inappropriate food storage or cooking methods can result in a reduction in nutrient content. Iron absorption depends on the source of the iron. Haem iron found in meat, liver, kidney, poultry and seafood is absorbed more readily than non-haem iron found in legumes, egg yolk, wholegrain foods, nuts, seeds and green leafy vegetables. Consuming foods rich in Vitamin C, for example a glass of orange juice, at the same time as non-haem iron foods enhances absorption. Anaemia may be an issue in older people with diabetes and renal disease, in whom anaemia occurs at an earlier stage in the decline in renal function than in non-diabetics.

The ability to absorb Vitamin B and folic acid is reduced with increasing age. Calcium absorption can be impaired by fibre and Vitamin D is required for calcium absorption. Older people are often deficient in Vitamin D and may require supplements to reduce the risk of osteoporosis. Zinc deficiencies affect taste sensation and may be a factor in poor food intake.

One of the simplest ways to increase the energy and nutrient content of the diet of older people is to provide nutritional supplements. However, before adding more substances, the risk of interactions and adverse effects needs to be considered carefully. Supplements are available as liquid, powder, capsules and tablets, often in combination preparations. It is important to realise that a daily intake of vitamins and minerals does not necessarily mean they are bio-available (Trusswell 2003). The American Heart Association (Kris-Etherton *et al.* 2002) recommended that doctors supervise omega-3 supplementation in people with heart disease and that if the required amount cannot be consumed by eating oily fish, supplements may be necessary to lower triglycerides. Some people may be put off by the fishy aftertaste, especially if more than 3 g per day are consumed. Gastrointestinal disturbances and worsening glycaemia also occur.

2.4.8   Sugar and non-nutritive sweeteners

'Sugar free' usually refers to the sucrose content of foods. Other sugars are often used to sweeten foods labelled 'sugar free', for example dextrose, fructose, maltose, lactose and galactose. These foods are not recommended. Non-nutritive sweeteners are an acceptable alternative to sugar, where it is important to control calories. The excessive use of sugar substitutes is not recommended and small amounts of sugar as part of a balanced meal may be appropriate. Some acceptable non-nutritive sweeteners are:

- Saccharin.
- Cyclamate.
- Aspartame (Equal).
- Isomalt.

Sorbitol, another sweetener often used in diabetic products, is not generally recommended because of its potential to cause diarrhoea in some people. In addition, it has the same calorific value as glucose and in significant amounts can increase the blood glucose level. Sorbitol is often used to sweeten 'diabetic foods', which are expensive and not recommended for people with diabetes.

Stevia (*Stevia rebaudiana*), a very sweet powder derived from a herb, is being promoted as a suitable sugar alternative for people with diabetes. Only very small quantities are required and it does not appear to affect blood glucose levels or have any side effects; however, it has not been extensively evaluated in clinical practice for people with diabetes. There is some evidence that stevia might reduce blood glucose.

2.4.9   Carbohydrate modified and 'dietetic' foods

Foods labelled 'carbohydrate modified' or 'dietetic' or 'diabetic' are often high in fat and are not generally recommended for people with diabetes.

2.4.10   Alcohol

Alcohol supplies considerable calories and provides little or no nutritional value so it contributes to malnutrition if consumed in excessive amounts. Alcohol consumption should be limited because of the changed metabolism in older people, its potential to affect blood glucose and contribute to, or mask, hypoglycaemia (see Chapter 4). Sweet alcoholic drinks can lead to hyperglycaemia. The alcohol itself leads to hypoglycaemia. Alcohol should never be consumed on an empty stomach.

In addition, alcohol clouds judgement and can lead to inappropriate decision making. Drunkenness resembles hypoglycaemia and thus treatment of hypoglycaemia may be delayed. Appropriate education about hypoglycaemia risk with alcohol consumption is essential, especially in settings where supervision and assistance are not readily available.

2.4.11   'Exchanges', 'portions' and 'serves'

Exchanges, portions and serves are ways of measuring the carbohydrate content of the food. They help to ensure an even distribution of carbohydrate when planning meals for individual people. The difference between the terms relates to the amount of carbohydrate measured. An exchange is equal to 15 g and a portion 10 g of carbohydrate. Exchanges are often used in the UK while Australia is increasingly using the Glycemic Index™.

2.4.12   Glycemic Index™

The Glycemic Index™ (GI) is a method of ranking foods based on their immediate effect on blood glucose levels. Foods that break down quickly are known as high Glycemic Index™ foods (high GI), e.g. sugars. Foods that break down more slowly are known as low Glycemic Index™ foods (low GI), e.g. cereals. The GI is the area under the glucose response curve measured after a test meal is consumed. Foods with a GI <55 are classified as low GI, GI 56–69 as moderate GI and GI >70 as high GI foods. In general, the lower the GI, the smaller the impact the food will have on the blood glucose level and satiety.

However, many factors affect the rate at which carbohydrate is absorbed, including the types of sugar and starch in food, the degree of processing, cooking method, the presence of other nutrients, such as fat and fibre, and the particular combination of foods consumed. Low GI foods are the preferred basis of a well-balanced diet. They slow food absorption from the gut so that the postprandial glucose load is reduced, help satisfy huger and assist with weight control, reduce HbA_{1c}, improve insulin sensitivity and help control lipids (Brand-Miller 1994).

Practice points

(1)   Low GI foods should be included in at least one meal each day for all people with diabetes. As indicated, simple sugars need not be excluded using the GI system.

(2)   Foods high in fat have a low GI because the fat delays their digestion and they are absorbed slowly. Therefore, high-fat foods are not recommended regardless of their GI score.

(3)   High-fat foods delay absorption and are not suitable to manage hypoglycaemia.

GI-based diets are not universally used and the GI system can be difficult for some people to understand, especially older people who are accustomed to other methods. Generally, if people are accustomed to working in portions, exchanges or serves and have reasonable metabolic control, they should not be expected to change, particularly if they are elderly.

2.4.13   Enteral feeding

An increasing number of older people, particularly those living in residential facilities, require enteral feeding due to impaired swallowing reflex or severe malnutrition.

Several medium to low GI enteral formulas are now available. It is important that OHAs/insulin are given and blood glucose tests performed prior to administering the enteral feed rather than according to routines for orally fed residents. Other medicines may need to be administered separately from feeds.

Enteral feeding can be achieved via nasogastric tubes, in the short tem, or gastroscopy, jejunostomy or PEG tubes, where enteral feeding is required long term. The aims of enteral therapy are to provide fluid and macronutrients to meet the individual's metabolic and nutritional requirements. Dietitian assessment to select the most suitable formula is essential to take account of:

- Medical and surgical history.
- Current health status, general and diabetes.
- Current intake and ideal nutrient intake based on height, weight, age, activity and biochemical factors such as urea and electrolytes, serum albumin and iron studies.

Enteral feeding is usually started slowly to prevent refeeding syndrome and other metabolic consequences that arise from commencing feeds in malnourished individuals. Electrolyte shifts associated with feeding affect a number of organs and can lead to congestive cardiac failure, cardiac arrhythmias and neuromuscular and respiratory consequences (Crook *et al.* 2001). The aim is to supply sufficient energy for growth and repair and physical activity, where relevant, and control blood and lipid levels.

If feeds are to be administered at home considerable education is needed to ensure feeds and medicine administration times match and the hang time of the feeds is appropriate.

Enteral formulas

A range of formulas are available that contain essential nutrients to sustain life but they need to be carefully selected, for example in relation to glucose tolerance, the need to reduce CO_2 production in respiratory disease where excretion is compromised, and the effect of medication on the formula and vice versa.

The formulas are produced as liquids or powders and have different ratios of carbohydrate, fat and protein. Types of formulas include:

- Standard, often used when enteral feeding first commences.
- Hypercaloric, used when fluid is restricted.
- Fibre +, used when constipation is a problem. It may have a role in gastroparesis.
- Speciality. A range of formulas exist for diseases such as renal, hepatic, IGT, respiratory disease, wound management and cancer states. Example speciality formulas for diabetes include Nutrison low energy for diabetes, Nutrison diabetes, Resource diabetes and Glucerna, which are generally low GI. High-GI feeds can predispose the person to osmotic diarrhoea, dehydration and hyperosmolar states. If high-GI foods are indicated they should be commenced slowly and increased slowly. Oral hypoglycaemic agents/insulin may need to be adjusted and the blood glucose should be monitored regularly.
- Elemental and subelemental formulas, which are easily digested and may be suitable for people with gastroparesis.
- Modular formulas, which contain single nutrients to allow a formula to be specially tailored.

Disadvantages of enteral feeding

As well as the advantages, there are a number of disadvantages to enteral feeding. These include:

- Loss of socialisation due to perceptions of having 'a tube', which leads to isolation and depression.
- May not prevent malnutrition, even when it is carefully tailored.
- Reduced healing.
- Development of pressure sores and infection around the tube insertion site.
- Aspiration.
- Reduced quality of life due to bleeding, infection, pulling the tube out, burden on carers, fear, false hope and incorrect administration of medicines, for example crushing enteric-coated, long-acting medicines.

Administering diabetes medicines with enteral feeds

The recommended process for administering medications via an enteral feeding tube is as follows.

(1) Liquid dose forms should be used if available. If tablets can be crushed to a fine powder they should be mixed with 10–15 mL of water. If capsules can be opened, the powdered contents should be mixed with 10–15 mL of water.
(2) When medicines need to be administered on an empty stomach, the feed should be stopped 30 minutes before the scheduled medication administration time. The feed should not be recommenced for a further 30 minutes after all the medicine has been administered.
(3) When there are documented drug/enteral formula incompatibilities, feeding should cease two hours prior to a single daily medicine dose and can recommence two hours later. For more frequent doses, allow one hour either side of the administration time. However, it should be noted that this method does *not* guarantee complete bio-availability.

Administration procedure

(1) Cease the enteral feed and flush the tube with 30 mL of water before administering the medicine.
(2) Remix the medicines by shaking the capped bottle or swirling the medication in the cup.
(3) The medicines should be placed in a needleless syringe.
(4) The medicines should be allowed to flow in by gravity. Gentle boosts (approximately one inch down) should be given with the plunger if the medication does not flow. Medicines should not be pushed through tubes because they can obstruct the tube.
(5) When other medicines are given, 5 mL of water should be introduced into the syringe between medicines. *Different medicines should never be mixed together in a syringe.*
(6) After administration, the tube should be flushed with 30 mL of water and clamped. The feeding can then be recommenced.

(7)   The amount of water used should be documented on fluid balance charts, especially when the person has oedema or renal disease.
(8)   A record should be kept of times of all medicines administered via the enteral tube to help determine whether subsequent problems are related to the medicine or administration process.

Consult a pharmacist before crushing medicines or opening capsules and administering them through enteral feeding tubes. Inappropriate crushing can increase toxicity, reduce efficacy and increase the chance of drug interactions. Where possible, alternative formulations such as liquid formulations, topical applications, intranasal sprays, patches, suppositories or injections should be used. Suggestions for administering medicines via enteral tubes include:

- Allow two hours between administering medicines and feeds where they cannot be administered simultaneously.
- Administer individual medicines separately and flush the tube with water between the administration of each medicine.
- Document and monitor the feeding regime so any food–drug interactions can be followed up.
- If medicines can be crushed, wash the mortar and pestle and any other equipment used between crushing each drug.
- Remember that crushing medicines or removing them from capsules and putting them in food to be administered orally can make the food unpalatable.

Hypoglycaemic, antihypertensive and hypolipidaemic agents that *should not* be crushed and administered via nasogastric or similar routes are listed below.

(1)   Oral hypoglycaemic agents:
   - glimepiride (Dimirel)
   - glyclazide MR.
(2)   Lipid-lowering agents.
   The following medicines should not be administered through a nasogastric tube:
   - colestipol granules (Colestid) swell in contact with liquid so must be separated from other medicines. Administer other medicines either one hour before or four hours after colestipol
   - ezetimibe – insoluble in water
   - metamucil – will obstruct the tube
   - cholestyramine (Questran Lite) – as for colestipol.
(3)   Antihypertensive agents:
   - Adalat Oros (nifedipine)
   - Adefin XL (nifedipine)
   - Agon SR (felodipine)
   - Atacand Plus (candesartan, hydrochlorothiazide)
   - Bicor (bisoprolol)
   - Cardizem CD (diltiazem)
   - Chem mart Diltiazem CD (diltiazem)
   - Corbeton (oxprenolol)
   - Cordilox SR (verapamil)
   - Diltahexal CD (diltiazem)
   - Dilzem CD (diltiazem)

- Felodur ER (felodipine)
- GenRx Diltiazem CD (diltiazem)
- Isoptin SR (verapamil)
- Natrilix SR (indapamide)
- Nifedipine-BC (nifedipine)
- Nifehexal (nifedipine)
- Plendil ER (felodipine)
- Terry White Chemists Diltiazem CD (diltiazem)
- Vasocardol CD (diltiazem)
- Veracaps SR (verapamil).

(Young 2004)

Practice point

During acute illness/trauma, blood glucose levels may be controlled more effectively with insulin.

It is important to check correct drug administration procedures with a pharmacist or the manufacturer's product information prior to administration because there may be specific requirements about the time of administration in relation to food, solubility, simplifying the dose regimen or ascertaining that the medication will still be delivered to the correct site of action when administered via the various enteral feeding routes. Some drugs need to be delivered to a specific area of the gastrointestinal tract to have a therapeutic effect.

Furthermore, new formulations/brands are constantly being marketed so the nature of pharmaceutical products available is constantly changing. The list above may not be current in the future and it is not appropriate to extrapolate between different brands of the same generic drug, because the formulation characteristics can sometimes be quite different.

It should be noted that there are no specific data about compatibility with the various enteral feeding products for many drugs. Therefore, patients should be monitored to ensure the desired pharmacological effect is still attained. Whilst medicines may not be contraindicated for enteral feeding, nurses/carers need to be aware that administration via enteral tubes may alter the bio-availability characteristics of some medicines; for example, crushing may increase the absorption and/or rate of absorption of some medications. Increased bio-availability may lead to an increased incidence of adverse effects (Engle & Hannawa 1999; Gilbar 1999; Young 2004).

Practice point

Medicines should not be mixed into a 'medicine cocktail' in a mortar prior to administration via an enteral tube. When multiple drugs are prescribed for administration at the same time, they should never be mixed together. Each drug should be given individually, separated by a flush.

2.4.14   Nutrition and dementia

Oral feeds or at least tastes should be used where possible to maintain normality, autonomy and dignity. Make eating easy by providing finger foods. If the appetite is poor supplements may be needed before meals to enhance the appetite at mealtimes.

2.4.15   Nursing responsibilities for nutritional management

Nutrition is a significant component of the care of older people with diabetes and nurses can make a major contribution to nutritional care, especially in acute and residential care facilities, by the following actions.

- Assessing dietary and nutritional characteristics to identify problems and refer to a dietitian as required, e.g. at a change from diet to tablets or tablets to insulin, if there are frequent high or low blood glucose levels, if a complication such as renal disease is diagnosed, if the patient displays inadequate knowledge or when the patient or carer requests a referral.
- Observing and, if necessary, recording food intake, with particular reference to the carbohydrate intake and daily distribution of carbohydrate intake for people on blood glucose-lowering medication.
- Promoting general dietary principles in accordance with accepted guidelines/ policies and procedures.
- Ensuring meals and carbohydrate content are evenly spaced across the day and are timed appropriately with respect to medications.
- Ensuring adequate carbohydrate intake for medications, fasting patients and those with diminished intake, to avoid hypoglycaemia.
- Administering medicines at an appropriate time in relation to food and the drug specifications.
- Knowing that the absorption of some medicines can be modified by food, including antibiotics, and their effectiveness may be diminished or increased. These medicines are detailed in Table 2.5. The pharmacological response to drugs is influenced by the individual's nutritional status. In turn, medicines can affect the nutritional status. The sense of smell and taste play a significant role in adequate dietary intake. Both these senses diminish with age and can be changed by disease processes and the effect of medicines. Gastrointestinal (GIT) disorders can lead to malabsorption while pH changes alter the bio-availability of nutrients and drugs, inhibit drug binding and chelation and impair the metabolism and excretion of drugs (National Health and Medical Research Council 1999).
- Observing the person for signs and symptoms of hyper- and hypoglycaemia and correcting these states by appropriate nutritional management as part of the overall treatment strategy (see Chapter 4).

2.5   Increasing mobility and exercise

Regular exercise has physical and mental benefits for people with diabetes of all ages. Exercise helps reduce the risk of developing diabetes and cardiovascular complications. However, exercise is difficult for many older people because of the decline in

Table 2.6 Relative and absolute contraindications to exercise in older people with diabetes.

Relative contraindications	Absolute contraindications
Labile hypertension	Unstable angina.
Autonomic neuropathy that causes postural hypotension	Uncontrolled cardiac arrhythmias, CCF, stenosis, heart failure.
Active foot pathology such as ulcers and untreated callus	Proliferative retinopathy, especially if it is not treated.
Heart disease such as stenosis, cardiomyopathy, arrhythmias	Retinal haemorrhage.
Electrolyte abnormalities such as hypokalaemia	Acute infections.
Low blood glucose levels	Significant renal failure.
Hyperglycaemic states	Current foot ulcer.
Moderate to high ketones in urine or blood	
Severe osteoporosis	
Musculoskeletal disorders such as arthritis	

muscle mass and general mobility, strength and energy. These factors increase the risk of falls, injury and fractures. Aerobic exercise for at least 30 minutes per day and strength exercises can help maintain muscle mass and energy. In addition, adequate nutrition, especially protein, is important.

Any movement of the body or limbs helps reduce cardiovascular fatalities by up to 50% and the chance of a second myocardial infarct by 25%, as well as reducing hypertension and stroke risk (Vicfit 2004). Despite these positives, there are a number of relative and absolute contraindications to exercise that are shown in Table 2.6. The benefits of exercise in older people, such as improving mobility, reducing falls and improving wellbeing, are now becoming apparent (Stessman *et al.* 2002; Vaitkevicius *et al.* 2002).

2.5.1   Commencing a physical activity programme

Planning is an important aspect of physical activity for older people and any activity needs to be safe for the individual and undertaken in a safe environment.

- A thorough physical assessment to determine vascular status and cardiac arrhythmias is required before commencing an exercise programme. Healthy older people in the community may require a graded exercise test. Blood pressure, lipid profile and assessment for autonomic neuropathy are required (Flood & Constance 2002).
- Assess for signs of peripheral neuropathy that could increase the risk of foot injury during exercise.

- Assess presence and status of retinopathy to reduce the risk of falls.
- Gait and balance need to be assessed.
- Monitor blood glucose levels and do not encourage activity if the blood glucose is below 6 mmol/L or above 10 mmol/L.
- Be aware that some of the signs of hypoglycaemia, such as sweating, faintness, weakness and dizziness, can be missed or attributed to the effect of the exercise or could have other causes such as angina.
- Some physical activity can lower blood glucose for up to 48 hours so people need to be observed for hypoglycaemia and have an adequate high GI intake.
- Clothing and footwear should be appropriate and should not restrict blood flow or breathing or put the feet at risk.
- Activity levels should be increased gradually.
- Warming up and cooling down activities are essential.
- Provide opportunities for activity within the usual daily routine.
- Counsel adequately about safety issues such as being attacked when out walking and taking care on poorly maintained footpaths.

Recommended exercises

The Society of Geriatric Cardiology recommends a physical activity programme that includes aerobic endurance exercises and strength training including:

- Tai chi, which has a number of benefits including reducing blood pressure, blood glucose and lipids, improving balance and wellbeing (Lan *et al.* 1998; Tsai *et al.* 2003).
- Walking 30 minutes/day or for 10 minutes three times/day.
- Resistance training, which can improve strength and make routine activities, such as carrying groceries and gardening, easier and reduce bone loss (Mueleman *et al.* 2000; Simkin 2004).
- Swimming and gentle water exercises. Socks or wetsuit bootees may be needed to protect at-risk neuropathic feet from trauma if the base of the pool is uneven.
- Dancing.
- Chair exercises.

2.5.2   Incidental exercise

A great deal of activity can be incorporated into usual activities such as playing with grandchildren, housework and gardening. Pedometers are readily available and can help older people measure their activity level and set personal goals.

2.6   Pharmacotherapeutic management

Only 15% of people with Type 2 diabetes are able to maintain an acceptable blood glucose range through dietary measures alone (UK Prospective Diabetes Study 1983) so medicines will usually be required. Medication management is an important nursing function and can be complex in older people because of the number of medicines required to manage primary diseases and comorbidities. Ten to twenty per cent of

Table 2.7 Common areas where medication errors occur. Sometimes an error may occur because of several of these factors or other factors may contribute.

Area where medication error can occur	Possible source of the error
When the medication is prescribed (56% of medication errors)	Prescriber is not up-to-date with current drugs.
	Similar sounding names of medicines.
	Diabetes complication screen not performed and/or medicines are not revised in light of changes, e.g. renal function decline or cardiovascular changes.
	History or possibility of allergies or intolerance not checked.
	Inappropriate dose form prescribed, e.g. Diamicron MR, which is crushed and added to enteral feeds.
	Illegible writing and transcription errors, e.g. taking telephone orders.
	Medications not communicated between community, residential care and acute care.
	Not asking about complementary therapy and over-the-counter medicines use.
Dispensing	Incorrect medicine or incorrect form dispensed.
	Consumer medicines information and education not provided.
Administration (34% of errors). Self-administration, carer, nursing staff or untrained carers in residential care, doctors	Incorrect medication or dose taken.
	Taken at the incorrect time or dose interval.
	Medicines crushed inappropriately.
	Administration not documented.
	Response not monitored.
	Complementary and over-the-counter medicine use not asked about/disclosed.

acute admissions of older people and 18% of deaths are the result of prescribed medicines (Ebbeson *et al.* 2001). Many of these admissions are the result of drug interactions.

The Quality Use of Medicines is a framework for promoting optimal outcomes from medicine use and reducing medicine-related adverse events (see Chapter 9). Medication errors can occur in any phase of medication management (see Table 2.7).

2.6.1   *Changes in drug metabolism and excretion in older people*

Normal ageing accounts for a number of age-related changes in liver and renal function, nutritional status and body composition that affect drug pharmacokinetics and pharmacodynamics (see Table 2.8). In addition, smoking affects blood vessels and possibly drug absorption, metabolism and distribution. Generally, using the lowest number of medicines at the lowest effective dose and using simple regimes can reduce

Table 2.8 Age-related changes that can affect drug pharmacokinetics and pharmacodynamics in older people and therefore have consequences for prescribing and monitoring medicines.

	Consequences
Nutrition changes Malnutrition with low serum iron and vitamin, mineral and protein deficits	• Decline in brain cells, which increases the effects of psychoactive drugs. • Reduced baroreceptor activity, which increases postural hypotensive effect of drugs. • Increased risk of gastrointestinal bleeding with NSAIDs and enhanced effects of anticoagulants.
Body composition changes • Weight loss • Reduced body water • Increased body fat • Low serum albumin	• Standard doses of drugs may have an increased effect. • Higher plasma concentration of water-soluble drugs and reduced plasma concentration of fat-soluble drugs. • Reduced protein binding, which means more free drug is available which produces an enhanced effect.
Liver changes • Reduced first-phase blood flow and drug metabolism • Decreased liver size, with a reduction in liver P450 enzymes	System and reduced hepatic drug metabolism.
Renal changes • Reduction in number of nephrons • Reduced glomerular filtration rate and tubular secretion	Serum creatinine may be normal despite reduced renal function. Increases the possibility that renally excreted drugs and their metabolites will accumulate.

medicine-associated morbidity and mortality and make it easier for people to manage their medicine regimens independently.

Regular medication review should be standard practice and should encompass physical and cognitive assessment. Dose adjustments are required for a wide range of drugs when renal impairment is present. Dose adjustments are required when the medicine is initiated and may also be necessary when other medicines are added to the regimen, especially renally excreted drugs and those with low therapeutic ratios, because of the reduced clearance rate (Howes 2001). Renal impairment alone may not represent a contraindication to a drug or mean that dose adjustments are necessary unless more than 50% of the drug is renally excreted or has active metabolites and renal function is reduced to <50%, with the exception of drugs with a low therapeutic index such as digoxin (Howes 2001). In addition, changes in body composition can change the volume distribution of the drug and result in higher steady-state plasma levels than required. Regular medication review is advocated (see Chapters 2 and 9).

Commonly prescribed medicines that may require dose adjustments in older people with mild renal impairment include oral hypoglycaemic agents, ACE inhibitors, calcium channel blockers, antiarrhythmics, beta blockers, ionotropes, NSAIDs and sedatives, which are all commonly prescribed for people with diabetes. Other drugs such as biguanides and potassium-sparing diuretics are usually relatively or absolutely contraindicated in people with established renal disease. Features of excess drug doses are specific to the particular drug, but common features include delirium, hypotension, respiratory depression, bradycardia and hypoglycaemia, which significantly contributes to falls risk, and behavioural changes that reduce self-care capacity. Some drugs reduce glucose tolerance and lead to hyperglycaemia, e.g. thiazide diuretics, beta blockers and glucocorticoids, which increase the risk of hyperosmolar states and ketoacidosis.

Practice point

Glomerular filtration rate (GFR) may be a more appropriate screen for renal failure in ambulatory older people than serum creatinine. People over 65 with low muscle mass can have significant renal impairment despite normal serum creatinine.

Recently some newer antipsychotics have been linked to IGT and diabetes, for example olanzapine. The increase in blood glucose is not due solely to weight gain (see Chapter 1). Development of diabetes symptoms and blood glucose should be monitored in patients treated with olanzapine. It is a more effective drug and is better tolerated than older antipsychotics and therefore the benefits may outweigh the diabetes risk.

Dose adjustments can be made by altering the dose interval and/or the amount of drug given per dose, depending on the toxicity of the drug. However, it is more common to reduce each dose and maintain the dose interval, unless toxicity is related to continuous exposure such as occurs with aminoglycoside antibiotics, which can contribute to peripheral neuropathy.

Practice points

(1) Serum creatinine is dependent on age, sex and body size.
(2) Serum creatinine may underestimate creatinine clearance in malnourished older people and women with low muscle mass. The serum creatinine may be lower for a given glomerular filtration rate (GFR) so the degree of renal impairment may be underestimated (Nankivell 2001). GFR rate may be a better screen for renal failure in older ambulatory people (MacGinley *et al.* 2004).
(3) It takes between three and five plasma half-lives for a drug to reach steady-state plasma levels and clinical effectiveness during regular administration. The time may be prolonged in older people with renal impairment.
(4) Drugs should be initiated at the lowest dose and increased slowly in small increments, depending on the clinical response.
(5) Regular, accurate blood glucose measurements are required when older people require oral hypoglycaemia agents or insulin.
(6) Multipractitioner prescribing is more likely to lead to adverse drug-related events.

2.6.2 Oral hypoglycaemic agents (OHAs)

Key points

- People with Type 2 diabetes benefit from OHAs before beta cell failure progresses to the stage where insulin is required.
- Lifestyle, blood glucose monitoring technique and self-care potential must be reviewed before commencing OHAs. Strategies to ensure regular blood glucose tests are performed need to be put in place if the individual cannot perform the tests themselves.
- Be aware of possible drug interactions, hypoglycaemia and falls potential.
- Hypoglycaemia symptoms may be atypical in people on OHAs.
- Renal and liver failure may be contraindications to OHAs.

Introduction

The original (first-generation) sulphonylureas first became available in the 1940s, followed by the biguanides in the 1950s. These drugs have been consistently improved over time and new generations of the original sulphonylureas introduced. Three new classes of OHA have been released in the last five years. It is possible that these newer OHAs will extend the life of the pancreatic beta cells and delay the need for insulin (Dornhorst 2001).

OHAs should be used to supplement diet and exercise programmes but they are not a substitute for poor dietary compliance. They are not suitable for people with Type 1 diabetes. Therefore, correctly diagnosing Type 1 diabetes in older people is essential.

Different types of OHAs target the different metabolic defects of Type 2 diabetes.

- Biguanides reduce insulin resistance and fasting blood glucose.
- Sulphonylureas and glitinides are secretagogues that stimulate insulin production.

Table 2.9 Oral hypoglycaemic agents, their dose range and dose frequency, possible adverse effects, the duration of action and main site of metabolism. Reproduced with permission from Dunning 2003.

Drug	Dose	Frequency	Possible side effects	Duration of action (DA)	Site of metabolism
(1) *Sulphonylureas* Chlorpropamide Diabinese 250 mg*	125–500 mg	Single dose taken with, or immediately after food	Hypersensitivity Hypoglycaemia (Rarely used in the elderly because of long duration of action and hypoglycaemia risk) Transient: nausea anorexia vomiting GIT discomfort *May produce a disulfiram reaction with alcohol*	DA: 20–60 h Peak: 5–7 h	Liver
Glibenclamide Daonil 5 mg Euglocon 5 mg Glimel 5 mg	2.5–20 mg	Up to 10 mg as a single dose >10 mg in divided doses Taken with, or immediately before food	Side effects rarely encountered include: nausea anorexia skin rashes Severe hypoglycaemia especially in elderly and those with renal dysfunction	DA: 6–12 h Peak: 6–8 h	Liver
Glipizide Minidiab 5 mg	2.6–40 mg	Up to 15 mg as a single dose >15 mg in a twice daily dosage Taken immediately before meals	GIT disturbances Skin reactions Hypoglycaemia (rare)	DA: Up to 24 h Peak: 1–3 h	Liver

Drug	Dose	Frequency	Side effects	Duration of action	Metabolism/excretion
Tolbutamide Rastinon 0.5 g/1.0 g	0.5–3.0 g	1–3 times/day Taken immediately before food	Mild GIT disturbances Hypoglycaemia (rare)	DA: 8–12 h Peak: 5–7 h	Liver
Diamicron MR (a sustained release preparation)	30–120 mg Dose increments should be two weeks apart	Daily	Hypoglycaemia	Released over 24 hours	Liver
Glimepiride (Amaryl)	1–4 mg	2–3/day	Hypoglycaemia	DA: 5–8 h	Liver
(2) *Biguanides* Metformin Diaformin 500 mg Diabex 500 mg Glucophage 500 mg	0.5–1.5 g May be increased to 3.0 g	1–3 times/day Taken with or immediately after food	GIT disturbances Lactic acidosis Hypoglycaemia with other OHAs Decrease B12 absorption	DA: 5–6 h	*Unchanged in urine*
(3) *Glitinides* (Repaglinide, Nataglitinide)	0.5–16 mg	2–3/day	Hypoglycaemia with other OHAs Weight gain GIT disturbance		Liver
(4) *Thiazolidinediones* (Rosiglitazone, Pioglitazone)	4–8 mg	Daily	Oedema Weight gain CCF, heart failure Raised liver enzymes Pregnancy risk in women with polycystic ovarian disease (Rosiglitazone)	DA: 24 h	Liver
(5) *Alpha-glucosidase inhibitors* (Acarbose)	50–100 mg	TDS with food	GIT problems, e.g. flatulence, diarrhoea Hypoglycaemia		Faeces and urine

* Diabinese is no longer used in Australia.

- Thiazolidinediones (TZD) reduce insulin resistance and daytime preprandial hyperglycaemia and have some effect on fasting blood glucose levels.
- Alpha-glucosidase inhibitors slow carbohydrate digestion, which reduces postprandial blood glucose levels (Braddon 2001).

These drugs effectively control blood glucose levels alone but they can be used in combination. In fact, combinations of different types of OHAs are often required because of their effects on the various underlying metabolic abnormalities of diabetes and the effects of ageing. OHAs can also be effectively combined with insulin.

Blood glucose monitoring is essential to determine when, and which, OHAs should be commenced or added to the regimen or doses reduced or the drug ceased. In other words, to monitor the individual's response to the drug and tailor the dose. Key testing times are:

(1) Before breakfast, which represents fasting levels and indicates the response of the liver to the prevailing insulin level.
(2) Postprandial, which usually means testing two hours after food and indicates how the glucose level has been cleared (glucose disposal). Postprandial glucose rise is an independent risk factor for death, cardiovascular disease, IGT and Type 2 diabetes. Performing postprandial tests is more important when the HbA_{1c} is <7.3%. Normal fasting blood glucose but elevated postprandial levels may indicate the need for a change of medications (Abrahamson 2004). Sometimes both fasting and postprandial testing is required.

Sulphonylureas

Sulphonylureas bind to high-affinity receptors on the pancreatic beta cells and inhibit the electrical activity of ATP-sensitive potassium channels, to reduce potassium efflux through these channels. As a result, voltage-dependent calcium channels on the beta cell membrane open, calcium enters the beta cell and insulin is released. Sulphonylureas are usually well tolerated but there is a tendency for people to gain weight because they stimulate the appetite. Hypoglycaemia is a considerable risk, especially in older people on long-acting agents and people with renal impairment. Sulphonylureas are usually used in a daily or b.d. regime depending on the duration of action and individual need.

A secondary sulphonylurea effect is to increase tissue sensitivity to insulin by unknown mechanisms. Normal and drug-induced insulin release is a biphasic response. The first phase occurs quickly in response to glucose. The second phase is slower and more prolonged. Type 2 diabetes is characterised by loss of the first phase.

Adverse side effects
Profound hypoglycaemia is the major adverse effect of all sulphonylureas due to accumulation of the drug if elimination is impaired, the dose increased, food is delayed, meals are missed, insufficient carbohydrate is consumed or activity is increased. Less commonly, weight gain occurs, which is particularly a problem in inactive and bed-bound older people. Liver dysfunction, nausea, vomiting, various skin rashes, increased appetite and, rarely, agranulocytosis and red cell aplasia may also occur.

Sulphonylureas are mostly metabolised in the liver and are renally excreted, therefore severe liver and renal disease are contraindications to their use. Caution should be exercised in people who are allergic to the sulphur drugs because the sulphonyl-ureas have a similar chemical composition and may cause reactions. Hyperglycaemia, with or without symptoms, initially (primary failure) or after a period of good control (secondary failure) commonly occurs and insulin therapy is required. Severe hyper-glycaemia inhibits food absorption from the GI tract due to gastroparesis caused by dehydration. The gastroparesis usually reverses once the blood glucose is controlled. If it does not, further investigation is warranted.

Recent research suggests sulphonylureas may attenuate the degree of ST-segment elevation during acute myocardial infarction, especially where protein kinase C levels peak between 500 and 1000 mg/L (Huizar *et al.* 2003). This could lead to under-use of thrombolytic therapy in older people and increase morbidity and mortality asso-ciated with cardiovascular disease. Another blood glucose-lowering agent or insulin may be required.

Active metabolites of sulphonylureas are produced in the liver but excreted by the kidney. In older people with renal impairment the hypoglycaemiac action may be prolonged. Gliclazide and glipizide may be the drugs of choice in these patients because they are converted to inactive metabolites in the liver. In particular, gliclazide MR is associated with fewer hypoglycaemic events because it has no active metabolites, the time course of action is slow (over six hours) and binding to the beta cell insulin receptors is reversible (Schernthaner *et al.* 2004).

Biguanides

Biguanides are the drug of choice in overweight people with Type 2 diabetes. Metformin is the only available form of biguanide. Biguanides can be safely combined with sulphonylureas.

The mechanisms of action of biguanides, listed below, are not as well understood as the actions of sulphonylureas.

- Delaying absorption of glucose from the gut.
- Inhibiting gluconeogenesis (glucose production by the liver).
- Increasing conversion of glucose to lactate in the gut.
- Enhancing glucose uptake into muscles and fat.
- Increasing effects of insulin at receptor sites.
- Reducing hepatic gluconeogenesis, which reduces the hepatic glucose output.
- Suppressing appetite (mild effect).

There is some evidence that biguanides cause malabsorption of Vitamin B_{12} but most of the studies are old and the clinical relevance is not yet established. Vitamin B_{12} malabsorption could be an important consideration in older people who are malnourished. Some studies indicate an association between Vitamin B_{12} mal-absoprtion and anaemia (Tomkin *et al.* 1971). Due to the importance of nutrition to wellbeing in older patients, regular measurement of Vitamin B_{12} serum levels in older patients on long-term metformin may be warranted. Biguanides should be ceased for two days before surgery and investigative procedures such as IVPs, angiograms and CAT scans, and investigations that require IV iodinated contrast media may be contraindicated (Calabrese *et al.* 2002). They are inappropriate in the presence of gastrointestinal disorders such as inflammatory bowel disease.

Practice points

Biguanides:

(1) Do not stimulate the production or release of insulin and therefore are unlikely to cause hypoglycaemia if they are used alone.
(2) Have favourable effects on the lipid profile and retard glucose absorption from the intestine.
(3) Do not generally stimulate the appetite and are less likely to contribute to weight gain.
(4) May reduce the appetite and assist weight loss.

Metformin is not metabolised and is excreted unchanged through the kidneys so is contraindicated in older people with renal impairment. The dose is not usually increased if the serum creatinine is 0.15 mmol/L and is ceased at 0.20 mmol/L. Metformin is usually administered before meals to reduce the GI effects.

Adverse effects of metformin
GI effects such as anorexia, nausea and/or diarrhoea and sometimes a metallic taste occur in 10–15% of patients. Some people report tiredness. Most patients tolerate biguanides if they are started at a low dose, the tablets are taken with or immediately after food, and the dose is titrated upwards gradually. However, adverse effects often limit the maximum tolerated dose (Jennings 1997).

Lactic acidosis is the most serious adverse effect of metformin and may occur if alcohol is consumed while taking biguanides. Lactic acidosis is rare but 57 cases have occurred since metformin was introduced in Australia; 16 were fatal and there were known risk factors present in 41 of the 57 cases (Jerrall 2002). The risk factors for lactic acidosis are discussed in Chapter 4.

The risk of lactic acidosis is increased in people with liver, renal and cardiac disease, which includes many older people.

Glitinides

Glitinides are non-sulphonylurea insulin-stimulating drugs that boost postprandial insulin release. They should only be taken with meals, usually 2–3 times per day. They are short-acting drugs and have a low hypoglycaemia risk, so may be useful for older people with erratic eating patterns. They target early-phase insulin release, which reduces the postprandial blood glucose rise and deals with the meal-related glucose load (Dornhorst 2001). In this way they initiate an insulin response pattern close to normal. They can be used in combination with biguanides and possibly TZDs. At present, glitinides are used as secondary agents in Australia because they are not subsidised through the Prescription Benefits Scheme.

Thiazolidinediones (TZDs)

The TZDs enhance insulin action and improve glucose tolerance by directly targeting insulin resistance and improving tissue sensitivity to insulin. They modify intracellular enzymes. It takes several days for their effects to show. They have a long duration of action with the main site of action being in adipose tissue. TZDs reduce muscle and liver insulin resistance, improve the blood glucose and lipid profiles, enhance insulin sensitivity and may restore the beta cell mass. TZDs can be combined with metformin or sulphonylureas. It may take up to three months for blood glucose improvements to occur.

An early form of TZD, troglitizone, was responsible for causing liver failure and was withdrawn from the market. This effect is unlikely with the currently available preparations but it is recommended that liver function be monitored regularly and caution exercised if they are used in people with liver damage or whose albumin excretion rate is elevated. This may mean TZDs are not suitable for many older people.

Hypoglycaemia is possible because TZDs reduce insulin resistance and enhance the effectiveness of the individual's endogenous insulin.

Adverse effects of TZDs

- Localised oedema.
- Congestive cardiac failure (CHF) and heart failure. They can be used in people with class I or II New York Heart Association (NYHA) heart disease categories who do not have signs of CHF, but at a lower dose. They are contraindicated in NYHA class III and IV.
- Reduced red and white cell counts.
- Weight gain, especially deposition of subcutaneous fat, while visceral obesity is reduced.
- Hypercholesterolaemia.
- Liver damage.
- Care should be taken in lactose-intolerant people, especially people from Asian backgrounds, because TZDs contain a small amount of lactose.

TZDs can be added to the insulin regime to improve glycaemic control (Raskin *et al.* 2001). In addition, they may have anti-inflammatory effects on endothelial function, monocyte and macrophage function, lipid abnormalities and fibrinolysis that have positive benefits for cardiovascular disease reduction.

Alpha-glucosidase inhibitors

These drugs competitively inhibit gastrointestinal alpha-glucosidase enzymes that metabolise disaccharides and complex carbohydrates to monosaccharides for absorption. They are often used with diet or OHAs.

They act by binding to alpha-glucosidase in the upper GI brush border, which delays the breakdown of complex carbohydrates to monosaccharides. There, they delay carbohydrate uptake from the gut and give normal glucose disposal mechanisms more time to deal with the postprandial glucose load, thereby reducing the postprandial glucose rise. They only have a small effect on fasting glucose levels. Acarbose itself is not absorbed. Because the site of action is the gut, gastrointestinal pathology may be a contraindication to their use.

Their major side effects occur in the GI tract due to the fermentation of undigested carbohydrate in the lower bowel. These effects include borborygmus, bloating, flatulence and diarrhoea. These symptoms can be distressing and embarrassing and people often stop their medications because of these side effects.

Taking the drugs with meals, starting with a low dose and increasing the dose slowly to tolerance levels and carefully explaining the likely effects to the individual can reduce these problems. Hypoglycaemia is possible if alpha-glucosidase inhibitors are combined with other OHAs.

Practice point

Alpha-glucosidase inhibitors prolong the absorption of simple sugar; therefore oral glucose may not be effective treatment for hypoglycaemia. IM glucagon is a recommended alternative or IV glucose if necessary.

Medication interactions with OHAs

OHA interactions are possible with many commonly used drugs and can lead to hypo- or hyperglycaemia. A number of mechanisms for the interactions are known.

(1) Enhanced hypoglycaemic effects:
- displacing drugs from binding sites, e.g. salicylates; usually a short-term effect occurs when commencing or stopping interacting drugs
- prolonging the half-life by inhibiting or reducing hepatic metabolism, e.g. warfarin and cimetidine
- delaying excretion, e.g. allopurinol, sulphonamides
- reducing insulin release. Exhibiting own hypoglycaemic action, e.g. alcohol.

(2) Hyperglycaemia:
- antagonising insulin action
- exhibiting own hyperglycaemic activity, e.g. corticosteroids, St John's wort. Potential drug–herb and herb–herb interactions should be considered when relevant.

Practice points

(1) The clinical relevance of some postulated drug interactions is not clear.
(2) Other miscellaneous interactions that should also be considered:
- beta blockers can mask tachycardia and other signs of hypoglycaemia and delay recognition and treatment of hypoglycaemia, which increases the risk of hypoglycaemia coma
- chronic alcohol consumption can stimulate the metabolism of sulphonylureas and delay their effectiveness.

Actual and potential interactions have yet to emerge for TZDs and the glitinides. Drugs that alter hepatic enzymes may cause interactions with these OHAs because they are metabolised in the liver.

Drugs that interact with alpha-glucosidase inhibitors can decrease their action by blocking their access to the gut mucosa, e.g. charcoal, digestive enzymes, cholestyramine and neomycin. In addition, GI problems, such as gastroparesis or irritable bowel syndrome, may be contraindications to using these drugs.

Combining OHAs together

There is no real benefit in combining two sulphonylureas because they both act by the same mechanism. Sulphonylureas can be used with biguanides for patients who have either primary or secondary OHA failure on sulphonylureas alone, especially if the person is overweight.

Practice point

Medication rounds should be planned so that OHAs and insulin are given with or before meals, or enteral feeds if these are given at different times from other meal-times, to reduce the risk of hypoglycaemia.

Combining OHAs and insulin

In some patients a combination of insulin and a sulphonylurea or biguanide may help control the blood glucose. The combination of insulin and biguanides is increasingly common, since the results of the UKPDS in 1998. The time of the day to administer insulin depends on the blood glucose profile. It is often commenced at bedtime to reduce fasting blood glucose levels and the OHA is given in the morning. Combination therapy allows people to become accustomed to the need for insulin and helps preserve beta cell function. In many cases a small dose of intermediate/long-acting insulin is given at bedtime to help control the blood glucose overnight, and thus reduce fasting hyperglycaemia in the morning, making it easier to control the blood glucose during the day. Psychological support is important for older people commencing insulin as is appropriate education to allay fears of hypoglycaemia and that insulin is a 'death sentence'.

The advantage of combination OHA/insulin therapy is that less insulin is required, which reduces peripheral hyperinsulinaemia, which may be less atherogenic than using insulin alone (Jennings 1997). However, the atherogenic role of insulin remains controversial. The disadvantages of using two potential harmful drugs together include the increased risk of hypoglycaemia and falls and a more complicated regimen. It does halt the beta cell decline that is a feature of Type 2 diabetes.

2.6.3 Lipid-lowering agents

An essential aspect of the diabetes management plan is reducing the cardiovascular risk. People with diabetes, especially Type 2, are at significant risk of cardiovascular disease unless the blood glucose and lipids can be kept within normal limits. Most management strategies aim to reduce cholesterol, especially LDL and triglycerides, and increase HDL. HDL aids in the removal of LDL cholesterol. A common lipid profile in people with Type 2 diabetes and hyperglycaemia is high cholesterol and triglycerides and low HDL, which significantly increases the risk of myocardial infarction. Other risk factors are also important and are often exacerbated by low levels of HDL (Colquhoun 2002).

Controlling blood glucose is integral to controlling lipids (Lipid Study Group 1998). Current lipid targets for patients with existing heart disease are:

- Total cholesterol <4 mmol/L.
- Triglycerides <2 mmol/L.
- LDL <2.5 mmol/L.
- HDL-c >1 mmol/L.
- Cholesterol/HDL-c ratio <4.5 mmol/L (National Heart Foundation 2001; Therapeutic Guidelines: Endocrinology 2004).

Lipid management

Lipid management strategies are set out in a number of guidelines and aim to lower the absolute cardiovascular risk rather than the lipid levels alone. Age and sex may also be relevant. Individual cardiovascular risk assessment includes the following.

- Previous cardiovascular events and current cardiovascular status, presence of hypertension, smoking and family history of hypercholesterolaemia and cardiac disease.
- Dietary modification including reducing salt, alcohol and fat but considering over-all nutritional needs.
- Low-dose aspirin to reduce platelet stickiness.
- ACE inhibitors are the agents of choice to control blood pressure. In some cases other antihypertensive agents may be required instead or to support ACE.
- Smoking cessation.
- Exercise/mobility programme.
- Lipid-lowering agents. Most people will be commenced on an HMG CoA reductase inhibitor (statin). Statins reduce recurrent coronary events, the need for revascularisation procedures and the incidence of thromboembolic stroke (La Rosa *et al.* 1999). Statins may be contraindicated in the presence of liver impairment and regular liver function tests are recommended. When triglycerides and cholesterol are raised, fibrates may be required.
- Coaching (see Chapter 5).

Recent research suggests that high cholesterol in people over 70 may produce better health outcomes (Simons *et al.* 2001). Some doctors are reluctant to commence statins in ageing older people despite the benefits outweighing the potential harm and guidelines advocating their use (Ko *et al.* 2004). Statins are very effective secondary cardiovascular risk prevention agents, even where cholesterol is not significantly elevated, and there is evidence of benefit in older people such as reduced number of coronary events. Table 2.10 depicts the major classes of lipid-lowering agents (Colquhoun 2002).

Adverse effects

The main adverse effects occur in skeletal muscle and include myositis, gastrointestinal disturbances (clofibrate) and myopathies.

Many people stop taking their lipid-lowering agents because they are not convinced they really need them, perceive that they have poor efficacy or dislike the associated adverse events. Nurses can play a key role in encouraging people to adhere to their medicines by explaining why they are needed as part of medicine education and suggesting ways to limit minor side effects.

Table 2.10   Lipid-lowering agents. Reproduced with permission from Dunning 2003.

Lipid-lowering drug and main action	Management considerations
HMG CoA reductase inhibitors: reduce LDL-c	Test liver function on commencing and in six months. Use caution if liver disease is present. Decrease the dose if the patient commences cyclosporine.
Fibrates: reduce cholesterol and triglycerides and increase HDL-c	Can be combined with HMG CoA after a trial on monotherapy. Monitor creatinine kinase and liver function at six weeks and then in six months.
Resins (cholestyramine, colestipol): enhance LDL-c lowering effects of HMG CoA agents	Allows lower doses of the resins to be used. Slows absorption of oral hypoglycaemic agents. Increases hypoglycaemia risk when used with these agents.
Low-dose nicotinic acid	Can be given with HMG CoA agents. Enhances reduction of triglyceride and HDL-c.
Statins: reduce LDL-c, have a moderate effect on triglycerides and increase HDL. Increase bone mineral density	They can be used with a resin. Monitor liver function.

Source: Nicholson 2002.

2.6.4   Insulin therapy in older people

Key points

- By the time a person with Type 2 diabetes is commenced on insulin therapy, they have usually had the disease for at least 10 years and have established complications of diabetes.
- Check dose and time of administration.
- Consider onset and duration of action when planning mealtimes and drug rounds.
- Monitor blood glucose profile.
- Reassurance is needed to allay the person's fears of insulin use.

Practice points

(1)   Type 2 diabetes is associated with progressive beta cell failure and insulin is ultimately required in the majority of people.
(2)   People with Type 2 diabetes on insulin report a lower quality of life than people not on insulin.

Type 2 diabetes is associated with progressive beta cell failure and insulin is required to control blood glucose and prevent mobilisation of lipid and protein glucose substrates to reduce the risk of morbidity and mortality. However, many people believe insulin means they have failed and they worry about having to start insulin. People are reluctant to start insulin for a number of reasons including weight gain, needle fears and phobias, fear of hypoglycaemia and the mythology about disease severity, e.g. 'insulin is the end of the line'. Health professionals often contribute to the myth that diet- and OHA-controlled diabetes are milder than insulin-treated diabetes (Dunning & Martin 1999). In addition, doctors often use insulin as a threat to motivate patients to comply with diet or OHA but are often reluctant to commence insulin, especially in older people. In turn, some older people perceive insulin to be 'the end of the road' and 'it means I have to go into a home' (personal experience).

Basic insulin action

Insulin is a hormone secreted by the beta cells of the pancreas. Normal requirements vary between 0.5 and 1.0 unit/kg/day. Insulin synthesis and secretion are primarily stimulated by the increase in the blood glucose level after meals. Once released, insulin attaches to insulin receptors on cell membranes and facilitates the passage of glucose into the cell via a number of mechanisms. Inside the cells, glucose is used as energy or stored as glycogen.

In addition, insulin reduces hepatic glucose production, stimulates the storage of fatty acids and amino acids, facilitates glycogen formation and storage in the liver and skeletal muscle, and limits lipolysis and proteolysis. Therefore, if insulin is deficient, protein, fat and carbohydrate metabolism are altered, producing hyperglycaemia and hyperlipidaemia which increase the risk of short- and long-term diabetes complications.

Exogenous insulin is a very effective drug. It is vital for people with Type 1 diabetes and eventually required by ≥50% of people with Type 2 diabetes. The possible need for insulin therapy should be raised early in the diabetes education process so the person understands that the progression to insulin is a natural process. Insulin is also the drug of choice if significant renal or liver impairment is present. Unfortunately, people with Type 2 diabetes are often given the impression that insulin is a last resort to be used when all else fails and they are to blame for the failure.

There is no doubt that insulin can be an added self-care burden and insulin management is an ongoing issue in residential care facilities, especially if more than one dose is needed per day and the individual needs assistance to prepare and administer the dose because they have limited manual dexterity, cognitive deficits or visual impairment. Family members or other care arrangements will be needed. Secondary causes of hyperglycaemia, such as intercurrent illness, thyroid disease and medicines, need to be determined and managed before starting insulin.

Objectives of insulin therapy

The objectives of insulin therapy are to:
- Achieve blood glucose and lipid levels in an acceptable range by replacing absent insulin secretion in Type 1 and supplementing insulin production in Type 2 diabetes, depending on individual hypoglycaemic risk, life expectancy and quality of life.
- Approximate physiological insulin secretion.
- Avoid hypoglycaemia and hyperglycaemia.
- Improve quality of life and reduce effects of long-term complications by achieving appropriate control.

- Continue diet and activity to maximise the effect of the insulin.
- Meet blood glucose targets: <6.1 mmol/L fasting and <7.8 mmol/L after meals, random 4–8 mmol/L to achieve HbA$_{1c}$ <7%. Note that these levels may be too strict for older people because of the risk of hypoglycaemia and consequent trauma.

Types of insulin currently available

A number of different brands of insulin are available, e.g. Novo Nordisk, Eli Lilly. Animal insulins are rarely used nowadays but are still available in some countries. Insulin is manufactured by recombinant DNA technology. The amino acid sequence of recombinant DNA insulin (HM insulin) is the same as insulin secreted by the beta cells of the human pancreas. HM insulin is now the only widely available insulin, regardless of the brand used.

In the past few years insulin analogues have been developed that produce a more 'normal' physiological response after injection and improve the blood glucose profile, e.g. Humalog and insulin Aspart. These insulins reduce postprandial hyperglycaemia and significantly lessen the risk of hypoglycaemia. Insulin glargine is a long-acting insulin analogue that gives a smooth, peakless glucose profile for 24 hours (Buse 2001). Insulin analogues allow greater management flexibility and insulin combinations that meet individual needs and reduce hypoglycaemia risk.

Rapid-acting insulins
Rapid-acting insulins should be clear and colourless in appearance. Examples are:

- Lispro (Humalog).
- Novorapid.

They have a rapid onset of action, usually within ten minutes, peak at 60 minutes and act for 2–4 hours. They are usually given immediately before meals but can be given immediately after eating. They are used in basal bolus regimes in combination with intermediate-acting insulin. They are also used in insulin pumps, but not many older people use this type of therapy because of the cost. Combining rapid-acting insulin with alpha-glucosidase inhibitors, which reduce glucose absorption from the gut, can increase the risk of hypoglycaemia. Peak times for hypoglycaemia are the first hour after injection and 2–3 hours after exercise.

Short-acting insulins
Short-acting insulins should be clear and colourless. Examples are:

- Actrapid.
- Humulin R or Humulin S.
- Hypurin neutral (beef), which starts working more slowly and lasts longer. It is rarely used.

They begin to take effect in 20–30 minutes after injection and act for about four hours. They can be used:

- Alone, two to four times a day.
- In combination with intermediate- or long-acting insulins.
- As IV insulin infusions in times of acute metabolic stress such as myocardial infarction, ketoacidosis and hyperosmolar states and surgery.

Intermediate-acting insulins

Intermediate-acting insulins must be mixed gently before they are used and should be milky after mixing. There are two broad types:

(1) Isophane insulin in which the protein protamine is used to slow the insulin absorption rate, e.g. Humulin NPH, Protaphane.
(2) Lente insulin in which zinc is used to slow the absorption, e.g. Humulin L and Monotard, which have been withdrawn from the market in some countries.

The onset of action of both types is 2–3 hours and the duration of action is 12–18 hours. However, Monotard can last for up to 24 hours. Intermediate-acting insulins are used:

- In combination with short-acting insulin, which is the usual method.
- Alone, for patients who are sensitive to short-acting insulin, or in combination with oral hypoglycaemic agents.

Long-acting insulins

Protamine or zinc is used in long-acting insulins to slow their absorption rate. These insulins must be combined by gently rolling the bottle or vial between the hands before use. Most should appear milky after mixing. Examples are:

- Hypurin Isophane (beef) (rarely used).
- Ultratard.
- Humulin UL.
- Insulin glargine (lantus), which acts for 24 hours with no peak action time.

Practice points

(1) Insulin glargine is *clear* but it is not short acting.
(2) It can be given at any time of the day but the time must be the same each day.
(3) It cannot be mixed with any other insulin.
(4) It must be injected into a different site from short- and rapid-acting insulins.

Long-acting insulins begin to act 4–6 hours after injecting, have their maximal effect between eight and 24 hours and continue to act for 30–36 hours. They are used in much the same way as intermediate-acting insulin and some have been withdrawn from the market in some countries, for example Humulin L and Ultralente. Long-acting insulins may significantly increase the risk of hypoglycaemia in older people which may be prolonged.

Biphasic or premixed insulins

Biphasic insulins are often prescribed for people with Type 2 diabetes. They make it easier for people to manage insulin injections themselves since it is not necessary to mix two types of insulins in syringes. Biphasic insulins include both short- and intermediate-acting varieties in various combinations. The bottle or vial must be gently rolled between the hands to ensure the insulin is correctly combined before using. Independent adjustment of the short and intermediate components of the mix is not possible; therefore it is difficult to achieve ideal blood glucose levels in some cases. These insulins always have protamine-containing intermediate insulin in the mix because the kinetics of the short-acting insulin component is not affected by protamine. Examples are:

- Mixtard 30/70.
- Mixtard 50/50.
- Mixtard 15/85 and 20/80.
- Insulin Aspart (NovoMix 30).
- Humulin 20/80.
- Humulin 50/50.
- Humalog Mix 25.

A range of devices are available to administer insulin. Some have large numbers to make it easier for visually impaired people to remain independent.

Storing insulin correctly

It is important to store insulin correctly in the home and care settings. Insulin should be stored according to the manufacturer's directions to maintain its efficacy. Unopened vials should be stored in the refrigerator at 2–8°C. Insulin vials currently in use can be stored out of the refrigerator, e.g. in the person's medication drawer or handbag, provided they are not stored near a source of heat (Campbell *et al.* 1993). Older people with diabetes need to be advised about correct storage and handling of insulin and to check expiry dates on the bottle as part of their education about insulin therapy.

Clinical observation

Hyperglycaemia associated with using incorrectly stored insulin and insulin that has passed the expiry date does occur.

Practice points

(1) Do not freeze insulin.
(2) Check the expiry date before use.
(3) Discard if out of date or the appearance has changed.
(4) Discard open bottles/vials one month after opening.

Administering insulin

Administer at the appropriate time before or with the meal depending on the insulin type. Sometimes it may be better to administer insulin after a meal when the amount of food eaten can be assessed and the insulin dose adjusted if necessary. The abdomen is the preferred administration site but upper arms, thighs and buttocks can also be used. However, sometimes there is little subcutaneous tissue in frail older people and the insulin profile will then be less predictable. Injection sites must be rotated to avoid lipoatrophy and lipodystrophy. Appropriate needle sizes are 12.7 mm for obese people, 8 mm if the weight is normal and 6 mm for lean people.

The insulin injection technique can influence insulin absorption and, therefore, its action. Insulin should be administered subcutaneously. Intramuscular (IM) injections lead to unstable blood glucose levels (Vaag *et al.* 1990). A number of injection devices are available (see Table 2.11). It might be more convenient for nurses to use insulin

Table 2.11 Commonly used insulin administration devices and some of the issues to be aware of with each device. Adapted with permission from Dunning 2003.

Device	Issues to be aware of
Syringes 30, 50 and 100 unit sizes	• There is still a place for using syringes. • Patients and carers need to be able to recognise different dose increments on different sized syringes. • Select syringe size appropriate for dose. • Needles are usually longer than other devices. • Can be used with all available insulins.
Insulin 'pens' There are two main manufacturers of insulin devices: NovoNordisk and Owen Mumford	• Insulin 'pens' are not suitable for people who need to mix insulins.
NovoPen 3	• Dose range 2–70 units. • Accurate dosing. • Uses 3 mL insulin cartridges. • Small, fine needles. • Replacing the insulin cartridge can be difficult. • Has a function to check the accuracy of the device. • Pen is reusable. • Use with Novorapid, Actrapid, Protaphane, Mixtard 30/80, 30/70, 50/80. • Different coloured pens are available, which can be used for different insulins. The colour can be matched to the colour on the insulin vial, e.g. Actrapid has a yellow band so choose a yellow pen.
NovoPen Demi	• Similar to NovoPen 3, but ½ unit dose increments are possible. • Useful for children and insulin-sensitive patients who require very small doses.
INNOVO	• Dose range 1–70 units. • Accurate dosing. • Uses 3 mL insulin cartridges. • Range of insulin available. • Battery operated; batteries last about four years and then the device needs to be replaced. • Small, fine needles. • A display indicates that insulin is being delivered, the number of units delivered, the dose given and time elapsed since the previous dose was administered. • Can be difficult to use, especially if large doses are needed. • May help people who forget whether they have taken their insulin. • Reusable device.

Table 2.11 (*cont'd*)

Device	Issues to be aware of
INNOLET	• Dose range 1–50 units. • Accurate dosing. • Small, fine needles. • Device is preloaded and disposable. • Only Protaphane and Mixtard 30/70 insulin available in Australia, at this stage. Protaphane is not available in the UK. • Contains 3 mL of insulin. • Clear, easy-to-see numbers on the dose dial, which is an advantage for vision-impaired people. • Easy to depress the plunger. • Larger than other devices – takes up storage space in fridge.
PenMate 3	• Automatic needle insertion device. • Used with NovoPen 3. • Hides needle and injects insulin quickly and automatically. • May benefit people with needle phobia and children.
NovoMix 30 FlexPen	• Contains 3 mL of insulin (1–60 units). • Disposable, preloaded device. • Small, fine needles.
Insulin pumps	• Provide continuous basal insulin with a facility for giving bolus doses with meals. • Use only short-acting insulin. • Use small, fine needles. • Expensive. • Require considerable expertise and time to be used effectively.
Jet injectors	• No needle required. • Not widely used. • Force insulin through skin under pressure. • Bruising common. • Sterilisation issues.
Humapen	• Non-disposable pen. • Takes 3 mL vials of Lilly insulins Humulin R, Humalog, Humulin NPH, 20/80, 30/70, Humalog mix 25. • Dials between 1 and 60 units. • Available in two colours.

syringes in hospital and residential care settings. However, if the person is able to, they should be encouraged to continue their insulin administration and blood glucose testing in these settings. To administer the injection:

(1) Pinch up a fold of skin (dermis and subcutaneous tissue) between the thumb and index finger.
(2) Inject at 90° angle. Pinch-up may not be needed and a 45° angle can be used in very thin people.
(3) Release the skin, remove the needle and apply pressure to the site.
(4) Document dose and time of the injection and monitor response.
(5) Injection sites should be regularly checked for swelling, lumps, bruising, pain or leakage of insulin, especially if the patient is on thrombolytic medications, salicylates and some herbs such as St John's wort.

Practice points

(1) A range of needle sizes is available. People with diabetes usually prefer small, fine-gauge needles (e.g. 30 or 31 gauge), which make the injections relatively painless.
(2) Giving the first injection is often very difficult for people with diabetes, especially older people. Encouragement and allowing them to take their time and inject at their own pace is important.
(3) If insulin leaks onto the skin after the injection, release the skinfold before actually injecting the insulin. Pressure from holding the skinfold sometimes forces the insulin back out of the needle track. Do not cover the injection site so that any insulin leakage can be observed. Check the individual's technique to ascertain that they leave the needle in the skin for about 10 seconds after injecting before removing the needle.
(4) Leaking even small amounts of insulin can cause unpredictable increases in the blood glucose and lead to inappropriate dose adjustment. Careful observation and estimation of the amount of insulin lost is necessary to make appropriate dose adjustments and help the individual correct their injection technique.
(5) The larger the volume of insulin injected, the greater the likelihood of some insulin leaking back along the needle track.
(6) Leakage can occur if the injection is too shallow or given intradermally.

Mixing short- and long-acting insulin

Mixing short- and long-acting insulins before injection may cause a reduction in the short-acting peak, especially if the insulin is left to stand for a long time before use. The effect is more marked when there is substantially more long-acting insulin in the mixture (as is usually the case).

The clinical significance of these changes is unknown. It is more likely to apply in home situations where home-based nurses or relatives draw up doses for several days for patients to self-administer. This practice is not ideal and not accepted in some places. However, it does allow people to retain a measure of independence if syringes are their chosen device.

Practice point

Long-acting and premixed insulins in vials and insulin pens must be mixed gently before administration.

Common insulin regimes

Daily injection
Daily injections usually consist of a combination of short- and long-acting insulin and are usually administered before breakfast but are often given at bedtime if combined with OHAs. Biphasic insulin is a common choice for morning daily regimes. Protaphane or NPH is often used at night for combination regimes.

Daily regimes are commonly used for:

- Older people.
- People who will only accept one injection.
- Situations where people are dependent on home nursing care.

Twice-a-day regime (b.d.)
These regimes usually consist of a combination of short- and long-acting insulin given before breakfast and before the evening meal. Biphasic insulins are commonly used but do not allow a great deal of flexibility in adjusting doses. There is a risk of nocturnal hypoglycaemia. Usually two-thirds of the total dose is given in the morning and one-third in the evening.

Figure 2.3 depicts the insulin profiles of the various insulin regimes and indicates the main hypoglycaemia risk times. It gives an indication of which insulin to adjust, when considered in conjunction with the blood glucose profile. Consideration should always be given to other factors that affect blood glucose levels.

Practice point

Rapid-acting insulins act very quickly so they should be given *immediately* before a meal to avoid hypoglycaemia. Sometimes they can be administered within 15 minutes after the meal when a person eats erratically or in palliative care settings.

Basal bolus regime
The aim of the basal bolus regime is to simulate the normal pattern of insulin secretion, i.e. a small amount of circulating insulin is present in the blood at all times and restrains gluconeogenesis and glycogenolysis. This is the basal insulin. In non-diabetics, a bolus amount of insulin is stimulated by the blood glucose rise after a glucose load. Bolus injections of short-acting insulin are given before each meal to mimic this response.

The longer-acting insulin is given before bed to supply the basal insulin requirement. The basal bolus regime offers more flexibility in insulin dose adjustment and mealtimes and therefore lifestyle is less restricted. The amount of insulin given at each dose is usually small so the likelihood of hypoglycaemia is reduced. The complexity of the regime is a disadvantage for many older people.

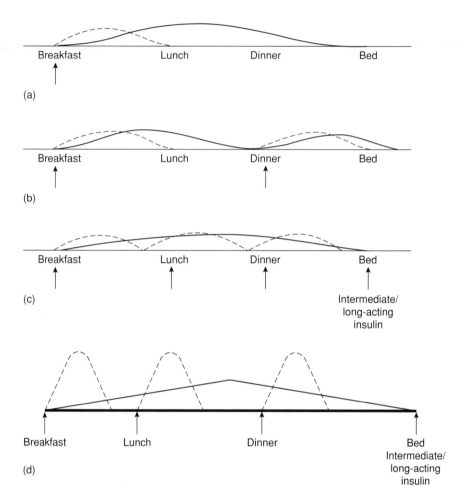

Figure 2.3 Diagrammatic representation of insulin action showing different regimes:
(a) daily, (b) twice a day, (c) basal bolus using short-acting insulins and (d) basal
bolus using rapid-acting insulins. Reproduced with permission from Dunning 2003.
Note: The broken line depicts short-acting insulin, the unbroken line intermediate/long-acting insulin.
The arrows indicate the time of injection.

Continuous subcutaneous insulin infusion (CSII)

Insulin pumps can be programmed to continuously deliver subcutaneous insulin at a
basal rate and set bolus doses before meals. They allow a more physiological insulin
profile to be attained and greater flexibility in meeting individual insulin requirements
but are not commonly used by older people. Insulin pumps are expensive and require
a great deal of commitment by the person with diabetes to use them safely and
effectively. They cannot be used if the person is cognitively impaired or has visual
or manual dexterity deficits.

The choice of insulin regime and insulin delivery system depends on personal
preference, the degree of blood glucose control aimed for and the willingness and

Table 2.12 Factors that affect insulin absorption and therefore the blood glucose profile.

Accelerated absorption	Delayed absorption
Exercise	Low body temperature, for example hypothermia.
High body temperature, e.g. during illness, after a hot bath	Poor circulation.
	Smoking, which constricts blood vessels.
Massage round the injection site	Intermediate- and long-acting insulins and OHAs.
IM injection	

ability of the patient to monitor their blood glucose. Many factors can influence insulin absorption and consequently the blood glucose profile. Some of these factors are shown in Table 2.12.

Sliding scale and top-up regimes

Sliding scales of insulin

A sliding scale of insulin refers to a regime where the amount of insulin administered is adjusted according to the immediate past blood glucose test result.

Subcutaneous insulin   Sliding scales address past events, rather than anticipate insulin needs. They do not consider future factors that might influence blood glucose results. In addition, the effect of the subcutaneous dose is not seen for at least 2–4 hours. Subcutaneous sliding scales are therefore not generally recommended. The use of subcutaneous sliding scales of insulin to control newly diagnosed or unstable, brittle or ill hospitalised diabetic patients is inefficient and delays the establishment of an appropriate insulin dose (Katz 1991). However, some flexibility is necessary to improve safety. Sliding scales may have a limited role for short periods after an acute event such as an AMI or surgery. However, prolonged sliding scales may make it difficult to achieve a stable blood glucose pattern.

Intravenous insulin   Insulin administered intravenously has a short half-life of 1–2 minutes, which allows acceptable blood glucose control to be achieved rapidly. Intravenous sliding scales are often used to manage:

- Diabetic ketoacidosis.
- Hyperosmolar coma.
- Surgery (perioperative).
- Acute cardiovascular and, increasingly, cerebrovascular events.
- Patients receiving nutritional support (TPN) in some hospital settings.

The particular sliding scale used varies depending on the underlying condition and established protocols. Blood glucose should be tested hourly initially and then two or four hourly when the condition is stable.

Adjusting the dose of intravenous insulin   The dose of insulin is ordered according to body weight and the previous blood glucose profile. It is important to establish the emerging blood glucose pattern to allow the appropriate insulin to be adjusted *prospectively.*

Ascertain the effects of other factors that influence blood glucose results.

- Insulin technique.
- Distribution of insulin doses over the day.
- Total dose of insulin to be given.
- Presence of pain, body temperature, emotional stress, infection/illness.
- Dietary intake.
- Timing of injection in relation to food intake.
- Activity/mobility level.
- Concurrent medications that affect blood glucose levels.
- Blood glucose monitoring technique.
- Condition of injection sites.
- The individual's preferred insulin delivery device may limit the choice of insulin.

Adjusting these factors may be more important than adjusting the insulin dose. The dose/s of insulin should then be adjusted for the *next* day and blood glucose monitored four hourly.

Intravenous (IV) insulin infusions   Intravenous insulin infusions are the optimal treatment method in metabolically hypotensive, compromised individuals to achieve insulin uptake into tissues. IV insulin limits:

- Hyperglycaemia, by limiting conversion of glycogen and fatty acids to glucose in the liver.
- Ketone formation, by reducing utilisation of fatty acids for glucogenolysis.
- Protein catabolism, which reduces the substrate available for gluconeogenesis.

Reducing hyperglycaemia lowers tissue resistance and facilitates glucose entry into the cells. The aim of the infusion is to gradually reduce the blood glucose concentration to a steady level between 10 and 12 mmol/L without causing hypoglycaemia. Satisfactory reduction in blood glucose is usually achieved using low-dose insulin infusions. Only clear, short-acting insulin is suitable for use in insulin infusions. Once the insulin is added to the IV fluid the solution must be gently mixed. It is usual to discard the first 50 mL through the giving set to allow insulin to bind to the plastic tubing and IV bag. All solutions must be discarded after 24 hours.

Other methods used to minimise insulin binding to plastic giving sets include:

- Adding the insulin to Haemaccel, which is expensive and is usually only used if a volume expander is required, which may be the case for older people.
- Flushing insulin solution through the infusion set to saturate the binding sites before the line is connected to the patient.

Insulin infusions are used during surgical procedures, including open heart surgery. Usually insulin is added to 4% dextrose in 1/5 normal saline or in a dextrose solution. The infusion should be administered through a burette or IMED pump usually at 120 mL/h (i.e. eight-hourly rate). Other instances where an IV insulin infusion is indicated are:

- Myocardial infarction where the IV insulin infusion is commenced on presentation to the emergency department and is continued for at least 24 hours, after which time subcutaneous insulin is commenced (Malmberg 1997). This is known as the DIGAMI protocol.

- Ketoacidosis.
- Hyperosmolar coma.
- Severe sepsis.

In some cases, where counterregulatory hormone levels are high, larger doses of insulin will be required, for example when a person with severe liver disease, such as fatty liver, is commenced on corticosteroid therapy, or in obesity.

Blood glucose must be carefully monitored because the results provide the basis for adjusting the insulin dose. That is, it indicates the efficacy of the infusion. Usually every 1–2 hours is adequate, changing to four hourly when the person is stable.

There are a number of adverse events associated with insulin infusions, the most common ones being:

- Hypoglycaemia.
- Cardiac arrhythmias, which may be precipitated by unpredictable, rapid changes in potassium as it moves between the intracellular and extracellular spaces.
- Sepsis at the IV site.
- Fluid overload leading to cerebral oedema, which is a serious, potentially fatal risk in older people. Hydration status and conscious state need to be closely monitored.

Top-up doses of insulin

Extra insulin may be required if the blood glucose is >18 mmol/L and urine or blood ketones are present prior to the next insulin dose. Where possible, blood ketone monitoring is preferred since this is an accurate reflection of the degree of acidosis (see Chapter 4). In acute care it is often helpful for the physician to receive an early morning telephone call from the ward so that the day's dose of insulin can be ordered on the basis of the previous 24 hours. In this situation short-acting insulin is used and is best added to the next prescribed dose of insulin. The insulin dose for the following day should be reviewed and adjusted if necessary, in the light of any top-up doses administered and the blood glucose pattern.

Practice points

(1) Vision often deteriorates when insulin is first commenced, which can be frightening for the individual and further limit their self-care potential and safety.
(2) People need reassurance to help them understand and accept these changes. Vision deteriorates because the lens absorbs excess glucose in much the same way as a sponge soaks up water. Changes in the amount of glucose in the lens can lead to blurred vision with both high and low blood glucose levels. Although it is frightening and can limit some functions temporarily, it is not a permanent threat to sight.
(3) The person's self-care capacity should be reassessed when the vision improves. This effect is quite different from diabetic retinopathy, which can threaten the sight.

Future treatment prospects

Inhaled insulin
The alveoli in the lungs are permeable to large polypeptides such as insulin and significant amounts of insulin can be absorbed through the nose, if enhancers are used. The technology is now available to create a dry powder insulin aerosol that can deliver insulin directly into the lungs. Although still under trial, inhaled insulin appears to be well tolerated and achieves acceptable glycaemic control in Type 1 and Type 2 diabetes, without causing short-term lung problems. The long-term effects on respiratory tissue are not known at this stage.

Inhaled insulin is administered using a spacer device and approximately 10% of the dose is absorbed systemically. The inhaler device is very large and may be unattractive to some people accustomed to small devices. However, the benefits of fewer injections might balance this concern and devices are likely to become smaller with time. It may be difficult for older people to learn the correct inhalation technique. The peak action and duration of effect are close to the rapid-acting analogues, i.e. shorter than subcutaneous injected insulin.

At present, subcutaneous long-acting insulin is still required because long-acting nasal insulin preparations are not available.

Insulin detemir
Insulin detemir is another long-acting, peakless insulin with a similar profile to glargine. It is available in some countries.

Pancreas transplants
Transplantation of the whole pancreas, isolated islet cells or the pancreas and kidneys is sometimes performed when end-stage renal failure is present and the organs are available. It requires major surgery and is usually reserved for people with Type 1 diabetes. Immunosuppressive therapy is required and if rejection does not occur, the response is good. The transplanted pancreas secretes insulin and HbA_{1c} normalises in about three months. Older people may not be given priority status for pancreatic transplants. However, they often ask about them.

2.7   Monitoring the effectiveness of management strategies and complication status

2.7.1   Blood glucose monitoring

Regular blood glucose monitoring is an important indicator of the effectiveness of the management strategy and is the basis for adjusting medication, food intake and activity levels.

- Follow correct procedure when performing blood glucose tests.
- Perform control and calibration tests on blood glucose meters regularly.
- Clean and calibrate meters regularly to ensure they give accurate results.
- Allow people to continue to self-test in hospital and residential facilities where they are capable of doing so. Supervision may be needed and it is an ideal opportunity to check their technique.

- Although some experts still recommend urine testing for some older people, it is inaccurate due to changes in the renal threshold for glucose and will not help to identify hypoglycaemia.

The role of blood glucose monitoring

Regular blood glucose monitoring provides important information about the effectiveness of the diabetes management plan and allows direct feedback to the individual about their prevailing blood glucose level and the emerging blood glucose profile.

Regular blood glucose monitoring can assist the person to reach management targets by:

- Detecting lack of control as indicated by elevated glycosylated haemoglobin (HbA_{1c}) levels.
- Achieving acceptable blood glucose levels that have a role in preventing short-term complications such as hypoglycaemia or delaying the onset of long-term complications.
- Establishing the renal threshold and therefore the reliability of urine testing in those cases where people still test their urine glucose. Although urine testing is no longer considered accurate or best practice, it can still have a place in self-care to assist the person to remain involved in their care and be independent.

In particular, blood glucose monitoring is essential when the person has:

- Frequent hypoglycaemic episodes, including nocturnal hypoglycaemia.
- Unstable diabetes, such as during prolonged stress or illness.
- Illnesses managed at home.
- Started a new treatment regime, for example OHAs or insulin are introduced, or when non-diabetic medicines are required for other conditions to detect drug interactions.
- Renal failure, autonomic neuropathy, cardiovascular disease or cerebrovascular insufficiency where hypoglycaemia can be masked or not recognised.

The target blood glucose range and frequency of testing should be established for the individual. Safety, comfort and preventing hypoglycaemia are important considerations.

Factors that influence blood glucose levels

It is important to realise that many factors affect blood glucose levels. The following need to be considered when interpreting blood glucose profiles.

- Onset, peak action and duration of action of medicines.
- Time of last food intake, quantity and type of food consumed.
- Injection site and state of the injection sites. The abdomen is the preferred site.
- Timing of exercise with respect to food and medicine, type of exercise and blood glucose level when the exercise began.
- Presence of intercurrent illness such as influenza, urinary tract infection, MI, CVA.

- Dose and dose interval of medications used for diabetes control.
- Use of other drugs, such as glucocorticoids, beta blockers and complementary and non-prescription medications, especially those that contain glucose, ephedrine, pseudoephedrine or alcohol, e.g. cold remedies.
- Consumption of alcohol, the type and relationship to food intake and amount consumed.
- The accuracy of the blood glucose monitoring technique, including not hand washing before testing if sweet substances have been handled.
- Presence of renal, liver and pancreatic disease.
- Possibility of other endocrine disorders such as thyroid disease, Cushing's disease.
- Parenteral nutrition.
- Presence of unrelieved pain.
- Unrecognised pathology such as asymptomatic MI and UTI.
- Injecting into oedematous tissue, which can delay insulin absorption.

Frequency of blood glucose monitoring

The following recommendations are suggestions only. Existing policies need to be taken into account as do the needs and capability of the individuals concerned.

Initially, blood glucose or urine tests are performed before meals and before bed (standard times are 7 am, 11 am, 4 pm and 9 pm), in order to obtain a profile of the effectiveness of diabetes therapy and to establish the renal threshold. Testing two hours after food, especially in Type 2 diabetes, is preferred in some cases to determine the rate of glucose clearance from the blood. Tests are sometimes required at 2 am or 3 am for 2–3 days to ascertain if nocturnal hypoglycaemia is occurring, when there are indications such as unusual snoring, bed wetting, cognitive changes, morning lethargy and hyperglycaemia.

Urine ketones should be monitored in all people with Type 1 diabetes and in some Type 2 people during severe stress, e.g. surgery, infection and myocardial infarction if blood glucose tests are elevated.

Practice point

The appropriateness of established testing needs to be revised regularly and adapted according to need; for example, in the presence of any of the factors outlined in the section on factors that influence blood glucose levels. These include staff safety when invasive procedures such as blood glucose testing provoke aggressive behaviour.

In care settings monitor initially for 48 hours, at 7 am, 11 am, 4 pm and 9 pm, to assess the effectiveness of current insulin therapy. Review after 48 hours and alter testing frequency if indicated. If the insulin regimen is altered, review again after 48 hours. Simpler regimens may be required in community settings.

Oral hypoglycaemic agents

Initial monitoring as for insulin-treated patients. Review after 48 hours and reduce monitoring frequency to twice a day, daily or once every second or third day, alternating the times of testing, as indicated by the level of control and the general medical condition of the patient.

Diet control

Initially, twice-a-day monitoring, then daily or once every second or third day, unless the person is having total parenteral nutrition (TPN) or diagnostic procedures, is undergoing surgery or is acutely ill. In the acute care setting, patients are usually ill and require at least four-hourly monitoring. The frequency can often be reduced in rehabilitation, mental health and residential care facilities. HbA$_{1c}$ should be checked every 3–6 months and the blood glucose monitoring frequency increased if elevated to enable timely adjustments to the management regime.

Special circumstances

(1) Insulin infusion: blood glucose tests are usually performed every 1–2 hours during the infusion and reviewed every two hours to decide whether dose adjustments are required. Reduce to 3–4 hourly when blood glucose levels are stable.
(2) People on glucocorticoids, some antipsychotics and other known diabetogenic drugs:
   ● non-diabetic people: there is no consensus on testing frequency, especially where the person does not have diabetes. A suggested regime is to test weekly in non-diabetics to screen for hyperglycaemia, unless results are elevated when more frequent testing is required
   ● people with diabetes: see protocols in the previous sections.
(3) Parenteral and enteral feeding guidelines:
   ● test at 7 am, 11 am, 4 pm and 9 pm for the first 48 hours after the feeds commence until the feeding routine is established and a blood glucose pattern emerges, then reduce the frequency. If the formula changes or new drugs are commenced, the testing frequency should be increased again.
   ● monitor urine and blood for ketones at 7 am, 11 am, 4 pm and 9 pm.

Practice point

Never prick the feet of an older person because it increases the risk of trauma and infection and predisposes the person to septicaemia and serious foot pathology, possibly requiring amputation.

Blood glucose meters

A range of blood glucose meters is currently available to monitor blood glucose in the home or in residential care. Staff should become familiar with the system in use in their area. A blood glucose meter quality management programme is essential to ensure that:

● Individual nurses demonstrate competence to use the meter.
● Regular control testing (at least daily) is carried out and meters are calibrated as required, usually when a new pack of strips is opened, are appropriately cleaned

and control tests are performed regularly. Meter maintenance should be a documented part of the quality management process.
- A procedure for dealing with inaccurate results and meter malfunction is in place.

Examples of blood glucose meters are Medisense PC, Precision PC$_x$ and Optium (Australia) and the Boehringer Advantage (Australia and the UK).

Practice point

Incorrect operator technique and inadequate meter maintenance and quality control testing are the major causes of inaccurate results using blood glucose meters. Many companies offer troubleshooting telephone support on freecall numbers.

Non-invasive/minimally invasive blood glucose testing

A non-invasive blood glucose monitoring method (the Glucowatch) was introduced in 2001. It is not yet widely used and may not be appropriate in acute illness. The Glucowatch is a watch-sized device that automatically monitors blood glucose through the skin as often as every 20 minutes.

The device works by reverse iontophoresis. An electric current stimulates sweat production. Glucose is absorbed from the sweat by an autosensor, which is a small disposable pad on the back of the device. The autosensor transforms the electrical signal to a glucose reading that can be displayed by pressing a button. The autosensor must be changed every 24 hours.

An alarm sounds if the blood glucose goes too low or too high. The Glucowatch holds up to 4000 tests in the memory and is only approved for adult use at present. Such devices may have particular benefit for older people in the future.

Practice points

(1) It is not necessary to swab the finger with alcohol prior to testing because it can dry the skin. Alcohol swabbing does not alter the blood glucose results (Dunning *et al.* 1994).
(2) The hands should be washed in soap and water and dried carefully before testing, especially if the person has been handling glucose, e.g. in an accident and emergency department/casualty, where the person presents with hypoglycaemia.

2.7.2   *Monitoring blood ketones*

A 30-second capillary blood ketone testing hand-held meter was launched in 2001. The meter measures capillary beta-hydroxybutyrate (B-OHB). Levels between 0.5 and 1.5 mmol/L indicate ketones are present. This may be due to fasting or indicate extra insulin is needed. The level should be checked after treatment. Levels >1.5 mmol/L indicate ketones are established and medical assessment is required. Possible underlying causes include infection, myocardial infarction or inadequate medicine doses. The presence of ketones indicates acute insulin deficiency and that fat stores have been mobilised in an attempt to provide energy. The main ketone bodies are:

- Acetoacetate, an end-product of fatty acid metabolism.
- Acetone, which is formed from spontaneous decarboxylation of acetoacetate. Acetone is volatile and is expelled in expired air, giving it the typical acetone smell of ketoacidosis.
- Beta-hydroxybutyrate (B-OHB) is a reduced form of acetoacetate and is the major ketone formed in acidosis.

Blood ketone testing for B-OHB is more reliable than urine ketone testing (Fineberg 2000). Currently available urine ketone test strips do not measure B-OHB. Laboratory ketone testing often does not do so either, unless it is specifically requested. Capillary ketone testing is increasingly being used in acute care settings. Type 1 patients with hyperglycaemia and HbA_{1c} >8.5%, in association with B-OHB, are insulin deficient and at risk of ketosis. Normal blood B-OHB is 0–0.5 mmol/L. While older people are more likely to develop HONK (see Chapter 4), ketoacidosis is still a significant risk. Ketone meters were developed for home use but are increasingly being used in health-care settings.

2.7.3 Monitoring urine glucose

In the presence of normal kidney function, glycosuria is correlated to the blood glucose concentration and occurs when the tubular maximum reabsorption has been exceeded, usually around 8–10 mmol/L blood glucose. This is called the renal threshold for glucose and varies within and between individuals. Urine tests reflect the average glucose during the interval since the person last voided, rather than the level at the time the test is performed. The renal threshold may be changed by increasing age, renal disease and long-standing diabetes.

In addition, fluid intake, hydration status and urine concentration influence the glucose concentration, and therefore the urine glucose test result, which means the blood glucose can be elevated without glycosuria being present. Importantly, urine glucose does not predict impending hypoglycaemia and a negative urine glucose finding does not indicate hypoglycaemia. While urine testing is not generally reliable, it *may* be a useful guide for older people who are not able or willing to monitor their blood glucose or where blood glucose testing provokes aggressive behaviour.

2.7.4 Additional health assessment

In addition to blood and urine testing, metabolic status can be assessed by:

(1) Regular weight checks, to estimate loss or gain and compare with the management goal.
(2) Regular testing of:
- blood pressure, lying and standing to detect any postural drop that could indicate the presence of autonomic neuropathy or dehydration

  - retinal screen and visual acuity
  - cardiac status
  - feet
  - kidney function
  - ADLs, quality of life and cognitive function.
(3) Regular assessment of knowledge about:
  - diet
  - self-monitoring techniques
  - injection sites
  - general diabetic knowledge.

Practice point

A recent Cochrane review indicates that fasting for long periods before surgery and procedures may be unnecessary (Brady *et al.* 2004). Brady *et al.* found people who were given a drink of water preoperatively had a significantly lower residual gastric volume than people who fasted and there was no increased risk of aspiration. When incorporating these findings into surgical policies, consideration must be given to the effects of hyperglycaemia, ketoacidosis, hyperosmolar states and diabetic gastroparesis on gastric emptying times.

2.7.5   Glycosylated haemoglobin (HbA$_{1c}$)

HbA$_{1c}$ is considered to be the 'gold standard' for assessing metabolic control. Circulating blood glucose attaches to the haemoglobin in the red blood cells and undergoes a chemical reaction (Armadori) whereby the glucose becomes permanently fixed to the haemoglobin. This is known as glycosylation. The glycosylated haemoglobin can be quantified to give an indication of the average blood glucose concentration over the preceding three months. HbA$_{1c}$ complements capillary blood glucose tests and the clinical assessment of the patient. The rate of haemoglobin glycosylation is influenced by chronic hyperglycaemia. Tests are usually performed at least three months apart but can be done sooner to gauge the effect of a treatment modification.

Practice points

(1) People who experience frequent hypoglycaemic episodes, have anaemia, recent blood loss, blood transfusion or large frequent blood glucose fluctuations and some abnormal types of haemoglobin may have satisfactory HbA$_{1c}$ results; therefore the HbA$_{1c}$ result should be considered as part of the total clinical picture and not viewed in isolation.
(2) Be aware that not all laboratory assays measure HbA$_{1c}$. A number of different assay methods are used and they have different degrees of precision and reference ranges. There are global moves to standardise assay methods.
(3) Fasting is not required.
(4) There is an international trend towards using the term 'A$_{1c}$'.

2.7.6 Serum lipids

Hyperglycaemia and elevated serum lipids are usually present together. Three classes of lipids are measured as part of assessing metabolic control. They are:

(1) Cholesterol.
(2) Triglycerides.
(3) Lipoproteins that consist of:
   - very low density lipoprotein (VLDL)
   - low density lipoprotein (LDL)
   - high density lipoprotein (HDL).

Fasting blood samples are most useful. In addition, alcohol should not be consumed for 24 hours before the serum lipid measurements are taken. High lipids, especially elevated triglycerides and LDL and low HDL, are known risk factors for cardiovascular disease (see Chapter 5). People with poorly controlled Type 2 diabetes frequently have such a lipid profile which is another reason to strive for normoglycaemia, even in older people provided they are not put at extra risk of hypoglycaemia. Elevated triglycerides may require medications such as fibrates, fish oil concentrates or nicotinic acid, depending on the type of lipid abnormality present.

2.7.7 C-peptide

C-peptide is a connecting peptide that determines the folding of the two insulin chains during insulin production and storage in the pancreas. It splits off in the final stages and can be measured in the blood to indicate whether endogenous insulin production is still occurring and to distinguish between Types 1 and 2 diabetes, if it is not clear in the clinical presentation. C-peptide is present in normal or elevated amounts in Type 2 diabetes. Because Type 1 diabetes can have a slower presentation in older people, C-peptide is sometimes indicated and fasting results are most useful (Cohen 1996). C-peptide is not changed by nor detects exogenous, injected insulin.

Two other tests are also used to confirm a diagnosis of Type 1 diabetes, which indicate that diabetes is an autoimmune disease.

(1) Islet cell antibodies (ICA) are present in the prediabetic state before clinical signs appear. ICA can also be present in first-degree relatives and indicate a high risk of developing diabetes.
(2) Glutamic acid dehydrogenase antibodies (GAD) are present in 80% of people with Type 1 diabetes and enable it to be distinguished from Type 2 diabetes (Cohen 1996). Determining whether the person has Type 1 or Type 2 diabetes is important so that appropriate management strategies can be implemented.

2.7.8 Creatinine clearance and urea

Creatinine is produced through metabolism of muscle creatinine and dietary creatine. Serum creatinine clearance and urea (blood urea nitrogen or BUN) are used to estimate renal function and nutritional status in relation to protein, to screen for renal decline and during TPN and dialysis. BUN may indicate impaired renal function but can also be increased if the patient is dehydrated, had internal bleeding or is on steroids. Anorexia, a low-protein diet and fasting can lead to a low BUN.

Creatinine is a more sensitive marker of renal function. The serum creatinine is compared with the urine creatinine clearance rate measured over the same period of time. An increased serum creatinine indicates renal impairment. A significant rise may only occur when up to 50% of kidney function is lost. Creatinine is measured regularly to note any increase in the creatinine level. Note the previous comment on pages 50–51 about the limitation of creatinine clearance in older people.

2.7.9   Tests of kidney function

Twelve- and 24-hour urine collections are used to detect early kidney damage by calculating creatinine clearance rates and microalbumin excretion rates. Microalbuminuria is the earliest marker of the onset of kidney and cardiovascular damage. Early diagnosis and treatment can delay the onset of nephropathy and therefore the need for dialysis by 2–4 years and increase life expectancy (Borch-Johnsen et al. 1993) and quality of life. Proteinuria occurs in 17% of people with essential hypertension despite satisfactory treatment (Ruilope et al. 1990).

Therefore, nurses have a role in screening and detecting declining renal function and educating the person about appropriate preventive measures. The procedure for collecting the urine should be explained to the patient carefully. Written and verbal instructions should be supplied if the collection is to be performed at home. Collections are best obtained during a period of good control and normal activity, not during illness; therefore the urine is usually collected on an outpatient basis. However, collections may occur during a hospital admission. In some cases 50 mL of the first early morning voided specimen will be collected. Micral-test, Micral-test II and Microbumin test are dipsticks that detect microalbuminuria.

2.7.10   Nursing responsibilities with respect to monitoring

It is important that nurses ensure:

(1) They know what the tests are for and entail in order to explain them to the individual.
(2) People who are required to fast for specific procedures, e.g. fasting lipids, are given appropriate written and verbal instructions about what to do about their medications and any other preparation required.
(3) The correct collection technique, appropriate amount of blood and correct tubes are used.
(4) The specimen reaches the laboratory within the appropriate timespan.
(5) The results are available for medical evaluation in acute and residential settings.
(6) They know the effects of illness and stress on the results of the test.
(7) Appropriate sterile blood collection technique is used.
(8) Appropriate disposal of used equipment and that patients are given their medication and something to eat after completing the test.

2.8   Mouth and dental care

Mouth and dental care is particularly important where people are unable to appropriately clean their teeth. People on some medications and enteral feeds are especially at risk of oral disease. Poor oral hygiene has been linked to cardiovascular disease and a range of infections. Oral assessment should be undertaken systematically and include risk factors for inadequate oral care such as:

- Usual mouth hygiene habits.
- The products used.
- How well dentures fit and whether the individual actually uses them to eat.
- Frequency of dental assessments.
- Medications.
- Smoking.
- Alcohol use.
- Usual metabolic control.
- Usual diet.
- Trauma from nasogastric tubes.

Systematic assessment needs to include the jaw, lips, tongue, buccal mucosa and teeth or dentures and breath odour. The state of the mouth can indicate underlying pathology such as hyperglycaemic states (dry mouth, acetone breath). Over time capillary blood flow to the buccal mucosa declines as part of generalised microvascular disease and predisposes the individual to a dry mouth, inflammation and cracks and fissures that can be portals for infection.

Vitamin deficiencies, as part of generalised nutrition deficits, predispose the person to cracked lips, painful swollen tongue, mouth ulcers and bleeding gums. Medications such as chemotherapeutic agents suppress the immune system and cause nausea and vomiting. Others inhibit wound healing and renewal of the cells of the buccal mucosa.

Periodontal disease is often overlooked as a site of infection in people with diabetes. Bacteria responsible for periodontal disease activate the immune system, initiate an inflammatory response and the production of cytokines (Iacopino 2001). Xerostomia and candida infection also occur. Periodontal disease contributes to hyperglycaemia as well as being triggered by it. In turn, periodontal disease affects food intake and nutritional status. The presence of renal disease and/or cancer contributes to the discomfort of periodontal disease.

2.8.1 *Managing oral hygiene*

Prevention

- An education strategy is necessary to ensure the person (or their carer) brushes their teeth and flosses regularly and has regular dental checks.
- Use antibacterial mouthwashes to destroy plaque-forming bacteria that damage teeth. Other strategies may need to be implemented if the person has a compromised gag reflex.
- Nurses may need to assist people to undertake appropriate dental care. This should include ensuring the teeth can be cleaned after eating, checking dentures still fit appropriately and food is not trapped under the plate.
- Ensuring the diet contains essential vitamins and minerals such as Vitamin C and the B group vitamins.

Table 2.13 Frequency of performing mouth care according to the degree of dysfunction.

Mild dysfunction	Assess twice per day. Provide mouth care after food, cleaning and mouth rinse and lip cream.
Moderate dysfunction, e.g. infection	Assess three times a day. Provide mouth care every 2–4 hours as indicated for mild dysfunction. Provide topical anaesthetic to manage pain.
Severe dysfunction, e.g. unconscious, on oxygen therapy, frequent suctioning	Assess three times a day. Provide mouth care every 1–2 hours. Administer analgesics and antibiotics as indicated.

- Softer oral swabs or 'toothettes' may be less likely to cause small scratches on susceptible gums. The tongue should also be cleaned and food removed from below the tongue or in cheek pouches.
- Observing the gums for tenderness, sores or bleeding, which could indicate infection, or white plaques that could indicate thrush.
- Ensuring water is available if xerostomia is a problem or providing ice to suck.
- Managing pain using ice, local anaesthetic mouthwashes or gels.
- Applying lubricant to the lips, including in the corners of the mouth, if they are dry and flaking.
- Observing the state of the saliva.

Managing dental dysfunction

The frequency of mouth care depends on the severity of the dental dysfunction and whether the person is self-caring at home or in care (see Table 2.13). Mouth swabs may be needed to determine whether infection is present.

Long-term use of chlorhexidine mouthwash is not recommended because it:

- May increase calculus formation.
- Causes tissue changes with long-term use.
- Alters taste perception with long-term use, which can affect the appetite and therefore intake, which may have consequences such as hypoglycaemia and malnutrition.
- Can cause excess tartar build-up and plaque.
- Is not metabolised by the body.

Lemon-glycerine swabs are not recommended because fibres can be left in the mouth and can be swallowed or inhaled, especially if cognition or conscious state is impaired. In addition, they can be a source of infection in susceptible individuals. Lemon juice is acid and long-term use can damage tooth enamel, stimulate excessive saliva production and irritate mucosa because of the acidity.

2.9 Preventive vaccinations

Regular vaccinations against influenza and pneumonia are recommended for older people. A recent report recommended vaccinating infants as young as six months if they are in contact with frail elderly grandparents/relatives to reduce the spread of infection (Rouse 2004). Interestingly, researchers found that, although people's immune response depends on the vaccination they received, the side of their brain that is most active also had an effect on the degree of the response (Davidson 2003). Davidson (2003) found that people aged 57–60 with left-sided brain activity in the prefrontal cortex developed stronger immunity. This part of the brain is associated with a positive outlook on life. While the study is small, it demonstrates the effect of psychological parameters on physical status. Another earlier study (Vedhara *et al.* 1999) demonstrated that chronic stress reduces immune function in older people and impaires antibody responses to influenza vaccinations. These findings also apply to older carers.

These studies suggest that chronically stressed older people, including carers, may be vulnerable to infection because they are not able to mount an adequate immune response. Therefore, infection control procedures and appropriate preventive measures must be in place.

Practice point

The drainage holes/slots in bath and shower seats can trap the genitalia of older people, especially males, and lead to cuts, lacerations, bruising, pain and extreme distress. The UK government drug and medical device safety department warned that the maximum weight should not be exceeded when using these seats because they bend under the weight and increase the risk of genital entrapment. Folded towels can be placed over the holes (Lowinger 2003). Bath seats are rarely used in Australia because of the safety risks.

2.10 Role of carers in diabetes management

The WHO (1983) emphasised the importance of helping older people live safe, dignified lives in society, if possible remaining with their families. Similarly, the Department of Human Services (2003) identified the important role carers play in maintaining the health of older people. Carers include family members, friends and other non-health professionals who should be involved in assessment, health planning and outcome monitoring processes. In addition, the burden on carers and the need to be mindful of their health and wellbeing must be acknowledged.

Caregivers report concern about not being consulted when their older relative is hospitalised even though they were often able to contribute important information (Li *et al.* 2004). Written action plans can support carers to manage older people in the community and could include strategies for managing:

● Diet and exercise/mobility programmes, including strategies for managing inter-current illness and food refusal.

- Hyperglycaemia.
- Hypoglycaemia.
- Blood glucose monitoring.
- Medicines.
- Foot care.
- Health-care appointments.

Having such strategies in place with the option of intermittent, or respite, care can relieve the burden of care and improve outcomes (Berthold *et al.* 1991). Managing an older person represents a significant health risk for the carers who need to feel supported, understood and acknowledged. Significant factors that contribute to carers presenting to emergency departments include:

- Concern about their own health, have long-standing health problems, experienced problems in the previous year.
- Experiencing a high level of frustration.
- Engaged in personal tasks such as bathing and dressing the older person and doing housework.
- Having difficulty communicating with the older person (Williams 1989, pp. 167–169).
- Inadequate respite care/support services.

In addition, the time devoted to caring for the older person increases the frequency of self-reported depression in carers. Therefore, carer burnout needs to be considered and respite care arranged as necessary (see Chapter 7) (Tokarski 2004).

Diabetes-specific social support is a strong determinant of self-care behaviour (Connell 1991). Encouragement, reassurance and having somebody to listen to concerns are extremely important to older people living in the community; however, many community-dwelling older people do not want or expect a great deal of 'physical help' from their family and friends (Connell 1991). When assistance is required it is usually for physical activity, foot care and blood glucose testing. Older people often receive help to follow a meal plan or take medicines but often report they do not want such help.

Providing support that is not wanted, even if it is needed, can result in negative outcomes and be perceived as interference. Carers often tread the fine line between support and 'interference' on a daily basis. An education programme for caregivers that included information about their relative's behaviour and complications associated with hospital admissions resulted in closer relationships between the carer and their older relative, fewer incidents of acute confusion and faecal incontinence during hospital admissions and fewer depressive symptoms (Li *et al.* 2004).

In addition to education programmes, modern technology such as email and mobile phones can transmit information such as blood glucose or blood pressure readings quickly to the person's doctor. Such devices allow timely interventions and may avert or reduce the severity of adverse events as well as reassuring the caregiver or older person that advice and support are readily available. One such device, the Personal Medical Phone (PMP4), has an inbuilt 12-lead ECG, blood glucose meter, blood pressure and other health monitoring options, including a stylus that doubles as a thermometer, as well as the ability to send text and pictures (Manktelow 2003). Such technology puts a new perspective on 'point-of-care testing'.

When the carers are older, it may be necessary to assess their ability to continue providing daily care tasks. Such assessments need to be approached diplomatically and from a supportive perspective.

References

Abrahamson, M. (2004) Optimal glycaemic control in Type 2 diabetes mellitus. Fasting post-prandial glucose in context. *Archives of Internal Medicine*, **164**, 486–91.

Australian Diabetes Educators Association (ADEA) (2003) *Guidelines for the Management and Care of Diabetes in the Elderly.* ADEA, Canberra.

Australian Institute of Health and Welfare (AIHW) (2002) *Australia's Health No. 8.* AIHW, Canberra.

Baines, S. & Roberts, D. (2001) Undernutrition in the community. *Australian Prescriber*, **24**(5), 113–15.

Bates, C., Leant, M., Mansoor, M. & Prentice, A. (2004) Nutrient intakes, biochemical and risk indices associated with type 2 diabetes and glycosylated haemoglobin in the British National Diet and Nutrition Survey of people aged 65 years and over. *Diabetic Medicine*, **21**, 677–84.

Berthold, H., Landahl, S. & Svanborg, A. (1991) Intermittent care and caregivers at home. *Ageing*, **3**(1), 51–6.

Borch-Johnsen, K., Wenzel, H., Vibert, G. & Mogensen, C. (1993) Is screening and intervention for microalbuminuria worthwhile in patients with IDDM? *British Medical Journal*, **306**, 1722–5

Braddon, J. (2001) Oral hypoglycaemics: a guide to selection. *Current Therapeutics*, **13**, 42–7.

Brady, M., Kinn, S. & Stuart, P. (2004) Perioperative fasting for adults to prevent perioperative complications. Cochrane review. The Cochrane Library, Issue 2, Oxford.

Brand-Miller, J. (1994) Importance of glycaemic index in diabetes. *American Journal of Clinical Nutrition*, **59**(suppl), 7475–535.

Brown, A., Mangione, C., Saliba, D. & Sarkisian, C. (2003) American Geriatrics Society guidelines. *Journal of the American Geriatrics Society*, **200**(51), S265–80.

Buse, J. (2001) Insulin analogues. *Current Opinion in Endocrinology*, **8**(2), 95–100.

Calabrese, A., Coley, K., DaPos, S., Swanson, D. & Rao, H. (2002) Evaluation of prescribing practice: risk of lactic acidosis with metformin. *Archives of Internal Medicine*, **162**, 434–7.

Callan, B. & Wells, T. (2003) Views of community-dwelling old-old people on barriers and aids to nutritional health. *Journal of Nursing Scholarship*, **35**(3), 257–62.

Campbell, J., Anderson, D., Holcombe, J. & Massey, E. (1993) Storage of insulin: a manufacturer's view. *Practical Diabetes*, **10**(6), 218–20.

Cohen, M. (1996) *Diabetes: A Handbook of Management.* International Diabetes Institute, Melbourne.

Colquhoun, D. (2002) Lipid lowering agents. *Australian Family Physician*, **31**(1), 25–30.

Connell, C. (1991) Psychosocial contexts of diabetes and older adulthood: reciprocal effects. *Diabetes Educator*, **5**, 364–71.

Crook, M., Hally, V. & Panteli, J. (2001) The importance of the refeeding syndrome. *Nutrition*, **17**, 632–7.

Davidson, R. (2003) Proceedings of the National Academy of Sciences, 5 September. Available online at: www.pnas.org/cgi/content/abstract/100/19/11148 (Accessed May 2004).

Davis, T. (2003) Patient-managed records: their use in diabetes care. *Diabetes Management Journal*, **5**, 18.

Department of Health (1992) *The Nutrition of Elderly People. Report on Health and Social Subjects No. 43.* Stationery Office, London.

Department of Health (2001) *National Service Framework for Diabetes Standards.* DOH, London.

Department of Human Services (2003) *Improving Care for Older People.* DHS, Melbourne.

Dornhorst, T. (2001) Insulinotropic meglitinide analogues. *Lancet,* **17**(358), 1709–16.

Drewnowski, A. & Warren-Mears, V. (2001) Does ageing change nutrition requirements? *Journal of Nutrition, Health and Ageing,* **5**(2), 70–4.

Dunning, T. (2003) *Care of People with Diabetes: A Manual of Nursing Practice.* Blackwell Publishing, Oxford.

Dunning, T. & Martin, M. (1999) Health professionals' perceptions of the seriousness of diabetes. *Practical Diabetes International,* **16**(3), 73–7.

Dunning, T., Rantzau, C. & Ward, G. (1994) Effect of alcohol swabbing on capillary blood glucose. *Practical Diabetes,* **11**(4), 251–4.

Ebbeson, J., Buajordet, I. & Eriksson, J. (2001) Drug-related deaths in a department of internal medicine. *Archives of Internal Medicine,* **161**, 2317–23.

Engle, K. & Hannawa, T. (1999) Techniques for administering oral medications to critical care patients receiving continuous enteral nutrition. *American Journal of Health-System Pharmacy,* **56**, 1441.

Esler, M., Hastings, J., Lambert, G., Kaye, D., Jennings, G. & Seals, D.R. (2002) The influence of aging on the human sympathetic nervous system and brain norepinephrine turnover. *American Journal of Physiology – Regulatory Integrative and Comparative Physiology,* **282**(3), R909-16.

European Diabetes Working Party for Older People (2004) *Clinical Guidelines for Type 2 Diabetes Mellitus.* www.euroage-diabetes.com (accessed November 2004).

Fineberg, W. (2000) Comparison of blood beta-hydroxybutyrate and urine ketones in 4 weeks of home monitoring by insulin-requiring children and adults. Paper presented at the American Diabetes Association Scientific Meeting, USA, June.

Flood, L. & Constance, A. (2002) Diabetes and exercise safety. *American Journal of Nursing,* **102**(6), 47–55.

Friedman, R. & Kalant, N. (1998) Comparison of long term care in an acute institution and in a long term care institution. *Canadian Medical Association Journal,* **159**(9), 1107–13.

Gilbar, P. (1999) A guide to enteral drug administration in palliative care. *Journal of Pain and Symptom Management,* **17**(3), 197–201.

Halter, J. (2001) Doctors wary of treating the elderly. Report of American Diabetes Association meeting. *Practical Diabetes International,* **18**(7), 251–2.

Howes, L. (2001) Dosage alterations in the elderly. Importance of mild renal impairment. *Current Therapeutics,* **42**(7), 33–5.

Huizar, J., Gonzalez, L. & Alderman, J. (2003) Sulphonylureas attenuate electrocardiograph ST-segment elevation during an acute myocardial infarct in diabetes. *Journal of American College of Cardiology,* **42**(6), 1017–21.

Iacopino, A.M. (2001) Periodontitis and diabetes interrelationships: role of inflammation. *Annals of Periodontology,* **6**(1), 125–37.

Ishida, Y. & Kawai, S. (2004) Comparative efficacy of hormone replacement therapy, etidronate, calcitonin, alfacalcidol, and vitamin K in postmenopausal women with osteoporosis: the Yamaguchi Osteoporosis Prevention Study. *American Journal of Medicine,* **117**(8), 549–55.

Jennings, P. (1997) Oral hypoglycaemics: considerations in older patients with non-insulin dependent diabetes mellitus. *Drugs and Ageing,* **10**(5), 323–31.

Jerrall, M. (2002) Warning over Metformin use. *Archives of Internal Medicine,* **162**, 434–7.

Katz, C. (1991) How efficient is sliding scale insulin therapy? Problem with 'cookbook' approach in hospital patients. *Postgraduate Medicine,* **5**(5), 46–8.

Ko, D., Mamdani, M. & Atler, D. (2004) Lipid lowering therapy with statins in high risk elderly patients: the treatment risk paradox. *Journal of the American Medical Association*, **291**, 1864–70.

Koch, S. & Garratt, S. (2001) *Assessing Older People: A Guide for Health Care Workers*. McLennan and Petty, Eastgardens, New South Wales.

Kris-Etherton, P.M., Harris, W.S. & Appel, L.J. (2002) AHA scientific statement: fish consumption, fish oil, omega-3 fatty acids and cardiovascular disease. *Circulation*, **106**, 2747–57.

Lan, C., Lai, J., Chen, S. & Wong, M. (1998) 12-month tai chi training in the elderly: its effect on health and fitness. *Medicine and Science in Sports and Exercise*, **30**(3), 345–51.

La Rosa, J., He, J. & Vupputuri, S. (1999) Effect of statins on risk of coronary disease: a meta-analysis of randomised controlled trials. *Journal of the American Medical Association*, **282**, 2340–6.

Li, H., Melnyk, B. & McCann, R. (2004) Review of intervention studies of families with hospitalised elderly relatives. *Journal of Nursing Scholarship*, **36**(1), 54–9.

Lipid Study Group (1998) The long term intervention with pravastatin in ischaemic disease. Prevention of cardiovascular events and death with pravastatin in patients with coronary heart disease and a broad range of initial cholesterol levels. *New England Journal of Medicine*, **339**, 1349–57.

Lowinger, J. (2003) Bath seat accidents: a major hazard for the elderly. *Medical Observer*, 23 September, 15.

MacGinley, R., Chipman, J. & Mathew, T. (2004) 40th Annual Scientific Meeting of the Australian and New Zealand Society of Nephrology. *Nephrology*, **9**(1), vii.

Malmberg, K. (1997) Prospective randomised study of intensive insulin treatment on long-term survival after acute myocardial infarction. *British Medical Journal*, **314**, 1512–15.

Manktelow, N. (2003) Mobiles put patient health online. *Medical Observer*, 28 March, 509.

Marks, S. (2000) Obesity management. *Current Therapeutics*, **41**, 6.

McTernan, C., McTernan, P. & Harte, A. (2002) Resistin, central obesity and Type 2 diabetes. *Lancet*, **359**, 46–7.

McWhirter, J. & Pennington, C. (1994) Incidence and recognition of malnutrition in hospitals. *British Medical Journal*, **306**, 945–8.

Mueleman, J., Brechue, W., Kubilis, P. & Lowenthal, D. (2000) Exercise training in the debilitated aged: strength and functional outcomes. *Archives of Physical Medicine and Rehabilitation*, **81**(3), 312–18.

Nankivell, B. (2001) Creatine clearance and the assessment of renal function. *Australian Prescriber*, **24**(1), 15–18.

National Health and Medical Research Council (1999) *Dietary Guidelines for Older Australians*. NHMRC, Canberra.

National Heart Foundation (2001) Lipid management guidelines. *Medical Journal of Australia*, **175**, 557–89.

Nicholson, G. (2002) Statins decrease fractures and increase bone mineral density. *Archives of Internal Medicine*, **163**, 537–40.

Peck, G. (2003) Community diabetes nursing in our ageing population. *Journal of Diabetes Nursing*, **7**(5), 181–3.

Persson, M., Brismar, K., Katzarski, K., Nordenstrom, J. & Cederholm, T. (2002) Nutritional status using mini nutritional assessment and subjective global assessments predicts mortality in geriatric patients. *Journal of the American Geriatrics Society*, **50**(12), 1996–2002.

Raskin, P., Rendell, M. & Riddle, M. (2001) A randomised trial of rosiglitazone therapy in patients with inadequately controlled insulin treated Type 2 diabetes. *Diabetes Care*, **24**(7), 122–3.

Reilly, H. (1996) Screening for nutritional risk. *Proceedings of the Nutrition Society*, **55**, 841–53.

Reuters health information (2004) Diabetics treated with diet only have more complications. http://www.medscape.com (accessed August 2004).

Rosenstock, J. (2001) Management of Type 2 diabetes in the elderly: special considerations. *Pulsebeat*, Oct.–Nov., 5.

Rouse, R. (2004) Free pneumococcal vaccine saves elderly. *Medical News*, 13 August, 17.

Ruilope, L., Alcazar, J., Hernandez, E. & Rodico, J. (1990) Does an adequate control of blood pressure protect the kidney in essential hypertension? *Journal of Hypertension*, **8**, 525–31.

Schernthaner, G., Grimaldi, A., Di Mario, U. *et al.* (2004) GUIDE Study: double blind comparison of once-daily gliclazide MR and glimepiride in type 2 diabetic patients. *European Journal of Clinical Investigation*, **34**, 535–42.

Simkin, B. (2004) Even frail elderly patients can benefit from exercise. *Geriatric Times*, **3**(4).

Simons, L.A., Simons, J., Friedlander, Y. & McCallum, J. (2001) Cholesterol and other lipids predict coronary heart disease and ischaemic stroke in the elderly, but only in those below 70 years. *Atherosclerosis*, **159**(1), 201–8.

Stessman, J., Hammerman-Rozenberg, R., Maaravi, Y. & Cohen, A. (2002) Effect of exercise on ease in performing activities of daily living and instrumental activities of daily living from age 70 to 77: the Jerusalem longitudinal study. *Journal of the American Geriatrics Society*, **50**(12), 1934–8.

Szoryi, G. (2004) Investigating weight loss in the elderly. *Medicine Today*, **5**(9), 53–7.

Therapeutic Guidelines: Endocrinology. Version 3. (2004) Therapeutic Guidelines Ltd, Melbourne.

Tokarski, C. (2004) Care-giving demands increase with depression symptoms in elderly. *American Journal of Psychiatry*, **161**, 857–63.

Tomkin, G., Hadden, D., Weaver, J. & Montgomery, D. (1971) Vitamin B12 status of patients on long term Metformin therapy. *British Medical Journal*, **2**(763), 685–7.

Trusswell, A. (2003) Nutrient supplements. *Australian Doctor*, 21 March, I–VII.

Tsai, J., Wang, W., Chan, P. *et al.* (2003) The beneficial effects of Tai Chi on blood pressure and lipid profile and anxiety status in a randomised control trial. *Journal of Alternative and Complementary Medicine*, **9**(50), 747–54.

UK Prospective Diabetes Study (1983) Effect of diet, sulphonylurea, insulin or biguanide therapy on fasting plasma glucose and body weight over one year: multicentre study. *Diabetologia*, **24**, 404–11.

Vaag, A., Handberg, A., Lauritzen, M., Henrisken, J., Pedersen, K. & Beck-Neilsen, H. (1990) Variation in insulin absorption of NPH insulin due to intramuscular injection. *Diabetes Care*, **13**(1), 74–6.

Vaitkevicius, P., Ebersold, C., Shah, M. *et al.* (2002) Effects of aerobic exercise training in community-based subjects aged 80 and older: a pilot study. *Journal of the American Geriatrics Society*, **50**(12), 2009–13.

Vedhara, K., Cox, N., Wilcock, G. *et al.* (1999) Chronic stress in elderly carers of dementia patients and antibody response to influenza vaccination. *Lancet*, **353**(9153), 627–31.

Vicfit (2004): www.vicfit.com.au/vicfit/DocLib/xPub/DocLibAll.asp

Visvanathan, R., Penhall, R. & Chapman, I. (2004) Nutritional screening of older people in a sub-acute care facility in Australia and its relation to discharge outcomes. *Age & Ageing*, **33**(3), 260–5.

Williams, E. (1989) *Caring for Elderly People in the Community*, 2nd edn. Chapman and Hall, London.

World Health Organization (WHO) (1983) *Guidelines for the Management of Diabetes in Older People*. WHO, Geneva.

Young, C. (2004) Pharmacy drug information paper prepared in response to a personal enquiry about administering commonly used diabetes medications via enteral tubes. St Vincent's Hospital, Melbourne.

Zembrzuski, C. (1997) A three dimensional approach to hydration of elders: administration, clinical staff, and inservice education. *Geriatric Nursing*, **18**(1), 20–6.

Chapter 3
Developing Care Systems for Older People

Angus Forbes

Key points

- Care systems are important to provide a framework for effective diabetes care.
- Older people with diabetes are a heterogeneous population with varying needs and care systems need to reflect the diabetes journey from prevention, through diagnosis to managing complications and palliative care.
- Comprehensive assessment of the older person includes functional status, social support systems and physical and psychological health.
- The aim of care is dependent on the individual's needs and the model of care adopted, but maximising quality of life and minimising risk are primary objectives.
- Ensuring equitable access to effective diabetes care for older people should be a primary objective of nursing care.

3.1 The challenge of developing effective care systems for older people

Explicit care systems are pivotal to effective diabetes management because of the complex nature of diabetes and its complications. Effective care systems increasingly follow evidence-based guidelines and a philosophy of consumer-centred care. The aim of care systems for older people with diabetes is to achieve optimal metabolic control to prevent acute and chronic complications. Many systems emphasise the need for a partnership model in which the individual is encouraged to actively participate in their care and indicate that health professionals' role is to support the individual through education and regular assessment.

Frail older people, those who are housebound or in institutional care may not receive optimal care (Croxson 2002). Diabetes is often undertreated in older people despite good evidence that optimal control delays the development of complications (Hendra & Sinclair 1997; Adler *et al.* 2000). Diabetes affects up to 10% of people over 75 and between 3% and 6% over 60 years in the UK (Croxson *et al.* 1991) and up to 17% over 65 in Australia. Most have Type 2 diabetes. The incidence of diabetes in older people is likely to increase due to the ageing of most populations.

Older people often have difficulty accessing services due to physical disabilities, diabetes complications and comorbidities (Hall 1992) and often receive a significantly poorer level of diabetes care than active, mobile individuals (Sinclair & Barnett 1993; Gadsby 1994; Farooqi & Sorrie 1999). Benbow *et al.* (1997) surveyed 109 people with diabetes living in residential care and found high levels of preventable complications such as amputations, a higher incidence of general practitioner (GP) consultations and hospital admissions and a low level of health surveillance. Only 18% had their feet examined and only 29% had their blood pressure checked, which suggests that older people miss out on fundamental components of diabetes care. For example, ophthalmic screening is inadequate despite high levels of vision deficits in older people (Sinclair *et al.* 2000). One reason is that no one health professional takes overall responsibility for the diabetes care of older people in most cases (Tong & Roberts 1994).

Inadequate management is likely to lead to emergency presentations and hospital admissions. Also, older people may present with atypical symptoms (Table 3.1) and the significance of the underlying cause may not be recognised (Caplan *et al.* 2004). Caplan *et al.* (2004) suggested that any presentation by an older person to an

Table 3.1 Atypical presentations of older people.

Underlying disease process	*Presenting symptom*
Almost anything	Confusion Delirium Depression Fatigue Weight loss Failure to thrive
Acute abdomen	Reduced appetite Constipation Unusual severe pain
Pneumonia	Vague chest pain Dry cough Fever
Infection with falls	Increased white cell count (WCC). Note: WCC is often raised in hyperglycaemic states and does not necessarily indicate infection
Sepsis and functional decline	Fever General weakness
MI	Dyspnoea Confusion Atypical chest pain ('indigestion') Hypoglycaemia
Heart failure	Fatigue Dyspnoea
Depression	Agitation

emergency department should be regarded as a 'sentinel event' that triggers a comprehensive geriatric assessment. They demonstrated that geriatric assessments improved overall health and cognitive functioning and reduced the risk of future hospitalisation. This finding is significant since older people have longer and more frequent admissions, especially for exacerbations of chronic illness and falls (Lee *et al.* 2004). In addition, 26% of hospitalised older people are discharged to another institution or home with significant home care services.

Practice point

If an older person presents to an emergency department a need for complete functional, physical, mental and social assessment is often indicated.

There is evidence that older people have limited access to diabetes education despite their willingness to learn about their condition (Keeson & Knight 1990; Silliman *et al.* 1996). Often diabetes advice is not sufficiently tailored to the needs of older people (Potter 1990; Forbes & Morris 1999). In addition, cognitive changes or a degree of fatalism may be barriers to health education messages (Forbes *et al.* 2004) (see Chapter 6). Indeed, one of the fundamental tenets of 'modern diabetes care', the promotion of self-management, may be at odds with the care of some groups of older people. In order to provide effective care for older people with increasing levels of dependency, it is necessary to locate their care within the web of relations that support them and include carers and other social structures in the care plan (Forbes *et al.* 2001).

The WHO St Vincent Joint Task Force for Diabetes highlighted the inadequate care of older people with Type 2 diabetes and called for the evolution of services and models of care to address the specific needs of older people. Additional impetus for the 'evolution' came from a number of recently published guidelines and policy initiatives such as the National Service Frameworks (NSF) for Older People (Department of Health 2001) and Diabetes (BDA 1999; Department of Health 2002) and *Guidelines for the Management of Diabetes in Older People* (ADEA 2003).

In Australia, changes to the Medicare system and the introduction of comprehensive medical assessments (CMA) of residents in federal government-subsidised residential aged care facilities occurred in 2004. Other government initiatives include home-based assessments, integrated medicine management guidelines for residential aged care (Australian Pharmaceutical Advisory Council 1997), comprehensive medicine reviews for residential and home-dwelling older people and guidelines for minimising adverse consequences of hospitalisation in older people (National Health and Medical Research Council 1994). These policies promote health professional collaboration, co-ordinated care and consumer involvement.

It is difficult to define the best approach to caring for older people with diabetes. Older people are often excluded from research surveys and trials that underpin most current practice, for example the United Kingdom Prospective Diabetes Study and the Diabetes Control Complications Trial, because of the difficulties researchers face working with older people (Forbes *et al.* 2002a, 2002b). Thus, developing effective care systems to support the diabetes care of older people is challenging and important. Nurses and other health professionals are responsible for meeting the challenge.

Some strategies that can be used to develop care systems for older people are described in this chapter, considering different models of care, and a protocol for assessing diabetes in older people is provided.

3.2   Defining 'old' – not a straightforward task

Older people are not a homogeneous group (Souder 1992). Therefore, each person should be assessed individually, ageist assumptions avoided and the special needs of older people considered to ensure effective, appropriate care. An important first step in developing effective care systems for older people is to identify how they should be classified. Common approaches include chronological age, place of domicile and the degree of frailty (see Chapter 1).

3.2.1   Chronological age

Chronological age seems to be the most obvious way to define old age; for example, anybody over 65 years is defined as 'old' and those over 75 years are often referred to as the 'older old'. While such an approach is useful for organisations to determine clear entry points into services, age alone does not account for the inherent differences between older people. As people age they tend to become more unique and diverse (Gueldner & Hanner 1989). In addition to the general socio-economic and ethnic differences found in any population, older people may vary in physical functioning, mental state and general health, often independently of their age. While there are biological ageing processes common to everybody, the levels and rate of disability and dependency vary considerably within each age cohort and within individuals (Hamerman 1999).

Diabetes impinges on many aspects of daily life and has a range of psychosocial implications. Therefore chronological age is not very helpful in understanding the needs of older people with diabetes. Age at diagnosis may also be significant, in that people diagnosed in childhood have a different view of their diabetes from people diagnosed in their 50s or 70s.

Practice point

'Chronological age is of little value for anything other than the pension or retirement. It is biologic age that determines the functional status of the individual.'

(National Health and Medical Research Council 1994, p. 3)

3.2.2   Place of domicile

Another common way of classifying older people is the relationship between where they live and their functional capacity. Specific services for 'housebound' older people with diabetes exist (Forbes et al. 2004). Early studies defined 'housebound' in terms of physical disease or disability (Buchanan & Chamberlain 1978). However, older people *choose* to remain in a particular type of housing, often because funding and specific services enable them to 'age in place', even when they become frail and dependent over time.

Other factors include loss of confidence or interest in the outside world. Mobility depends on mechanical, motivational and environmental factors. For example, a steep staircase may make going out difficult. Regional differences such as living in rural areas and isolated villages and farms, where transport and services are not readily available, may limit access to services. In inner-city areas social issues such as the fear of crime may predominate (Bowling & Browne 1991). These issues make it difficult to define a population on the basis of where they live.

Lindesay & Thompson (1993) identified three 'housebound' levels, based on degrees of impaired mobility:

(1) Completely housebound people who have not left their homes for at least one month.
(2) Blockbound people who live in multiple housing units such as blocks of flats, who have been outside their flat but not beyond the boundary of the block for at least one month.
(3) People who can only venture outside their homes with the assistance of others.

Lindesay & Thompson's criteria are objective regarding the person's actual or reported behaviour, actual age or the judgement of health professionals. However, they do not account for the mechanisms that define housebound behaviour such as:

● Physical disability.
● Mental motivation.
● Social, e.g. fear of crime.
● Environmental, e.g. stairs.
● Individual changes in health status or due to participation in rehabilitative therapies.

Practice points

(1) 'Houseboundness' is the extreme point on a continuum of mobility. It is not always clear where the individual fits on the continuum.
(2) The concept of houseboundness is useful when planning diabetes care because it helps to identify problems in accessing services and the need to provide care on a domiciliary basis.

The type of residence, for example supported housing, low-level or high-level residential care, is an alternative domicile-based criterion. Explicit criteria usually control the entry into accommodation options, where the most frail and dependent people live in residential aged care facilities. Older people with diabetes in institutional care require special consideration, but there is evidence that the level of diabetes-specific care is often inadequate in these settings.

3.2.3 Frailty

Hamerman (1999) defined frailty as 'the complex and cumulative expression of altered homeostatic responses to multiple stresses'. Despite a primary focus on the biological processes that promote frailty, Hamerman usefully located frailty within the 'geriatric functional continuum' as the mid-point between independence and predeath and identified a range of factors that can cause frailty:

● Physical: advanced age, allostatic load, disease, disability and functional decline.
● Social: dependence on others.
● Psychological: cognitive impairment and depression.

In contrast, Chin et al. (1999) defined frailty as inactive (physical activity <210 min/week) in relation to other variables such as weight loss, low energy and low BMI. Interestingly, Chin et al. found the relationship between weight loss and frailty was the strongest predictor of mortality (odds ratio 4.1, confidence interval 1.8–9.4). Sinclair et al. (2000) more recently extended the concept of frailty by suggesting that appropriate metabolic targets could be set for frail older people with diabetes. They defined frailty as the presence of two or more of the following:

● Age >80 years.
● Difficulty performing ADLs.
● Mobility disorder.
● Significant additional comorbidity.
● Little evidence of functional decline (the single disease model).

The first four states require symptomatic control and prevention of iatrogenic complications. The last requires optimal therapy to achieve metabolic targets (Sinclair et al. 2000).

Forbes et al. (2004) identified three frailty subgroups in older people with diabetes by observing a small group of 12 older people with diabetes. The subgroups highlight the subtle distinctions within Sinclair's general frailty model.

Older frail independent

These people were generally quite independent and able to do their own shopping and access care outside their own homes independently. However, they were also deemed 'frail' by virtue of their extensive comorbidity and the presence of diabetes complications, particularly retinopathy (Sinclair 2000).

Older frail dependent

This group also had multiple comorbidities and were reliant on others for physical care and support. They had extreme difficulty accessing services outside their homes without help.

Older frail highly dependent

People in this group had global mental and physical impairment that gave rise to cognitive and communication problems, which was the greatest challenge to delivering diabetes care. Older frail dependent people are likely to live in high-dependency care environments or be heavily supported at home. In these circumstances carers often require support and access to respite care (see Chapter 2).

3.3 Models of care

The single disease and frailty models provide a basis on which to develop care plans for older people. While it is still important to provide care on an individual basis, these models can inform the objective nature and context of care.

3.3.1 Single disease model

The objective of care using the single disease model is the same as for everybody else with diabetes where the aim is to achieve optimal glycaemic and metabolic targets (see Chapter 2). The care should focus on empowering the individual to take responsibility for their diabetes within their capacity, for example by monitoring their blood glucose levels and managing their diet and medicines to achieve optimal control. However, in the presence of complications, particularly kidney damage, contraindications to medicines need to be considered.

In most cases the individual can be managed in primary care in collaboration with specialist diabetes and geriatric services. Home-based health assessments can help maintain older people in independent living and have small positive effects on quality of life. However, they do not prevent deaths and may increase the probability of placement in residential care (Byles *et al.* 2004). It is not clear if the findings apply to older people generally, since the study by Byles *et al.* only involved veterans and war widows. It may be that early detection of inability to cope meant that admission to residential care occurred sooner.

3.3.2 Frailty model

Older frail independent

The objective of care is to achieve good glycaemic and metabolic control while minimising the associated risks, for example hypoglycaemia and falls, and promoting quality of life. One of the key challenges to providing care to this group of people is ensuring that the care, particularly the information and health education provided, is meaningful to the individual. These patients may have other pathology such as arthritis that they consider more important than the often 'invisible' problems that result from their diabetes. People may also exhibit a degree of fatalism and lack the motivation to make lifestyle changes or manage their diabetes independently. Thus education must be specific and targeted, involve carers and, when appropriate, provide additional support to meet diabetes targets if required.

Given the multiple pathology associated with frailty, a collaborative specialist service provided by diabetologists, diabetes educators and geriatricians may be necessary. In the absence of multidisciplinary residential care, either primary care or specialist diabetes care may suffice, provided the care addresses the additional factors relevant to this group of older people.

Older frail dependent

The primary objective of care for older frail dependent people is to minimise the risk associated with poor metabolic control and medicines use and promote quality of life.

A key element of care in this model is to include significant others, such as current formal and informal carers who support the individual to fulfil their daily living requirements, in care decisions otherwise it is likely that the care may fail. Care delivery in this model may include domiciliary nurse visits, either by a community nurse or a diabetes nurse specialist, or providing organised transport to day-care facilities and appointments. Domiciliary care enables a full assessment of the person in their home environment and improves accessibility to diabetes care.

Older frail highly dependent

The objective of care for highly dependent older people is principally palliative to ensure quality of life and minimise adverse symptoms such as excessive thirst and polyuria. It is important to control the blood glucose to avoid these symptoms and acute complications such as diabetic ketoacidosis (DKA) or hyperosmolar non-ketotic diabetic coma (HONK) (see Chapter 4). The care should be similar to that provided for older frail dependent people; however, the care is often provided in institutions such as a nursing home. Hence, educating the care staff is an important aspect of care.

These models apply generally. In reality there may not be a clear indication of which model the individual fits into. The onus is on the nurse to ensure that decisions about care are based on the desires of the individual and their carers, as well as those of the multidisciplinary team. Advance directives need to be taken into account where they exist. In addition, the application of these models may be dependent on local factors, particularly the availability of resources.

Practice points

(1) Nurses need to consider all the issues related to the care of older people and be aware of any limitations in current systems.
(2) There is only very limited research on which to base the care of older people with diabetes.

3.3.3 Care pathways

In addition to identifying models of diabetes care for older people, it is important to recognise that they change frequently when diabetes or comorbidities advance or the individual becomes frailer. People often need to transfer from one model to another, which alters the focus of treatment from optimal control to palliative care. Therefore, people need to be systematically reassessed at strategic intervals or at least annually. Likewise, collaboration and good communication between services are vital to ensure a smooth transition between facilities (Lee *et al.* 2004).

Managing diabetes in older people includes primary prevention of the disease and the need to identify the large numbers of older people who have IGT and are undiagnosed through screening initiatives (see Chapters 1 and 2). Arguably, this includes everyone over 60, although such a course may be expensive and ineffective. In essence, nurses should seek to promote health, identify and screen people at risk of diabetes and ensure that those with diabetes are entered into a lifelong care pathway based on regular, appropriate, holistic assessment.

3.4   Assessing diabetes in the older person

The principles of assessing diabetes in older people are fundamentally the same as for any other person with diabetes. The aim is to identify and minimise the risk of complications and promote health. However, the assessment needs to be broader and include actual functional mental or physical deficits, medication regime and the current care and services that support the older person in their daily lives (see Chapter 2). There is also a need to consider the overall focus of care in order to identify the model of care most appropriate for the individual (Silliman *et al.* 1996).

Simply adopting a more traditional assessment approach and focusing on key indicators such as HbA_{1c} and blood pressure may be inappropriate in older people. These parameters have been very successful in improving the care of younger people with diabetes but they are mechanistic and inflexible, may alienate an older person or miss factors that affect their capacity to absorb and act on advice and accept treatment, which is often interpreted as non-compliance/adherence. Non-adherence in older people is complex and is usually related to:

- The side effects, adverse events and level of inconvenience associated with the medication regimen, e.g. insulin therapy.
- Deficits in the functional, cognitive, physical and social abilities necessary to ensure adherence, rather than a lack of willingness to comply. For example, adherence to dietary advice may depend on who does the shopping and cooking.
- Cognitive and physical function.

Practice point

Assessing older people requires an individual approach that reflects the wider social networks that enable older people to cope.

It is also important to identify deficits in the person's support network so that alternatives can be instigated, for example Meals-on-Wheels. As a result there is a move away from systematic 'conveyor belt care' to individualised care programmes (Department of Health 2001) (see Figures 2.1 and 2.2 in Chapter 2). Details of diabetes-specific assessment factors are outlined in other chapters, particularly 2, 5 and 7.

Assessment consists of four basic stages:

(1) Preparation.
(2) Subjective assessment.
(3) Objective assessment.
(4) Decision making.

3.4.1   *Preparation*

Preparation is very important. Ensure that the individual and their carer are aware of the purpose of the assessment and how long it will take. The assessment can take up to an hour and should not be attempted in less than half an hour, unless there is no other choice. More than one episode may be needed to avoid exhausting the individual. Assessment can be undertaken in a clinic, on the ward or in the person's home.

Home-based assessment may be particularly useful for frail older people in familiar surroundings, to allow observation in 'real' situations. For example, I observed a 75-year-old woman dial up her insulin using a pen system perfectly. She then expressed all the insulin from the pen onto the floor, before injecting herself with nothing.

All the equipment needed to undertake an assessment should be available before commencing the assessment (Forbes & Morris 1999). Ensuring any necessary investigations are performed in advance and the results are available saves time and enables the results to be discussed during the review. Fasting is necessary for some blood tests and the person/carer needs to be adequately instructed about exactly what to do so they are not put at risk of events such as hypoglycaemia.

The assessment should be undertaken in the light of previous reviews. Therefore, it is important to have access to any previous assessments, such as podiatry and hospital specialists, so progress can be assessed and changes noted and to avoid continuing the same care, if no change has occurred.

There are many assessment proformas with standardised assessment guidelines, in electronic form. However, Forbes *et al.* (2001, 2004) developed a domiciliary assessment tool for older people with diabetes, which was used as the basis for this chapter. Adopting a formal process to guide and record the assessment findings accurately is advisable and the focus should be on the person rather than on a mechanical checklist. In addition, the proforma used must provide appropriate and adequate information to enable clinical decision making. Many available proformas do not have demonstrated validity or reliability for the target population or user group.

3.4.2 Subjective assessment

The underlying aim of any assessment is to develop a relationship with the person and their carer(s), to try to understand diabetes from their perspective. Thus, active listening is crucial. Often the most important factors are the subtle cues a person provides; for example, do they appear anxious or seem removed from events? Are they depressed, angry or in denial? To facilitate active listening it is useful to begin by engaging in a fairly open conversation by asking general questions before focusing on the diabetes.

Note any concerns and come back to them at the end of the review to ensure they have been adequately addressed. Explore any significant lifestyle changes such as a change in diet or a reduction in activity, perhaps following a recent fall. Explore any social changes and issues such as bereavement or changes in the pattern of care, such as new home help. Make a careful and concise record of these issues so they can be considered when the diabetes status is assessed. Throughout the interview you should involve the carers to help validate the individual's response and identify any independent concerns the carer may have.

3.4.3 Objective assessment

Once the subjective history is complete a more systematic and objective physical, mental and functional assessment can be made considering the issues discussed in

Chapter 2. In addition, it is important to reinforce the importance of lifestyle factors and key safety advice about issues such as injection sites, hypoglycaemia, falls and medicine use. Any potential obstacles or motivational factors that may promote or retard positive health behaviours should be noted.

Functional assessment

An impression of the individual's functional capacity can be derived subjectively, but it is important to confirm their status objectively. A number of clinical tools can be used to assess physical functioning. Commonly used instruments include the Bartel Index and the Nottingham Extended Activity of Daily Living Scale (Nouri & Lincoln 1987) and nutritional assessment scales (see Chapter 2).

These tools assess areas such as mobility and upper limb functioning, which are important factors to consider when choosing insulin pens and the ability to complete daily living tasks such as washing and dressing. Mental state can be assessed using tools such as the Abbreviated Mini-Mental Test (Tombaugh & McIntyre 1992). This test assesses cognitive ability and memory and this information is important when assessing the likely safety and effectiveness of care. It is also possible to detect depression, for example using the Philadelphia Geriatric Morale Scale (PGMS) (Lawton 1975) and the Brief Case Finding for Depression (BCD) (Clarke & McKenzie 1996) (see Chapter 8). The BCD forms part of the Australian ANDIAB diabetes complication screening process.

The assessment must be undertaken sensitively so the person is not offended and does not become confused. The hospital ward is not an appropriate setting for most assessments because privacy is important and noise and distractions can influence the outcome. Figures 2.1 and 3.1 are proformas that can be used to assess the social network and identify the sources of support the person utilises. Given that comorbidity is common in older people and is a key determinant of the care needed, it is important to take a full medical history to identify all relevant health problems.

Lifestyle factors

Lifestyle factors contribute to diabetes control and complication status. It is important to take a detailed history of the person's diet, smoking behaviour, alcohol intake and the amount of exercise they undertake (see Chapter 2). Diet is clearly crucial and a detailed verbal history can be difficult to obtain and is often unreliable, particularly in cases of mental frailty. A diet diary can be useful, but people need to be motivated and able to keep such records.

Involving their carers may be necessary. As an alternative, the person can be shown pictures of food and asked how much they eat of each food per day or they can be asked to describe what they ate yesterday. The aim of these questions should not be punitive but to identify food value and overall proportions of carbohydrate, protein and fat in the diet. Asking who does the shopping and cooking helps to target the advice. Determining whether the person is at risk of under- or overnutrition and malnourishment is an essential basis for referral to a dietitian.

Assessing weight and fat distribution is important in relation to identifying cardiovascular risk and planning appropriate treatment and was described in Chapter 2. Obesity is strongly associated with coronary heart disease, which is the main cause

Carer network

	Shopping	Cooking	Blood glucose monitor	Gives insulin	Gives medication
Self-care					
Neighbour					
Relative					
Friend					
Home help					
District nurse					
Other (specify below) _____					
Meals on Wheels					

Figure 3.1 Proforma to assess an older person's social support network and who provides assistance with specific tasks.

of death in people with Type 2 diabetes. Low body mass suggests a failing beta cell mass, which increases the risk of acute complications such as DKA and HONK (see Chapter 4). HONK is common in older people, especially those in nursing homes, and is associated with a high level of mortality.

Blood glucose levels are an important part of the assessment. Only very limited data about what comprises optimal glycaemic control for older people are available but in general it is appropriate to use accepted targets for good, borderline and poor control. Assuming all the necessary blood results are available, the assessment should focus on the blood glucose pattern and potential causes of suboptimal results. Home blood glucose monitoring is important to obtain a profile of results across the 24-hour period. Fasting results are an important indicator of overall control and the risk of hypoglycaemia. Older people are particularly at risk of hypoglycaemia, which can precipitate a fall and result in trauma (see Chapter 4).

HbA_{1c} provides useful information about the overall blood glucose control over the previous 30–60 days and is a useful benchmark for glycaemic control and monitoring progress. Optimal control is HbA_{1c} <7% but every percentage point reduction, even from quite high HbA_{1c} levels, reduces the risk of short- and long-term complications. Blood glucose targets need to be appropriate; for example, in the frailty model care is geared toward alleviating symptoms such as polyuria and polydipsia that can aggravate behavioural problems rather than achieving tight control. The symptoms may also exacerbate other common problems such as urinary incontinence, which may only become apparent in discussion with carers.

Physical assessment

Physical assessment is outlined in Chapters 2, 5 and 7. Additional assessments include the following.

Vision

- Any recent visual changes such as loss of vision, blind spots, floaters.
- History of glaucoma or cataract, macular degeneration.
- Visual acuity with and without 'pinhole' glasses.
- Dilation fundoscopy.
- Retinal photography.
- Low vision support such as welfare benefits and equipment (see Chapter 5).

Assessing vision is vitally important but very complex so optometrists, ophthalmologists or an ophthalmic nurse should undertake detailed eye assessments.

Practice point

Nurses can identify sudden or recent changes in vision, such as the emergence of floaters or blind spots, which are unlikely to be the result of normal visual deterioration.

Visual acuity is tested using an eye chart. The person reads the eye chart with each eye in turn, wearing their normal glasses, standing at the appropriate distance from the eye chart, usually six metres. A three-metre chart is available. Note which line number the person can read down to. On a Snellen chart the line numbers are 60, 36, 24, 18, 12, 9, 6 and 5. The result is written as the line number by the distance away from the chart, e.g. 12 (line)/6 (distance).

Vision is rechecked by pinhole glasses, which are cardboard glasses with a 1 mm hole in them. In the absence of any pathology, visual acuity should improve with the pinhole because it focuses a narrow shaft of light onto the eye, which compensates for refractive or lens problems. If the vision does not improve, pathological changes in the eye are likely and referral to an ophthalmologist is advisable. A score of below 12/6 on a Snellen chart indicates that ophthalmic assessment is needed. Ideally, where available all people should have either dilation fundoscopy or retinal screening.

If the person has significant visual impairment it may be to their advantage to be registered 'blind' so they can claim additional benefits, such as talking books and various household gadgets. However, this also has implications in other areas such as driving.

Cardiovascular assessment

Cardiovascular risk is extremely high in older people with diabetes and is the biggest cause of death, affecting both men and women. People with diabetes often have 'silent myocardial infarctions' which may accompany hypoglycaemia. Therefore any abnormal symptoms warrant an ECG. It may be useful to routinely perform an ECG in people with hypertension, a high BMI or abnormal lipid profiles.

Hypertension increases the cardiac, kidney, cerebral and peripheral vascular disease risk. Therefore, the implications of hypertension need to be considered more globally rather than for cardiac health alone. The UKPDS (1998) recommended that tight blood pressure control, systolic below 140 and diastolic below 82, significantly reduces mortality and morbidity.

Practice points

(1) Taking the blood pressure with the arm in a horizontal position rather than with a bent elbow or the arm by the person's side is important to achieve accurate results.
(2) The horizontal position most closely approximates the heart level.
(3) Measuring the blood pressure on a dependent arm could lead to overdiagnosis of hypertension and subsequently inappropriate treatment.
(4) Using the appropriate cuff size is also important.

Achieving blood pressure targets in the older person is likely to require antihypertensive therapy as well as lifestyle changes which are often less effective or appropriate in older people. Lipids should be assessed. Lipid targets are shown in Chapter 2. Key dietary strategies include reducing saturated fat (high in LDL) intake and increasing monounsaturated fat (high in HDL) intake, increasing exercise and reducing alcohol consumption.

Foot assessment

Foot assessment is of the utmost importance and both feet should be assessed to detect problems early to help avoid the risk of foot ulceration (see Chapter 5). Foot ulceration is often associated with multiple bacterial infections, which increase the risk of septicaemia and amputation.

The ability to self-care for the feet can be compromised by low vision, reduced manual dexterity, inability to reach the feet, inadequate knowledge, cognitive deficits and depression. If foot self-care is inadequate alternative strategies need to be incorporated into the care plan.

Renal assessment

Renal function changes are common in older people with diabetes and can affect the clearance of medicines. The principal problem in kidney damage is that microvascular damage reduces the glomerular filtration rate. The glomerulus then begins to leak protein. Unfortunately most of the current routine assessment methods only detect protein loss once a significant reduction in kidney function has occurred. Detection of protein using Multistick urine test strips indicates renal damage is likely to be advanced. Nevertheless, the urine should be tested for protein and leucocytes, which may indicate a urine infection, in which case the urine should be sent for laboratory culture and sensitivity assessment.

Neurological assessment

Diabetes affects both the autonomic and sympathetic nervous systems. Foot assessment will detect peripheral nerve damage, but it is important to also ask about finger sensation. Sitting and standing blood pressure measurements are used to assess the autonomic nervous system function. A systolic drop of 30 mmHg or more on standing suggests postural hypotension that is likely to be caused by autonomic neuropathy and may represent a falls risk.

Another neurological symptom is persistent diarrhoea. Other causes of diarrhoea include constipation with overflow, laxative abuse or endocrine disease. Bladder dysfunction should be explored. Urge and overflow incontinence are the most common problems. A bladder scanner, which is often available through a local continence service, can be a useful assessment tool.

Sexual function should also be discussed sensitively with men and women. Do not assume that because the person is older, they are not sexually active and do not have sexual needs. Erectile dysfunction is a common problem for men and referral to a genitourinary clinic may be appropriate (see Chapter 10).

Skin assessment

The skin of people with diabetes is often thickened due to the formation of glycated end-products which can restrict joint movement, particularly in the fingers, and lead to Garrod's knuckle and Dupuytren's contracture. The skin also tends to be dry due to reduced sweating as a result of autonomic neuropathy. In addition, a number of specific skin disorders are associated with diabetes.

- Diabetic dermopathy or shin spots is one of the most common skin conditions in diabetes. The early lesions are oval, up to 1 cm in diameter, developing into brown scaly scars. They usually develop on the shin but can be found on the forearms, thighs and bony prominences.
- Necobiosis lipoidica diabeticorum is rare. Lesions are irregular in shape with indurated plaques and central atrophy and can become ulcerous. It is more common in Type 1 diabetes.
- Acanthosis nigricans is a hyperpigmented velvety overgrowth of the epidermis usually found in the axilla, groin and neck.
- Skin infections are common and are often a presenting symptom of diabetes. Boils, often due to *Staphylococcus aureus*, occur especially if immunity is compromised.
- *Candida albicans*, often in the vagina and glans penis, can occur and can affect intertriginous areas.
- Chronic infection of the nail folds (paronychia) is also a problem.

The assessment process represents an opportunity for providing some important health education and safety messages. These include management of hypo- and hyperglycaemia, insulin administration technique, blood glucose monitoring, driving, medication self-management, diet, exercise, smoking, alcohol, available welfare benefits and the contact details of relevant health professionals and national or local diabetes associations.

Assessing fitness to drive

Practice points

(1) The ability to drive is a cornerstone of independence for many older people. It may be the only way they are able to take part in activities outside the home such as shopping and attending health appointments. In addition, many older grandparents are the main child carers and drive their grandchildren to a range of activities.
(2) Chronological age is not necessarily a barrier to driving.
(3) The focus should be on assessing the risks to the individual and other people when making decisions about fitness to drive and encompass physical status and cognitive functioning.
(4) Older people with diabetes need to know that they may still be permitted to drive but that restrictions might be placed on their licence.
(5) Driving regulations differ. Health professionals need to be familiar with the regulations in their area and their responsibility regarding notifying motoring authorities when safety concerns arise.
(6) If a driver's licence is cancelled the person's life may be changed dramatically.

Higher rates of traffic accidents per kilometre travelled occur in people over 70 years. Fatalities resulting from car accidents also increase with increasing age. Identifying which older driver is at greatest risk is not clear cut. Some older people voluntarily put 'restrictions' on their driving, others cite their long record of safe driving as a reason to continue driving without restrictions. In addition, older people may drive older cars that are not well maintained or roadworthy because of financial constraints.

Diabetes affects a person's ability to drive safely by:

- Reducing vision or development of tunnel vision (reduction in peripheral vision) as a result of laser treatment.
- Reducing sensation in the feet that makes feeling brake and accelerator pedals difficult.
- Making it difficult to operate pedals and steering wheel following limb amputations, stroke or carpal tunnel syndrome.
- Reduced cognitive functioning as a result of age or medicines, including insulin and oral agents that cause hypoglycaemia.
- Slowed reflexes and lethargy as a consequence of hyperglycaemia.
- Risk of silent myocardial infarction whilst driving.

Some important issues to consider when assessing fitness to drive include:

(1) Medicines, especially those that alter blood glucose, blood pressure and level of consciousness or cognition.
(2) Visual acuity. Vision deficits have a number of consequences as described by Miller (1999) which include:
    - longer adaptation time between light and dark conditions
    - reduced peripheral vision
    - changed perception of speed

- changes in visual accommodation that can affect the ability to read the dash-board controls and then accommodate to the road or roadside signs
- conditions such as tinted car windows, glare from sun, snow or rain and fog may affect the clarity of vision
- changed colour perception, for example perception of red and green, may en-hance glare at sunset and sunrise and make it difficult to distinguish road signs.

(3) Hearing.
(4) Neck, upper body and limb strength and range of movement.
(5) Reaction times.
(6) Attention and concentration span.
(7) Insight, judgement, thought processing and problem-solving abilities.
(8) Memory.
(9) The individual's need to be able to drive and what alternatives can be put in place.

Counselling may be necessary. For example, cancelling the licence of an older man may represent a 'loss of manhood or status as head of the household'.

Isolated physical deficits may not be sufficient reason to cancel or restrict driving. However, the presence of several physical and cognitive deficits may mean the individual's driving capacity should be formally assessed and driver rehabilitation programmes may be necessary, for example following a stroke or medical event (Austroads 2003).

3.4.4 Making nursing decisions and choosing a model of care

It is beyond the scope of this chapter to provide a detailed account of all the potential actions that could arise from assessing the older person with diabetes. The focus is placed on some key principles that a nurse should observe when constructing a care plan with the individual and their carers. In essence, the nurse needs to assimilate all the data from their assessment in order to identify the way forward – the most challenging aspect of the assessment. Frequently, many issues need to be discussed with the other professionals. Key decisions include:

- Determining which care model to use, based on the characteristics of the individual and on their personal preferences.
- Locating problems. It is useful to identify any problems or issues arising from the assessment in three domains: physiological, psychological and social (see Figure 3.2). The obstacles to achieving health targets also need to be identified and addressed if possible. Type 2 diabetes is a chronic and deteriorating condition. The person may be doing everything 'right' but their beta cells have become less effective over time. In such circumstances it is important to reassure the individual and explain what may be happening, and change their treatment accordingly.
- Finding solutions to presenting problems involves identifying where the problems arise and how much of the care the individual or their carer can undertake and whether treatment can be adjusted sufficiently to address the problem. Referral to other health professionals may be necessary. Care pathways or guidelines can help identify the appropriate action (see Figure 3.1).
- Minimising risks. It is important to try to gauge the degree of risk involved, including risks associated with treatment. Sometimes quantifying risk is difficult and a

Locating the problem

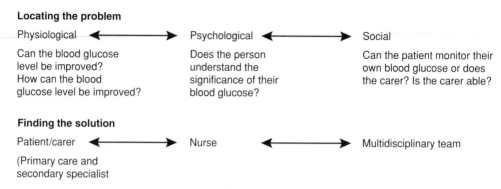

Figure 3.2 A schematic representation of how to locate presenting problems in the physiological, psychological or social domain and find an acceptable management strategy.

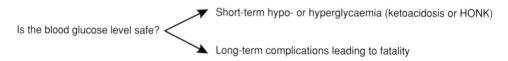

Figure 3.3 A suggested proforma for gauging the level of risk presented by the person's current situation and represented by any proposed care plans.

case discussion with the relevant team or specialist colleagues is needed before taking action. The decision to discuss risks with individuals is difficult to make; for example, the risk of hypoglycaemia if the OHA is increased may motivate some people and dishearten others (see Figure 3.3).

3.5   Promoting quality of life and optimal mental health

The need to maximise the older person's quality of life has been a recurrent theme throughout this chapter. In considering treatment options it is important to ensure that there is a balance between achieving clinical targets and the happiness and wellbeing of the individual. It is possible to undertake a more formal assessment of quality of life using standardised instruments as part of wider assessment. One instrument that has been used in older populations is the ADDQoL (Bradley & Todd 1999) (see Chapter 8).

One aspect of quality of life is a person's ability to undertake positive health practices. A number of factors predict positive health practice (Yarcheski *et al.* 2004).

- Moderate effect: loneliness, social support, perceived health status, self-efficacy, future time perspective, self-esteem, hope, depression.
- Small effect: stress, education, marital status, age, income and sex.

Patient ←————————→ Negotiation Clarity of understanding ←————————→ Nurse

Figure 3.4   Proforma for setting and reviewing goals.

3.6   Setting targets

Once the relevant issues are identified, management targets need to be discussed and agreed by the individual and a time for review set. The person must be very clear about what is expected of them (see Figure 3.4). If a medicine is changed within an agreed protocol, make sure the person receives a prescription for the new drug or dose and it is amended on their repeat list. Check that the patient fully understands what the changes are. If a patient-held record system is used, write the care in simple terms in that record so it can be followed at home. If the patient does not speak English it is necessary to use an advocate or interpreter and provide materials in the appropriate language.

Targets need to be realistic and achievable so the individual does not become disheartened. Ensure there is a balance between what they can achieve and more testing targets but proceed slowly and change one thing at a time. Finally, check whether the person understands everything and agrees with the review period.

3.7   Reducing the costs of diabetes

Having diabetes can be expensive and represents a significant financial burden for many older people. Diabetes costs include:

- Extra food costs, for example low Glycemic Index™ foods, the difference between the price of 'no-brand' bread and a brand name bread.
- Blood glucose meters, strips and lancets (and sometimes diaries to record blood glucose levels).
- Medications, insulin pens, pen needles and syringes.
- Diabetes-related health costs such as appointments with GPs, endocrinologists, diabetes educators, dietitians, podiatrists and optometrists. More frequent visits may be needed.
- Appropriate footwear, orthotics, socks and hosiery.
- Recommended foot moisturisers and foot-care equipment.
- Diabetes association membership.
- Diabetes education/ongoing support group.
- Diabetes complications, for example wound products, dialysis.
- Complementary therapies.
- Purchasing books and videos about diabetes or accessing IT sites.

In the UK many of these products are supplied freely by the NHS, and in Australia some processes are in place to reduce these costs. The National Diabetes Services Scheme (NDSS) is an Australian Commonwealth Government programme whereby people with diabetes can register free of charge and access a variety of diabetes products free or at a reduced price. Subsidised products include:

- Blood glucose testing strips and electrodes.
- Urine glucose testing strips.
- Urine ketone testing strips.
- Insulin pump consumables.

Products provided free of charge include:

- Insulin syringes.
- Insulin pen needles.

In Australia the cost of blood glucose meters is not subsidised. However, older people who hold a Department of Veteran Affairs (DVA) Gold Card can receive their meter free of charge or receive full reimbursement from the DVA if they have already purchased a meter. Other people with diabetes who have private health insurance may receive partial or full reimbursement from their fund depending on the type of fund, type of policy (for example if they hold an 'extras' policy) and policy level.

Public health services are usually free of charge but in some Australian states cost retrieval policies have been implemented and people are required to pay to access community services such as podiatry and group education. Interestingly, there is a growing body of work suggesting that if they have to pay for health education, participants place greater worth on it and are more likely to be compliant.

Accessing private services can be costly, although this is not an issue in the UK where diabetes health care is provided freely through the NHS in primary care facilities and in specialist diabetes centres. Some medical specialists charge in excess of the Medicare item number and private health funds do not always cover the entire costs. Accessing podiatry services can be particularly expensive. Some people with diabetes are forced to do this without having private health insurance due to the enormous waiting list attached to public services. People with diabetes who hold a DVA Gold Card can access a variety of private sector health professionals free of charge. This is particularly useful in terms of podiatry services, freeing up public waiting lists. Private health funds may also cover the costs of consumer membership of Diabetes Australia. Membership of such consumer organisations can have additional benefits in terms of receiving free education and reductions in equipment, educational material and food items.

3.8   Conclusion

Clearly developing care systems for older people involves more than the actions of any one individual nurse or discipline. The multidisciplinary team must support this endeavour. However, nurses can and should take a lead role in identifying populations of older people with diabetes, considering ways of determining the individual and collective needs of those populations and in developing care systems that are sympathetic to the needs of older people.

References

Adler, A.I., Stratton, I.M., Neil, H.A. *et al.* (2000) Association of systolic blood pressure with macrovascular and microvascular complications of type 2 diabetes (UKPDS 36): prospective observational study. *British Medical Journal*, **321**(7258), 412–19.

Australian Diabetes Educators Association (ADEA) (2003) *Guidelines for the Management of Diabetes in Older People*. ADEA, Canberra.

Australian Pharmaceutical Advisory Council (1997), *Integrated Best Practice Model for Medication Management in Residential Aged Care*. APAC, Canberra.

Austroads Incorporated (2003) *Assessing Fitness to Drive*. Austroads, Sydney.

Benbow, S.J., Walsh, A. & Gill, G.V. (1997) Diabetes in institutionalised elderly people: a forgotten population. *British Medical Journal*, **314**, 1868–9.

Bowling, A. & Browne, P. (1991) Social networks health and emotional well-being among the oldest old in London. *Journal of Gerontology*, **46**, 530–2.

Bradley, C. & Todd, C. (1999) The development of an individualised questionnaire measure of perceived impact of diabetes on quality of life: the ADDQoL. *Quality of Life Research*, **8**(1–2), 79–91.

British Diabetic Association (BDA) (1999) *Guidelines for Practice for Residents with Diabetes in Care Homes*. British Diabetic Association, London.

Buchanan, J. & Chamberlain, M. (1978) *Survey of the Mobility of the Disabled in an Urban Environment*. Royal Association for Disability and Rehabilitation, London.

Byles, J., Tavener, J., O'Connell, R. *et al.* (2004) Randomised controlled trial of health assessments for older Australian veterans and war widows. *Medical Journal of Australia*, **181**(4), 186–90.

Caplan, G.A., Williams, A.J., Daly, B. & Abraham, K. (2004) A randomized, controlled trial of comprehensive geriatric assessment and multidisciplinary intervention after discharge of elderly from the emergency department – the DEED II study. *Journal of the American Geriatrics Society*, **52**(9), 1417–23.

Chin, A., Paw, M.J., Dekker, J.M. *et al.* (1999) How to select a frail elderly population. A comparison of three working definitions. *Journal of Clinical Epidemiology*, **52**(11), 1015–21.

Clarke, D.M. & McKenzie, D.P. (1996) Brief screening for depression. *Journal of the American Geriatrics Society*, **44**(2), 212–13.

Croxson, S.C. (2002) Diabetes in the elderly: problems of care and service provision. *Diabetic Medicine*, **19**(suppl 4), 66–72.

Croxson, S., Burden, A., Bodington, M. & Botha, J. (1991) The prevalence of diabetes in elderly people. *Diabetic Medicine*, **8**, 28–31.

Department of Health (2001) *National Service Framework – Older People*. Department of Health, London.

Department of Health (2002) *National Service Framework – Diabetes*. Department of Health, London.

Farooqi, A. & Sorrie, S. (1999) Monitoring of elderly housebound and mobile diabetics in 31 Leicestershire practices: a comparative study. *Practical Diabetes International*, **16**(4), 114–16.

Forbes, A. & Morris, L. (1999) Housebound older people are missing out on diabetes care. *Nursing Times*, **95**(14), 30–1.

Forbes, A., Berry, J. & While, A. (2001) A critical examination of a clinical protocol to support district nurses in the domiciliary annual review of older frail people with Type 2 diabetes. *British Journal of Community Nursing*, **6**(12), 652–60.

Forbes, A., Berry, J., While, A., Hitman, G. & Sinclair, A. (2002a) Issues and methodological challenges in developing and evaluating health care interventions for older people with diabetes mellitus. Part 1. *Practical Diabetes International*, **19**(2), 55–9.

Forbes, A., Berry, J., While, A., Hitman, G. & Sinclair, A. (2002b) Issues and methodological challenges in developing and evaluating health care interventions for older people with diabetes mellitus. Part 2. *Practical Diabetes International*, **19**(3), 81–4.

Forbes, A., Berry, J., While, A., Hitman, G. & Sinclair, A. (2004) A pilot project to explore the feasibility and potential of a protocol to support district nurses in the assessment of older frail people with Type 2 diabetes. *Nursing Research*, **9**(4), 282–94.

Gadsby, R. (1994) Care of people with diabetes who are housebound or in residential care. *Diabetes in General Practice*, **4**(3), 30–1.

Gueldner, S.H. & Hanner, M.B. (1989) Methodological issues related to gerontological nursing research. *Nursing Research*, **38**(3), 183–5.

Hall, K. (1992) Care of the housebound diabetic. *Practice Nurse*, **December**, 539–42.

Hamerman, D. (1999) Toward an understanding of frailty. *Annals of Internal Medicine*, **130**(11), 945–59.

Hendra, T.J. & Sinclair, A.J. (1997) Improving the care of elderly diabetic patients: the final report of the St Vincent Joint Task Force for Diabetes. *Age & Ageing*, **26**, 3–6.

Keeson, C. & Knight, P. (1990) *Diabetes and Elderly People*. Chapman and Hall, London.

Lawton, A. (1975) The Philadelphia Geriatric Center morale scale: a revision. *Journal of Gerontology*, **30**, 85–9.

Lee, K., Westley, C. & Fletcher, K. (2004) If at first you don't succeed: efforts to improve collaboration between nursing homes and a health system. *Topics in Advanced Nursing Practice e-journal* 4(3).

Lindesay, J. & Thompson, C. (1993) Housebound elderly people: definition, prevalence and characteristics. *International Journal of Geriatric Psychiatry*, **8**, 231–7.

Miller, C. (1999) *Nursing Care of Older Adults*. Lippincott, Philadelphia.

National Health and Medical Research Council (1994) *Minimising Adverse Consequences of Hospitalisation in the Older Person*. NHMRC, Canberra.

Nouri, F. & Lincoln, N.B. (1987) An extended activities of daily living scale for stroke patients. *Clinical Rehabilitation*, **1**, 301–5.

Potter, J. (1990) Diabetes in the day hospital. *Care of the Elderly*, **2**(1), 11–13.

Silliman, R., Bhatti, S., Khan, A., Dukes, K. & Sullivan, L. (1996) The care of older persons with diabetes mellitus: families and primary care physicians. *Journal of the American Geriatrics Society*, **44**(11), 1314–21.

Sinclair, A. (2000) Diabetes in old age – changing concepts in the secondary care arena. *Journal of the Royal College of Physicians of London*, **34**(3), 240–4.

Sinclair, A. & Barnett, A. (1993) Special needs of elderly diabetic patients. *British Medical Journal*, **306**, 1142–3.

Sinclair, A., Girling, A. & Bayer, J. (2000) Cognitive dysfunction in older subjects with diabetes mellitus: impact on diabetes self-management and use of care services. *Diabetes Research and Clinical Practice*, **50**, 203–12.

Souder, J.E. (1992) The consumer approach to recruitment of elder subjects. *Nursing Research*, **41**(5), 314–16.

Tombaugh, T.N. & McIntyre, N.J. (1992) The Mini-Mental State Examination: a comprehensive review. *Journal of the American Geriatrics Society*, **40**, 922–35.

Tong, P. & Roberts, S. (1994) Diabetes care in the frail elderly. *Practical Diabetes International*, **11**(4), 163–4.

UK Prospective Diabetes Study (UKPDS) Group (1998) Intensive blood-glucose control with sulphonylureas or insulin compared with conventional treatment and risk of complications in patients with type 2 diabetes (UKPDS 33). *Lancet*, **352**(9131), 837–53.

Yarcheski, A., Mahon, N., Yarcheski, T. & Canella, B. (2004) A meta-analysis of predictors of positive health practices. *Journal of Nursing Scholarship*, **36**(1), 102–7.

Chapter 4
Short-term Complications of Diabetes

Michelle Robins

Key points

- Short-term complications can cause considerable morbidity and mortality.
- Treatment strategies for complications may differ in older people.
- The significant risk of short-term complications is often not recognised in older people with diabetes.
- Short-term complications increase the risk of falls and trauma and admission to hospital.
- Hypo- and hyperglycaemia can cause confusion.

4.1 Introduction

Diabetes-related complications are generally divided into two groups for all people with diabetes regardless of diabetes type or age: short-term and long-term complications. What constitutes a short- or long-term complication for an older person with diabetes can be quite different from that of younger people with diabetes. For example, a newly diagnosed older person with Type 2 diabetes may already have microvascular complications, such as renal impairment, and macrovascular disease including hypertension, hyperlipidemia, ischaemic heart disease, peripheral vascular disease or a previous myocardial infarct or stroke.

Other conditions such as profound eye disease are often also present and include age-related macropathy, glaucoma and cataracts. A decline in renal function is a normal part of the ageing process. Postural hypotension, normally associated with autonomic neuropathy in people with diabetes, may occur in the older person who is dehydrated. Erectile dysfunction occurs in approximately 90% of men, with and without diabetes, over the age of 80 years. Foot ulceration may already be present at the time of diagnosis and if it was slow to heal, should have been a warning sign that diabetes could be present in the undiagnosed person with diabetes. Long-term complications are discussed in detail in Chapter 5.

4.2   Short-term diabetes-related complications

- Hypoglycaemia.
- Hyperglycaemia-related emergencies.
- Dehydration caused by hyperglycaemia.
- Delayed wound healing.
- Falls.
- Postural hypotension.
- Constipation.
- Increased risk of infection, for example urinary tract infections.
- Changes in skin condition such as a propensity to dryness and trauma.
- Acute changes in mental status.

4.3   Hypoglycaemia

Key points

- Hypoglycaemia is the most serious short-term complication of diabetes in older people.
- Hypoglycaemia can cause significant morbidity and mortality.
- May present with atypical or absent symptoms.
- Must be treated immediately regardless of whether symptoms are present or not.
- First-line treatment is glucose, which may be administered in a variety of ways to meet individual needs.
- Follow up initial glucose treatment with slowly digested carbohydrate.
- Document the event carefully.
- Prevention strategies, proactive treatment and follow-up are vital in residential facilities.

4.3.1   What is hypoglycaemia?

Hypoglycaemia is usually defined as a blood glucose level less than 3.0 mmol/L (Dunning 2003). However, in older people the level may need to be revised to <4–5 mmol/L or higher as part of hypoglycaemia risk management.

Preventing hypoglycaemia is one of the most significant issues in managing diabetes in older people. Older people have sustained lasting injuries and died as a result of hypoglycaemia. Therefore, from a safety viewpoint, blood glucose levels in older people, especially if they are frail and unwell, should be maintained above 5 mmol/L. Anecdotally, many health professionals and carers who fear the adverse effects of hypoglycaemia in older people with diabetes maintain the blood glucose in the hyperglycaemic range, which itself contributes to a reduced quality of life, morbidity and mortality. Therefore, a balance needs to be struck between preventing hypoglycaemia and controlling hyperglycaemia to reduce the negative effects on health and wellbeing.

Understanding the causes of hypoglycaemia is fundamental to developing preventive strategies and treatment protocols. Older people with diabetes can achieve stable glycaemic control with education and supportive clinical policies in acute and residential care facilities.

Practice point

Blood glucose levels in older people, especially if they are frail and unwell, should be maintained above 5 mmol/L as part of an overall strategy to reduce the risk of hypoglycaemia.

4.3.2   Causes of hypoglycaemia

Not all people with diabetes experience or are at risk of hypoglycaemia. Hypoglycaemia occurs in people with diabetes treated with insulin, sulphonylureas or meglitanides. Hypoglycaemia is rare in people treated with metformin but it can occur. Hypoglycaemia is more common in older people who:

- Miss or delay meals.
- Eat insufficient amounts of carbohydrate.
- Administer too much insulin or oral hypoglycaemic agents.
- Consume alcohol on an empty stomach. Even small amounts of alcohol significantly increase the risk of hypoglycaemia.
- Reduce oral steroid dosage without reducing their insulin or OHA.
- Suddenly lose weight without reducing their insulin or OHA.

4.3.3   Particular issues associated with hypoglycaemia in older people

As part of normal ageing, the counterregulatory hormones associated with the normal physiological response to low blood glucose levels are impaired. Even when hypoglycaemia is induced under controlled research conditions, older people who do not have diabetes exhibit a prolonged recovery from hypoglycaemia and reduced ability to secrete glucagon, which in turn increases the blood glucose levels (Marker *et al.* 1992).

The other main issue is that older people with diabetes often fail to exhibit 'textbook' symptoms of hypoglycaemia or the symptoms that do occur are mistaken for coexisting medical conditions. For example, tingling in the lips and tongue is usually absent in older people having a hypoglycaemic event. Sudden dizziness is often confused with frailty and postural hypotension. Shaking may be too difficult to distinguish from the characteristic rigid movements of Parkinson's disease. Confusion, behaviour change or vagueness can be considered a normal part of ageing or part of dementia (Whitehead & Finucane 1995).

Sudden verbal or even physical aggression may be mistaken for dementia behaviour rather than hypoglycaemia. If an individual has a brain injury, for example from a stroke, the normal neural pathways that indicate blood glucose levels may be disrupted, thus diminishing identifiable symptoms of hypoglycaemia. For the client who cannot verbally communicate with carers, symptoms may be experienced but not expressed.

Practice point

Hypoglycaemic episodes must always be treated in older people, even if symptoms are absent.

4.3.4   Older people with diabetes at high risk of hypoglycaemia

Hypoglycaemia prevention strategies are particularly important for older people who:

- Live alone, especially if they are unable to shop or prepare food.
- Rely on home-delivered meal services, such as Meals-on-Wheels. In these situations the person may make one meal last over two different mealtimes.
- Are depressed.
- Have impaired cognition or dementia.
- Have established diabetes complications such as autonomic neuropathy, renal and cardiovascular disease.
- Have concurrent conditions and illnesses that profoundly affect their ability to perform activities of daily living. Unexpected decline in renal function can explain hypoglycaemia (Parmar 2004).
- Have no teeth or poor oral hygiene.
- Have a diminished swallow reflex or require soft or vitamised meals.
- Require enteral feeds.
- Require palliative care.
- Are prescribed long-acting sulphonylureas such as glibenclamide, glimepiride and gliclazide MR.
- Are prescribed intermediate- and long-acting insulins such as Protaphane.
- Drive.

Increasing chronological age is associated with a higher risk.

Several oral hypoglycaemia agents are contraindicated in older people with diabetes especially if they are at high risk of hypoglycaemia. Glibenclamide can cause prolonged hypoglycaemia, often lasting for several hours, because of its prolonged half-life in older people. This means that older people prescribed a daily morning dose of glibenclamide (with breakfast) may in fact become hypoglycaemic later in the evening when the drug is acting at its peak long after it would have been metabolised and excreted in a younger person. One study identified a higher prevalence of unconscious hypoglycaemia in older people taking glibenclamide compared to insulin therapy (Ben-Ami *et al.* 1999). Tolbutamide, a short-acting oral agent previously used extensively in older people, has been withdrawn from the market in Australia. It is still available in the UK but not used widely.

Hypoglycaemia occurs less frequently and is less severe if shorter-acting agents such as gliclazide are used (Van Staa *et al.* 1997). Longer-acting sulphonylurea agents are now available, such as glimepiride and gliclazide MR. Data about their propensity to cause hypoglycaemia in older people are limited. Therefore they should be used with caution, especially in the frail elderly with labile dietary intake (Sinclair

Table 4.1 Comparison of hypoglycaemic symptoms in younger and older people with diabetes.

Younger people with diabetes	Older people with diabetes
Early symptoms	
Sudden dizziness	Sudden dizziness
Sudden shaking	Sudden weakness
Profuse sweating	Changes in behaviour
Sudden blurred vision	Tachycardia/palpitations
Tingling of lips and tongue or fingers	Falls
Frontal headache	Poor concentration
Tachycardia/palpitations	
Hunger	
Later symptoms	
Changes in behaviour	Changes in behaviour
Poor concentration	Poor concentration
Reduced conscious state	Reduced conscious state
Very late symptoms	
Fitting	Unconscious/coma
Unconscious/coma	Myocardial infarction

& Finucane 2001). However, gliclazide MR has a lower incidence of hypoglycaemia because it has no active metabolites, and a different action profile and binding activity from other oral agents (Schernthaner *et al.* 2004) (see Chapter 2).

4.3.5   *Differences in the presentation of hypoglycaemia in older people with diabetes*

Older people with diabetes may present with unusual hypoglycaemic symptoms. For example, tingling in the lips and tongue is rare in older people experiencing hypoglycaemia but common in younger people with diabetes. Older people with diabetes often describe a feeling of sudden 'weakness', which may be confused with the lethargy caused by raised blood glucose levels (see Table 4.1). Absence or unrecognised symptoms in older people represents a significant risk for adverse events such as falls. In addition to conditions that can mask hypoglycaemic symptoms, other conditions or medications that may contribute to non-recognition of symptoms include people who are unable to communicate and those taking sedatives.

One of the many challenges faced by those caring for older people with diabetes is being able to distinguish hypoglycaemia from other concurrent conditions. Older people with dementia and diabetes who experience hypoglycaemia may exhibit physically aggressive behaviour, not dissimilar to very young children with diabetes demonstrating naughty behaviour during hypoglycaemia. Table 4.2 outlines the differences between hypoglycaemia symptoms and other concurrent conditions.

Table 4.2 Different presenting symptoms in older people with hypoglycaemia and concurrent conditions.

Hypoglycaemia symptoms	Other concurrent conditions
Sudden dizziness	Postural hypotension due to dehydration, antihypertensive medication
Sudden shaking or tremor	Parkinson's disease
Change in behaviour – especially aggressive	Dementia
Tachycardia/palpitations	Other cardiac conditions – atrial fibrillation, panic attacks associated with dementia

4.3.6   Consequences of hypoglycaemia in older people

Hypoglycaemia is dangerous for older people when sudden dizziness and confusion occur. Falls are common and often result in severe injuries requiring hospitalisation. If an older person falls and fractures a hip they may require admission to a residential care facility from hospital and may never return home (Stepka *et al.* 1993).

As a result of the profound stress placed on the body during a severe hypoglycaemic episode, heart attacks can occur.

4.3.7   Managing hypoglycaemia

Practice point

There are four components to the management of hypoglycaemia.

(1) Detection.
(2) Immediate management.
(3) Ascertaining why it occurred.
(4) Prevention of further episodes.

First-line management

● Assure safety; for example, if the person is standing, assist them to sit or lie down.
● Perform a blood glucose test.
● Assist the person to ingest glucose. Choose the highest Glycemic Index™ food (see Table 4.3).

Glucose alone will only maintain blood glucose levels between 4 and 10 mmol/L for up to one hour. Therefore prompt follow-up is required to prevent the blood glucose levels from falling again and hypoglycaemia recurring. If longer-acting insulin or oral agents caused the hypoglycaemia, the first-line treatment strategies may need to be repeated twice or even three times before the blood glucose levels start to increase. Repeating the glucose quantities suggested in Table 4.3 rather than repeating the follow-up foods, until symptoms subside and blood glucose levels increase, will 'put a lid on' the extent of the blood glucose rise. Repeating follow-up slowly digested

Table 4.3 First-line hypoglycaemic management of older people with specific feeding issues and the Glycemic Index™ score of the relevant options.

Specific feeding issue	Management options	Glycemic Index™ score
Normal swallow reflex	2 teaspoons of glucose dissolved in water	GI score – 100*
	OR	
	5–6 glucose jelly beans	GI score – 78*
	OR	
	half bottle Lucozade	GI score – 95*
Impaired swallow reflex requiring thickened fluids and/or vitamised meals	1 tube of glucose paste	GI score – more than 80
	Vitamised pears in natural juice	GI score – 43
	Vitamised peaches in natural juice	GI score – 38
	Custard	GI score – 38
	Low-fat mousse	GI score – 34
	Yoghurt	GI score – 14–40
Enteral feeding	2 teaspoons glucose powder dissolved in water and delivered through a PEG or nasogastric tube	GI score – 100*

* Taken from Brand-Miller & Foster-Powell 2002.

carbohydrate until symptoms resolve and/or the blood glucose levels start to rise often equates to three or four serves of carbohydrate, which raises the blood glucose levels very high and keeps them high for some hours.

Long-acting agents that can cause profound and often prolonged hypoglycaemia include:

- Oral agents: chlorpropamide, glibenclamide, glimepiride, gliclazide MR.
- Long-acting insulin and insulins containing a longer-acting component: Protaphane, Humulin NPH, Mixtard 20/80, 30/70, 50/5, Humulin 20/80, 30/70, Novomix 30, Humalog Mix 25, Monotard, Lente, Ultratard, Ultralente, Glargine, Levemir.

Follow-up treatment

- Measure blood glucose level.
- Repeat first-line treatment if blood glucose level is less than 4 mmol/L and do not leave the person alone.
- Help the person to consume slowly digested low Glycemic Index™ carbohydrate (Table 4.4).

4.3.8 Unconscious hypoglycaemia

If hypoglycaemia is severe enough to cause unconsciousness, it is a medical emergency. In home situations and residential aged care facilities:

Table 4.4 Suggested low Glycemic Index™ follow-up carbohydrate food to use after the initial treatment of hypoglycaemia.

Specific feeding issue	Management options	Glycemic Index™ score
Normal swallow reflex	Glass of milk with a flavour additive, e.g. Milo OR	GI score – low 32*
	piece of fruit OR	GI score – low to medium Banana – 52*, pear – 32*, orange – 42*
	immediate next meal OR	GI score – variable
	multigrain toast – 1 slice	GI score – low 31*
Impaired swallow reflex requiring thickened fluids and/or vitamised meals	Vitamised fruit or milk-based dessert	GI score – low
Enteral feeding	Immediate or extra serve of enteral feed	GI score – low

* Taken from Brand-Miller & Foster-Powell 2002.

- An ambulance should be called immediately.
- Place the person in a safe coma position (lying on their side).
- At no stage should anything be given orally because it may cause aspiration and ultimately pneumonia.
- Stay with the person.
- Perform baseline observations, such as blood pressure, respirations, conscious level, blood glucose, if possible.

Some people with diabetes have family members and carers trained to administer glucagon. Some residential facilities have written orders from a medical officer enabling glucagon to be administered in situations where it is unsafe to give anything orally to treat severe hypoglycaemia. In acute facilities, treatment may vary from administering glucagon to inserting an intravenous line and/or administering 50% dextrose intravenously. The latter treatment option can prove quite difficult in older people who often have poor venous access, which is further compromised by peripheral shutdown that occurs during hypoglycaemia. Intramuscular glucagon may in fact be a much quicker treatment mode if venous access is limited.

Managing hypoglycaemic unconsciousness in older people also includes performing a 12-lead ECG once consciousness returns. The stress associated with an unconscious hypoglycaemic state in older people is significant and heart attacks can result. Older people have an increased frequency of severe and fatal events compared to younger people with diabetes (Stepka *et al.* 1993).

4.3.9 Why treat hypoglycaemia initially with glucose?

Traditionally, many health professionals have been instructed to treat hypoglycaemia with sucrose or fructose, for example lollies, soft drinks or fruit juice. The problem with using these substances is that 'blood sugar' does not actually exist in a physiological sense in the body; that is, there is no such entity as blood sugar. It is blood *glucose* which, in the case of hypoglycaemia, requires an immediate boost. The quickest way to increase the blood glucose level is to ingest glucose. Sucrose- or fructose-based products can take considerable time to be digested and absorbed. Products high in sucrose and fat may take even longer to be absorbed, for example chocolate.

Other traditional hypoglycaemic treatment products such as hard lollies may carry additional risks for the older person during hypoglycaemia; for example, barley sugar can easily get under false teeth or caught in the back of the throat, particularly if the person is shaking as a consequence of their hypoglycaemia or another disease process. Refer to Chapter 2 for further information about the Glycemic Index™.

It is important to:

- Treat hypoglycaemia even if it is asymptomatic.
- Not delay treatment until the next meal is served. It may be a low Glycemic Index™ meal and therefore take considerable time to be digested. Older people may lose consciousness before finishing a low Glycemic Index™ meal.
- Administer glucagon or instigate the medical emergency procedure if the person cannot swallow safely.
- Try to ascertain the cause of the hypoglycaemia to prevent future events.

4.3.10 Preventing hypoglycaemia

Hypoglycaemia is preventable in most cases. By ensuring older people with diabetes eat regularly, snack if they are hungry and eat meals or snacks that contain at least one slowly digested carbohydrate, sudden low blood glucose levels can usually be avoided. Being aware of when diabetes medicines begin to act after administration, their peak time of actions and duration of action is also useful. For example, rapid-acting insulins start working often within 10 minutes of being injected. Therefore, they can even be administered after meals, which is another strategy that can be used to reduce the risk of hypoglycaemia. Rapid-acting insulins include:

- Humalog.
- Humalog Mix 25.
- Novorapid.
- Novomix 30.

Therefore, older people using rapid-acting insulins need to be aware that they must eat within a few minutes after injecting. Older people prescribed these insulins will need to have very regular meals and snacks. If they are self-caring, they may need to be assessed regularly to ensure they do not become confused about their medicines and put themselves at risk of hypoglycaemia. Sometimes frequent insulin adjustments will be necessary, for example during intercurrent illnesses and dialysis treatments.

When monitoring blood glucose levels it is important to try to identify trends. For example, if blood glucose levels are gradually falling and are getting close to what would be considered hypoglycaemic levels in one part of the day, consideration should be given to whether medications need to be reduced or carbohydrate intake increased to prevent hypoglycaemia from becoming a recurring problem.

Education is a vital part of the prevention of hypoglycaemia in older people. Educating the person and their family, carers and health workers helps reduce the occurrence and severity of hypoglycaemia. Research has demonstrated deficits in older people's knowledge about hypoglycaemic events, symptoms and treatment (Thomson *et al.* 1991) and some older people experience symptoms of hypoglycaemia without recognising the condition (Mutch & Dingwall-Fordyce 1985).

One strategy that can be used in residential facilities, which may increase staff awareness of hypoglycaemia and the different presenting symptoms, is to place coloured dots beside the names of residents who are at risk of hypoglycaemia. This may also assist casual staff to adopt risk management strategies.

Regular complication assessment, particularly of renal function, is essential (see Chapter 5) and regular medicines review should occur to identify people at risk of interactions that cause hypoglycaemia and to monitor renally excreted medicines.

4.3.11   Nocturnal hypoglycaemia

Blood glucose levels can drop overnight without necessarily waking the individual. Nocturnal hypoglycaemia can occur at all ages for people with diabetes. The liver slowly releases stored glucose in response to hypoglycaemia. Unfortunately, the response is often 'heavy handed' and the person experiencing overnight hypoglycaemia often wakes with a very high blood glucose level. The very real concern about this situation, called the Smogyi phenomenon, is that the person or medical officer may increase the evening diabetes medication in the belief that an inadequate dose is causing morning hyperglycaemia.

Strategies to detect overnight hypoglycaemia include:

- Testing blood glucose levels prior to bedtime, then at 2 am or 3 am and again prior to breakfast to identify overnight trends.
- Identifying some suggestive symptoms such as awaking with a headache, awaking very sweaty and hungry, nocturia, disturbed sleep.
- Partners may comment about the individual being very hot or sweating and being restless during the night.

Sometimes the evening diabetes medication dose does not need to be reduced. Ensuring that a slowly digested carbohydrate food is eaten prior to bedtime is often sufficient to prevent overnight hypoglycaemia. For older people such suppers could contain:

- A glass of whole milk warmed with cocoa or chocolate-flavoured milk powder added.
- A bowl of ice cream.
- Toasted heavy fruit loaf.

Suppers that increase the risk of overnight hypoglycaemia include those that have no carbohydrate in them at all, such as a cup of tea or coffee, or insufficient carbohydrate, including a couple of biscuits with cheese or tomato.

Interestingly, dogs have been shown to exhibit behaviour changes that alerted their owners to their hypoglycaemia, enabling them to treat it earlier (Chen *et al.* 2000).

4.4 Hyperglycaemia

Key points

- Hyperglycaemia is usually present at time of diagnosis and will persist if management is suboptimal.
- Symptoms can present differently in older people with diabetes compared to younger people with diabetes.
- Ageist attitudes, absence of 'textbook' hyperglycaemic symptoms and a fear of hypoglycaemia can often result in suboptimal treatment.
- Hyperglycaemia can increase the risk of further morbidity and mortality and has a direct influence on quality of life.
- Dehydration and the associated clinical consequences produce a range of problems that need to be addressed.

4.4.1 Introduction

Hyperglycaemia is defined as blood glucose levels above 10 mmol/L. Symptoms of hyperglycaemia usually occur when blood glucose levels are elevated over 15 mmol/L. Hyperglycaemia can be transient or continuous in which case it has significant short- and long-term consequences.

4.4.2 Causes of hyperglycaemia

- Undiagnosed or newly diagnosed diabetes.
- Inappropriate or insufficient dietary changes.
- Inappropriate or insufficient medication treatment.
- Immobility.
- Infection or acute illness, which is the most common cause.
- Stress.
- Corticosteroid and other diabetogenic medicines such as olanzapine (Koller & Doraiswamy 2002; Livingstone & Rampes 2004) (see Chapter 2).

4.4.3 Risk factors for hyperglycaemia

Older people most at risk of hyperglycaemia are those who:

- Receive limited or suboptimal treatment.
- Have secondary failure of OHAs. Secondary failure means OHAs are no longer effective at keeping the blood glucose in an acceptable range and the person requires insulin. People's fear of hypoglycaemia and health professionals' belief that older people are incapable of self-administering insulin compound the issue.
- Have had none or limited access to diabetes education.
- Are prescribed diabetogenic drugs such as corticosteroids.
- Have none or insufficient capillary blood glucose monitoring performed.
- Are older women with dementia residing in nursing homes (Wachtel *et al.* 1987).

4.4.4   Presentation of hyperglycaemia in older people

Hyperglycaemia often presents differently in older people (see Table 4.5).

4.4.5   Treating mild hyperglycaemia

Mild hyperglycaemia is defined as blood glucose levels often reaching 15 mmol/L in a relatively healthy older person. Raised blood glucose levels should be treated using standard diabetes management strategies:

- Reviewing the diet.
- Maximising mobility.
- Reviewing and changing medication.
- Screening for an intercurrent illness, pain or psychological stress.

The person with mild hyperglycaemia living at home requires education to manage their diabetes. They should be encouraged to perform home blood glucose monitoring and their progress should be regularly reviewed. Regular review and changes to their medication regimens may be required.

When people with diabetes are admitted to an acute hospital they often become hyperglycaemic. It is important to determine whether this phenomenon is common outside the hospital or occurred as a result of the hospitalisation. Anxiety, reduced mobility, pain, especially angina, infection and some medications or treatments can increase blood glucose levels. An admission to hospital represents an opportunity to assess diabetes management, practices, knowledge and complication status. Referral to a diabetes educator, dietitian or endocrine unit may be required.

Similarly, some of these issues can account for hyperglycaemia detected in a person newly admitted to a residential care facility. People entering residential aged care facilities experience considerable stress, which may include the loss of a spouse, selling the family home or loss of independence due to illness and the move. Vigilant and regular capillary blood glucose testing should be initiated. Suboptimal diabetes management, particularly if the new resident had been quite isolated in the community, may also account for hyperglycaemia. Optimal management and monitoring should be instituted.

4.4.6   Treating moderate and severe hyperglycaemia

Moderate hyperglycaemia accompanying acute illness or infection and severe hyperglycaemia require immediate medical management. Residents in aged care facilities may need to be transferred to an acute facility for specialised care. The person's doctor must be notified of the condition and the need for immediate intervention. Information that can be useful to relay when contacting medical officers includes:

- Capillary blood glucose levels.
- Temperature and vital signs.
- Urinalysis to detect the presence of glucose, ketones, nitrates.
- Existence of a productive cough, increased shortness of breath, audible consolidation.

Table 4.5 Differences in the presenting symptoms of hyperglycaemia between younger and older people with diabetes.

Younger people with diabetes	Older people with diabetes
Thirst	Thirst is usually absent.
Polyuria	Polyuria may present as urge incontinence or urinary incontinence, nocturia or be confused with prostatism.
	Sleep disturbance as a result of polyuria and nocturia, which increases the risk of falls and results in changes in mental status.
Fatigue	Fatigue – often viewed as part of normal ageing.
Weight loss	Weight loss – often viewed as 'positive' in term of diabetes management. Weight loss due to reduced mobility and metabolic rate is unusual.
Increased risk of diabetic ketoacidosis	Increased risk of diabetic ketoacidosis.
Increased risk of hyperosmolar states	Increased risk of hyperosmolar states.
Increased risk of microvascular complications	Increased risk of microvascular complications.
Increased risk of macrovascular complications	Increased risk of macrovascular complications.
	Dehydration – related to polyuria and inability to detect thirst.
	Constipation related to dehydration.
	Dry fragile skin related to dehydration, which increases the risk of skin breakdown especially if incontinence is present.
	Postural hypotension related to dehydration – increasing the risk of falls.
	Electrolyte imbalance related to dehydration – causing changes in mental status and cardiac function.
	Increased risk of urinary tract infections.
	Dry mucous membranes.
	Increased risk of thrombosis.
	Confusion due to electrolyte imbalance associated with dehydration.

- Signs of infection or marked deterioration observed in a wound.
- Chest pain, more frequent or unresolved angina.
- Sudden change in mental status.
- Inability to eat and drink.
- Urine output.

4.4.7   Why is it important to manage hyperglycaemia in older people?

Hyperglycaemia increases the risk of mortality in older people by increasing the possibility that they will develop diabetic ketoacidosis (DKA) or hyperosmolar states (HONK). Although DKA primarily occurs in Type 1 diabetes it must be considered in older people with Type 2 diabetes, who are likely to be more acidotic and require longer treatment to reverse the acidaemia (Newton & Raskin 2004). In addition, hyperglycaemia predisposes the person to:

(1)   Increased risk of morbidity:
   ● dehydration-related problems such as postural hypotension, electrolyte imbalance and changed mental status
   ● thrombosis formation, increasing the risk of stroke, myocardial infarction and pulmonary embolus
   ● increased risk of infections such as urinary tract infections and candida
   ● poor wound healing and increased risk of skin breakdown and pressure areas.
(2)   Increased risk of developing chronic diabetes complications:
   ● diabetic retinopathy
   ● diabetic renal disease
   ● diabetic neuropathy
   ● cardiovascular disease
   ● cerebrovascular disease.
(3)   Reduced quality of life:
   ● dry mucous membranes
   ● dry skin
   ● development of painful peripheral neuropathy, which limits mobility and social activities
   ● constipation
   ● urinary frequency, urge incontinence, urinary incontinence, sleep disturbance and therefore impacts on mental status
   ● fatigue affecting the ability to perform activities of daily living and increasing the risk of depression.
(4)   Safety problems due to an increased risk of falls resulting from:
   ● polyuria – especially frequent trips to the toilet at night
   ● postural hypotension caused by hyperglycaemia-induced dehydration
   ● painful neuropathy of the feet, making walking difficult
   ● diminished sensory neuropathy to the feet, making walking difficult
   ● visual changes.

4.4.8   Preventing hyperglycaemia

Hyperglycaemia prevention is a priority in the management of diabetes. Eating a healthy diet that reflects current recommendations and maximising activity can help stabilise blood glucose levels. Home blood glucose monitoring alternating pre- and postprandial times assists with the day-to-day evaluation of glycaemic control. Regular three-monthly blood glucose average measurements (HbA$_{1c}$) enable health professionals to gain an overall view of diabetes management, but do not replace capillary monitoring.

Compliance with diabetes medicines and optimal prescribing is paramount. The UKPDS (1998a) demonstrated that beta cell failure eventually occurs in the majority of people with Type 2 diabetes who require insulin therapy with increasing duration of diabetes. In addition, other complications, especially renal failure, may necessitate the change to insulin. Commencing insulin therapy in older people can be challenging. Planning and incorporating a team approach makes the transition more achievable and less stressful for the patient and their carers. Failure to prescribe insulin when secondary failure of OHAs is evident increases the morbidity and mortality of older people with diabetes.

Reduced thirst sensation and an increased threshold for removal of glucose by the kidneys is a consequence of normal ageing. Even healthy older people may not exhibit the symptoms of polyuria and polydipsia when hyperglycaemia is present (Terpstra & Terpstra 1998). Polyuria in older people may present instead as urge incontinence, urinary incontinence or prostatism and therefore not be generally recognised as a symptom of hyperglycaemia. Lethargy is also often considered to be 'normal' in older people. Poor wound healing is generally readily identified as a symptom of hyperglycaemia but in older people, it is often viewed as part of normal ageing or a result of other barriers to wound healing such as malnutrition, other concurrent medical conditions and immobility. Recognising and managing hyperglycaemia early reduces the associated morbidity and mortality.

Practice point

Urine testing for glucose is inaccurate in older people with hyperglycaemia due to the raised renal threshold for glucose; that is, *a raised blood glucose level is often not detected in urine*. Capillary and laboratory blood glucose testing is the only accurate way to determine the presence of hyperglycaemia.

4.4.9 Dangers of hyperglycaemia in older people

Acute or prolonged hyperglycaemia in older people can precipitate hyperglycaemic emergencies that result in higher rates of morbidity and mortality compared to younger people with diabetes.

4.4.10 Hyperglycaemia emergencies

Diabetic ketoacidosis

Diabetic ketoacidosis (DKA) usually occurs in younger people with Type 1 diabetes. However, there is increasing recognition that people with Type 2 diabetes also present with DKA (Bagg *et al.* 1998; Balasubramanyam *et al.* 1999; Newton & Raskin 2004). Studies have shown that relative insulin deficiency in the face of mounting insulin resistance can cause DKA in people with Type 2 diabetes (Carroll & Schade 2001). Latent autoimmune diabetes in adults (LADA) is now recognised as a distinct entity. Older adults who are slim and have a history of weight loss may be misdiagnosed with Type 2 diabetes and commenced on OHAs. However, they may not achieve acceptable blood glucose control because they require insulin, often within weeks or months. Antibodies associated with Type 1 diabetes can be detected in these people. Therefore, it is important to consider the possibility of DKA, regardless of the person's age and the fact that they have a diagnosis of Type 2 diabetes.

The presentation of DKA in the early stages includes:

- Blood glucose level greater than 17 mmol/L.
- Arterial pH less than 7.3.
- Ketones in blood and urine. There may be an acetone smell on the breath.
- Marked diuresis.
- Nausea and vomiting.
- Abdominal cramping.
- Tachycardia.
- Fast shallow breathing. Kussmaul's respiration.

Later symptoms can include reduction in respiratory (respiratory distress) and heart rates, reduction in core body temperature and conscious state that can lead to coma. Older people are more likely to die during hyperglycaemic states than younger people with diabetes (Malone *et al.* 1992).

Practice point

Diabetic ketoacidosis can occur in people with Type 1 and Type 2 diabetes.

Pathophysiology of DKA

When the beta cells in the pancreas fail to release sufficient insulin, counterregulatory hormones such as glucagaon, epinephrine, cortisol and growth hormone are released, all of which further increase the blood glucose levels. Catecholamines induce lipolysis and mobilise free fatty acids and induce protein catabolism in an attempt to maintain an energy source (energy in the form of glucose enters cells in the presence of insulin). The toxic byproducts of lipolysis, ketones, are produced when fat stores are used as an alternative energy source in the absence of insulin. In the ketotic state, blood pH, bicarbonate, sodium and carbon dioxide are all reduced. Potassium is increased. Such an acute metabolic destabilisation is a medical emergency.

Managing DKA

Managing DKA constitutes a medical emergency. Immediate aims include:

- Correcting dehydration without causing fluid overload, correcting the electrolyte imbalance and reversing ketone production and hyperglycaemia.
- Preventing thrombosis and myocardial infarction. Note that a myocardial infarction may be the precipitating cause for DKA.
- Preventing respiratory distress.
- Preventing the development of pressure ulcers.
- Identifying the cause of the DKA.
- Providing education.

Ideally, initial treatment should be undertaken in either an intensive care or high-dependency unit with one-to-one nursing. Two decades ago, 65% of older people admitted with a hyperglycaemic coma died within the first two days of hospitalisation (Gale *et al.* 1981). This figure has been significantly reduced with modern management.

The specific management of DKA includes:

- Intravenous fluid replacement, preferably via a central line, titrated to measure blood volume and prevent circulatory overload.
- Intravenous insulin delivered via either a continuous infusion pump or syringe driver.
- Intravenous anticoagulant therapy may be required to prevent thrombosis. If myocardial infarction has already occurred, a glycerine trinitrate infusion will usually also be required and managed according to the relevant procedures and protocols.
- Continuous cardiac monitoring and regular ECG recordings.
- Indwelling urinary catheter to measure hourly urine output.
- Hourly blood ketone measurements, for example using the Optium™ meter, which is more accurate than urinary ketone measurements. It may be more accurate than some laboratory ketone measures depending on which ketone body is measured.
- Hourly or second hourly blood glucose measurements.
- Regular potassium and other electrolyte levels.
- Regular pH via arterial blood gases.
- Regular urine specific gravity.
- Measure and record conscious and mental status.
- Oxygen therapy as required.
- A nasogastric tube, to prevent inhalation of vomitus and aspiration pneumonia, may be needed.
- Hourly vital signs, central venous pressures and oxygen saturation levels.
- Intravenous antibiotics if infection is present.
- Antiembolic stockings.
- Mouth care.
- Regular repositioning to avoid venous stasis and pressure areas.
- Chest physiotherapy as required.

Once the patient's condition has improved treatment can change to:

- Ceasing the intravenous insulin and change to regular subcutaneous insulin. Insulin is often required at this stage even if the person has Type 2 diabetes, to prevent hyperglycaemia.
- Encouraging light diet and fluids in order to reduce the need for intravenous fluids.
- Fourth hourly blood glucose testing (including overnight) once intravenous insulin has been ceased.
- Changing intravenous anticoagulation therapy to subcutaneous injections.
- Measuring blood ketone levels until they are no longer present.
- Changing intravenous antibiotics to oral preparations if possible.
- Encouraging mobilisation.
- Daily electrolytes measurement.
- Referral to the diabetes educator.

If DKA is the first known presentation of diabetes, intensive education will be required. Diabetes education can be challenging in older people who have just recovered from such a life-threatening episode, mainly due to some residual cognitive impairment that may last days or even weeks. The patient will need to learn about diabetes, blood glucose monitoring, insulin administration (including people with Type 2 diabetes because beta cell functioning may not return for several weeks, if at all), hypoglycaemia detection, treatment and prevention, and diet.

Education takes time, even when applying a similar 'survival skills' approach to that adopted for younger people. 'Survival skills' refer to the skills a person needs to have for the first few weeks after being diagnosed with diabetes in order to maintain some stability and safety. Therefore, health professionals and family members need to be patient in terms of the person's ability to learn and retain new information. Often a greater emphasis needs to be placed on family members performing the diabetes management tasks until the individual is able to manage by themselves. In addition, if other adverse outcomes have occurred as a consequence of DKA, such as a heart attack or stroke, these will directly affect the person's ability to start to take care of their own diabetes.

HONK

Hyperosmolar non-ketonic coma (HONK) is an acute result of hyperglycaemia and is characterised by markedly raised blood glucose levels and serum osmolarity, severe dehydration and the absence of ketones (Dunning 2003). In addition, neurological symptoms such as confusion, cerebral oedema and seizures can be present. HONK in older people is a life-threatening metabolic emergency and has a mortality rate between 10% and 63%. HONK (just like DKA) can be the first presentation of diabetes in up to 50% of all reported cases (Braaten 1987). Mortality is commonly associated with thrombosis, particularly in the lower limbs, lungs, heart and brain. Older people with Type 2 diabetes at the highest risk of developing HONK:

- Have a urinary tract infection.
- Have pneumonia.
- Are commenced on or have dose increases of corticosteroid therapy.
- Are over the age of 80 years.
- Reside in residential care (Wachtel *et al.* 1991).
- No longer respond effectively to oral agents.
- Are on peritoneal dialysis.
- Are on diuretic therapy.

Treatment primarily centres on correcting the dehydration as quickly and safely as possible, which can be difficult to do in frail older people. Treatment is similar to that for DKA.

Hyperglycaemia requires correction with intravenous insulin, initially. However, prevention of thrombosis is also a priority and can be achieved using intravenous or subcutaneous anticoagulation therapy, antithrombotic stockings and physiotherapy.

Managing fluid replacement and preventing circulatory overload is similar to the management of DKA. The mental status of older patients with HONK can take some time to resolve and so education can be difficult and challenging. Subcutaneous insulin may be required for some weeks after the resolution of HONK, especially if the patient is insulin deficient. If secondary failure of OHAs or contraindications to continuing OHAs (renal or liver impairment) are present, insulin therapy will be required for the rest of the person's life. Obtaining an HbA_{1c} result and a detailed history from the patient assists the diabetes team to identify whether OHAs or insulin will be required.

4.5 Lactic acidosis

Key points

- Lactic acidosis differs from diabetic ketoacidosis (DKA) and hyperosmolar non-ketonic coma (HONK).
- Although rare, lactic acidosis occurs when metformin is prescribed when contraindications are present.
- Impaired renal function is a contraindication for metformin; in particular, a serum creatinine ≥ 0.2 mg/L is not uncommon in older people.
- Lactic acidosis has a reported mortality rate of up to 50%.

Metformin has become the first-line drug treatment of Type 2 diabetes (UKPDS 1998b). Metformin is the most effective OHA and the only one not associated with weight gain. Even when secondary failure to combined OHA regimens occurs and insulin is required, metformin is usually continued in order to reduce the overall amount of insulin required and to minimise weight gain. Metformin has been shown to be effective for older people with Type 2 diabetes but should only be prescribed if the contraindications are not present. These include:

- Renal dysfunction (serum creatinine ≥ 0.2 mg/L). Note that metformin dosage should not be increased if serum creatinine is ≥ 0.15 mg/L.
- Chronic heart failure requiring medication, especially biventricular failure.
- Hepatic impairment, for example hepatitis or alcohol abuse.
- People with diabetes over the age of 80 years (Calabrese *et al.* 2002).

Lactic acidosis is a life-threatening condition and is characterised by a low arterial pH <7.1 and elevated lactate levels ≥ 5.0 mM or an anion gap ≥ 18 mM (Sinclair & Finucane 2001). Usually ketones are not present and hyperglycaemia is often mild.

4.5.1 *Management*

Management involves intravenous fluid replacement and administration of often large amounts of bicarbonate to correct the acidosis. Regular subcutaneous insulin may be sufficient to control the hyperglycaemia.

4.5.2 *Metformin and tests involving radiocontrast media*

Metformin must be omitted 48 hours prior to any radiological contrast test, for example, a coronary angiogram, in order to reduce the effect on renal function.

4.6   Diabetes and urinary tract infections

Urinary tract infections (UTI) can be short-term complications or become chronic long-term complications associated with autonomic neuropathy (see Chapter 5). The incidence of UTIs in people with diabetes is higher compared to the wider community. Within the community setting uncomplicated UTIs are among the most common infections in women of all ages (Gupta *et al.* 2001). Women with UTIs who have diabetes experience more urinary symptoms, present with more severe infections and are at higher risk of hospitalisation for pyelonephritis (Nicolle *et al.* 1996). In fact, UTIs often trigger hyperglycaemia requiring hospitalisation.

UTIs may also occur as a consequence of sexual intercourse, poor perineal hygiene and anatomical dysfunction. There is an increased prevalence of asymptomatic UTI in older people (Fonda *et al.* 2002). However, incontinence, an indwelling catheter, history of antibiotic treatment and impaired functional status, especially dementia, are linked to UTI in older women in residential care facilities (Stamm & Raz 1999).

Diabetes-related risk factors for UTIs include long duration of diabetes and the presence of autonomic neuropathy, which reduces the ability to completely empty the bladder, leading to residual urine, especially if large amounts of glucose are present. However, many older people have high levels of residual urine and do not experience UTIs (Fonda *et al.* 2002).

There is controversy about the most appropriate treatment of asymptomatic UTIs, especially given the increasing rate of antibiotic-resistant organisms. The term 'asymptomatic UTI' refers to the absence of urinary symptoms. Yet hyperglycaemia occurs regardless of whether symptoms are present or not and can be a consequence of the UTI or contribute to the development of a UTI. A range of antibiotics is suitable for symptomatic UTIs, especially when more extensive renal infection is present. Preventive treatment is important.

Recent research suggests that 300 mL of cranberry juice daily in women with diabetes reduces the rate of UTIs. However, it is not effective for established UTIs (Griffiths 2003). Cranberry tablets may be more cost-effective and easier to manage than heavy juice bottles (Stothers 2002).

Practice point

The symptoms of UTI include:

- Offensive mouse-like odour.
- Cloudy urine.
- Presence of nitrates on urinalysis.
- Often hyperglycaemia.
- Confusion.
- Loss of appetite.
- Increased incidence of falls.
- Urinary incontinence.

Frequent urination, fever and flank pain are rare in older people.

References

Bagg, W., Sathu, A., Streat, S. & Braatvedt, G. (1998) Diabetic ketoacidosis in adults at Auckland Hospital, 1988–1996. *Australian & New Zealand Journal of Medicine*, **28**(5), 604–8.

Balasubramanyam, A., Zern, J.W., Hyman, D.J. & Pavlik, V. (1999) New profiles of diabetic ketoacidosis: type 1 vs type 2 diabetes and the effect of ethnicity. *Archives of Internal Medicine*, **159**(19), 2317–22.

Ben-Ami, H., Nagachandran, P., Mendelson, A. & Edoute, Y. (1999) Older patients are at particular risk of drug-induced hypoglycaemia. Glibenclamide induced hypoglycaemic coma in 51 older patients with Type 2 diabetes mellitus. *Journal of the American Geriatrics Society*, **47**, 631–3.

Braaten, J. (1987) Hyperosmolar non ketonic diabetic coma: diagnosis and management. *Geriatrics*, **42**, 83–92.

Brand-Miller, J. & Foster-Powell, K. (2002) *The New Glucose Revolution*. Hodder, Sydney.

Calabrese, A.T., Coley, K.C., DaPos, S.V., Swanson, D. & Rao, R.H. (2002) Evaluation of prescribing practices: risk of lactic acidosis with metformin therapy. *Archives of Internal Medicine*, **162**, 434–7.

Carroll, M. & Schade, D. (2001) Ten pivotal questions about diabetic ketoacidosis. Answers that clarify new concepts in treatment. *Postgraduate Medicine*, **110**(5), 89–92.

Chen, M., Daly, M., Williams, N., Williams, S. & Williams, G. (2000) Non-invasive detection of hypoglycaemia using a novel, fully biocompatible and patient friendly alarm system. *British Medical Journal*, **321**, 1565–6.

Dunning, T. (2003) *Care of People with Diabetes*. Blackwell Publishing, Oxford.

Fonda, D., Benevenuti, F., Cottenden, A. *et al.* (2002) Urinary incontinence and bladder dysfunction in older persons. In: *Second International Consultation on Incontinence. Paris 1–3 2001* (eds P. Abrams, S. Cardozo, A. Khoury). Health Publications, Plymouth, UK.

Gale, E., Dornan, T. & Tattersall, R. (1981) Severely uncontrolled diabetes in the over-fifties. *Diabetologia*, **21**, 25–8.

Griffiths, P. (2003) The role of cranberry juice in the treatment of urinary tract infections. *British Journal of Community Nursing*, **8**(12), 557–61.

Gupta, K., Hooton, T.M., Roberts, P.L. & Stamm, W.E. (2001) Patient-initiated treatment of uncomplicated recurrent urinary tract infections in young women. *Annals of Internal Medicine*, **135**(1), 9–16.

Koller, E. & Doraiswamy, P. (2002) Olanzapine-associated diabetes mellitus. *Pharmacotherapy*, **22**(7), 841–52.

Livingstone, C. & Rampes, H. (2004) Atypical antipsychotic drugs and diabetes. *Practical Diabetes International*, **20**(9), 237–331.

Malone, M., Gennis, V. & Goodwin, J. (1992) Characteristics of diabetic ketoacidosis in older versus younger adults. *Journal of the American Geriatrics Society*, **40**, 1100–4.

Marker, J., Cryer, P. & Clutter, W. (1992) Attenuated glucose recovery from hypoglycaemia in the older. *Diabetes*, **41**, 671–8.

Mutch, W. & Dingwall-Fordyce, I. (1985) Is it a hypo? Knowledge of the symptoms of hypoglycaemia in older diabetic people. *Diabetic Medicine*, **2**, 54–6.

Newton, C. & Raskin, P. (2004) Diabetic ketoacidosis in type 1 and type 2 diabetes mellitus. Clinical and biochemical differences. *Archives of Internal Medicine*, **164**, 1925–31.

Nicolle, L.E., Friesen, D., Harding, G.K. & Roos, L.L. (1996) Hospitalization for acute pyelonephritis in Manitoba, Canada, during the period from 1989 to 1992; impact of diabetes, pregnancy, and aboriginal origin. *Clinical Infectious Diseases*, **22**(6), 1051–6.

Parmar, M. (2004) Recurrent hypoglycaemia in a diabetic patient as a result of unexpected renal failure. *British Medical Journal*, **328**, 883–4.

Schernthaner, G., Grimaldi, A., Di Mario, U. *et al.* (2004) GUIDE study: double-blind comparison of once-daily gliclazide MR and glimepiride in type 2 diabetic patients. *European Journal of Clinical Investigation*, **34**(8), 535–42.

Sinclair, A. & Finucane, P. (2001) *Diabetes in Old Age*, 2nd edn. John Wiley and Sons Ltd, Chichester.

Stamm, W.E. & Raz, R. (1999) Factors contributing to susceptibility of postmenopausal women to recurrent urinary tract infections. *Clinical Infectious Diseases*, **28**(4), 723–5.

Stepka, M., Rogala, H. & Czyzyk, A. (1993) Hypoglycaemia: a major problem in the management of diabetes in the older. *Aging*, **5**, 117–21.

Stothers, L. (2002) A randomized trial to evaluate effectiveness and cost effectiveness of naturopathic cranberry products as prophylaxis against urinary tract infection in women. *Canadian Journal of Urology*, **9**(3), 1558–62.

Terpstra, T. & Terpstra, T. (1998) The older Type 2 diabetic: a treatment challenge. *Geriatric Nursing*, **19**(5), 253–9.

Thomson, F., Masson, E., Leeming, J. & Boulton, A. (1991) Lack of knowledge of symptoms of hypoglycaemia by older diabetic people. *Age & Ageing*, **20**, 404–6.

UK Prospective Diabetes Study Group (1998a) Intensive blood-glucose control with sulphonylureas or insulin compared with conventional treatment and risk of complications in patients with type 2 diabetes (UKPDS 33). *Lancet*, **352**, 837–53.

UK Prospective Diabetes Study Group (1998b) Effect of intensive blood-glucose control with metformin on complications in overweight patients with type 2 diabetes (UKPDS 34). *Lancet*, **352**, 854–65.

Van Staa, T., Abenhaim, L. & Monette, J. (1997) Risk factors for hypoglycaemia in users of sulphonylureas. Rates of hypoglycaemia in users of sulphonylureas. *Journal of Clinical Epidemiology*, **50**, 735–41.

Wachtel, T., Silliman, R. & Lamberton, P. (1987) Predisposing factors for the diabetic hyperosmolar state. *Archives of Internal Medicine*, **147**, 499–501.

Wachtel, T., Tetu-Mouradjian, L., Goldman, D., Ellis, S. & O'Sullivan, P. (1991) Hyperosmolarity and acidosis in diabetes mellitus: a three year experience in Rhode Island. *Journal of General Internal Medicine*, **6**, 495–502.

Whitehead, C. & Finucane, P. (1995) 'Is it just my age doctor?' Separating normality from pathology in old age. *Modern Medicine of Australia*, **163**, 94–101.

Chapter 5
Long-term Complications of Diabetes

Trisha Dunning

Key points

- Older people can present with a long-term complication of diabetes at diagnosis.
- Complications may present differently in older people.
- Complications affect quality of life and optimal functioning, including self-care.
- Identifying and managing complications is important to reduce the associated morbidity and mortality.
- Managing lipids and blood pressure may be more important than blood glucose control.
- Diabetes complications and comorbidities are interrelated.
- Preventive screening and management are often suboptimal in older people, especially in residential care facilities.
- Many complications represent falls and pressure area risks, over and above the usual risk factors and are not included on current falls risk assessment tools.

5.1   Introduction

The long-term complications of diabetes are responsible for significant morbidity and mortality and reduced quality of life. Long-term complications occur as a consequence of several interrelated factors, including prolonged hyperglycaemia, which results in a range of pathological, metabolic and mechanical changes that exacerbate normal ageing. A range of underlying causative mechanisms arising from chronic hyperglycaemia has been described.

- Oxidative damage occurs through unclear mechanisms and may weaken the antioxidant defences or increase free radical generation. Reactive oxygen species generated as a result of hyperglycaemia may contribute to diabetes complications such as nephropathy, retinopathy and neuropathy.
- Increased tissue glycolysation. Glucose enters the polyol pathway in hyperglycaemic states where it is primarily converted to fructose, which increases the rate of glycolysation. Substances called advanced glycated end-products (AGE) develop and accumulate over time and are irreversible. The higher the blood glucose, the more AGE are formed. AGE are a significant factor in glucose-derived cross-tracking

that alters the function of the vascular wall and stimulates cytokine growth factors.

- Inflammatory disease, which promotes the production of cytokines, chemokines and adhesion molecules. Oxidative stress increases the expression of AGE, which results in a positive feedback loop of continued oxidative stress and inflammation.
- Although hyperglycaemia appears to be a prerequisite for the development of complications, genetic susceptibility also plays a role and differs significantly from patient to patient and may determine the impact of the hyperglycaemia on the individual. Three broad levels of susceptibility exist:
    (1) Five per cent of people with diabetes are destined to develop complications, even with relatively brief, mild hyperglycaemia.
    (2) Twenty per cent tolerate prolonged hyperglycaemia.
    (3) Five per cent have moderate degrees of susceptibility. In this group, intensive blood glucose and blood pressure control may prevent or delay the onset of complications (Ruskin & Rosenstock 1992).

Long-term complications are:

- Macrovascular disease, such as myocardial infarction (MI) and stroke, which is not peculiar to diabetes but having diabetes increases the risk of these comorbidities occurring.
- Microvascular disease, such as nephropathy and retinopathy, which is specific to diabetes.
- Neuropathy:
    (1) peripheral, leading to foot pathology.
    (2) autonomic, causing a range of pathologies such as gastroparesis, unrecognised hypoglycaemia, erectile dysfunction (ED), silent MI, silent UTI.

Many complications such as foot pathology and ED are multifactorial and involve both blood vessel and nerve damage.

In turn, the long-term complications of diabetes, short-term hyperglycaemia and hypoglycaemia predispose older people to a range of other problems such as falls, nutritional deficits and pressure ulcers and significantly reduce quality of life and increase morbidity and mortality. In addition, a range of other disease processes is common in older people, such as osteoporosis and thyroid disease, which complicate management.

5.2 Cardiovascular disease

Key points

- Cardiovascular disease is the leading cause of death in industrialised countries.
- Chest pain may be atypical in older people with diabetes, the so-called 'silent' myocardial infarction.
- Weakness, fatigue, increased blood glucose and hypoglycaemia may indicate myocardial infarction.
- Smoking increases micro- and macrovascular damage.

Cardiovascular disease, including heart failure and MI, is a major cause of hospital admissions and mortality in people with diabetes and is often associated with diabetic renal disease and ED. People with diabetes have more extensive coronary and cerebral blood vessel atherosclerosis than non-diabetics. Complex metabolic abnormalities are present, especially with MI, and the need for surgical intervention is high. Autonomic neuropathy can give rise to atypical presentations of cardiovascular disease and heart attack and lead to delayed treatment. Recent data from the Australian Institute of Health and Welfare suggest that objective diagnostic tests for heart failure are underused. Only 3.8 per 100 new heart failure problems are being referred for diagnostic imaging. In addition, men who survive MI are more likely to develop heart failure.

Cardiac disease is a common complication of diabetes and carries a higher mortality rate than in non-diabetics. Cardiac disease in people with diabetes is associated with diffuse atherosclerosis, coexisting cardiomyopathy, autonomic neuropathy, hyperglycaemia and hyperlipidaemia. The resultant metabolic consequences include hypercoagulability, elevated catecholamines and insulin resistance. Until recently, atherosclerosis in people with diabetes was considered to be part of normal ageing and cardiac disease was inevitable. Atherosclerosis is now regarded as a disease process in its own right and cardiovascular disease is preventable. Age is the most important determinant of cardiovascular disease (Bush 1991), which is the most common cause of death in older people.

Disordered breathing during sleep and sleep apnoea appear to be associated with cardiovascular disease (Merritt 2004). Sleep apnoea leads to acute and chronic haemodynamic changes when the person is awake, including reduced stroke volume and cardiac output, increased heart rate, elevated sympathetic tone and changes in hormones that regulate fluid volume, blood pressure and vasoconstriction and vasodilation. Sleep apnoea is associated with obesity and hyperlipidaemia, which are known risk factors for heart disease. Thorough investigation and treatment of sleep apnoea appears to be warranted.

Cardiac disease accounts for >50% of deaths in Type 2 diabetes (Standl & Schnell 2000; Huang *et al.* 2001) and half of these people die before they reach hospital. The mortality rate for people with diabetes has not been reduced despite new therapeutic measures and preventive health screening and education programmes. The mortality rate may be partly due to the silent nature of the disease. Recent research suggests that the blood glucose level on admission predicts the long-term mortality after an MI. If this is the case, the admission blood glucose may be a tool to stratify risk and the possible impact of treatment (Stranders *et al.* 2004).

The major, general risk factors for cardiovascular disease are shown in Table 5.1, and Table 5.2 shows the diabetes-specific risk factors. Recently, researchers have suggested that poor oral health may be linked to cardiac disease (Barclay 2004). A number of clinical trials demonstrate the importance of reducing lipids, blood pressure and blood glucose to reduce the risk of cardiovascular disease (Hansson *et al.* 1995; Hansson 1998; UKPDS 1998). Hypertension is a consistent risk factor for heart disease and stroke. Diabetes increases the risk of MI. Hypertension adds to the risk and is also a risk factor for renal disease. Conversely, the coexistence of diabetes, MI and renal disease increases the blood pressure. There is a linear relationship between the diastolic blood pressure and morbidity and

Table 5.1 Cardiovascular disease is multifactorial. Major risk factors for cardiovascular disease in diabetes in older people, in addition to the risk factors for the general population. Some of these risk factors can be modified and significantly reduced.

Risk factor	Effects
Hypertensive and taking antihypertensive medicines (Simons *et al.* 2003)	High prevalence of hypertension in ages 65–74 years in both sexes. Thickened, less elastic blood vessels. Increased strain on the heart.
Smoking	Relative low prevalence in older people, but high prevalence of former smokers. Increased risk of cardiac disease, especially in women. Increased risk of cancer. Constricts blood vessels.
Total cholesterol Hyperlipidaemia	Elevated cholesterol, LDL, significant positive predictors of cardiovascular disease in older men and women.
Coagulopathies	Plaque formation. Emboli.
Family history of cardiovascular disease	Increases the risk of cardiovascular disease.
Hyperglycaemia	Increased platelet aggregation. Micro- and macrovascular disease.
Psychosocial factors	Some psychosocial factors are associated with increased cardiovascular risk. These include: ● depression ● social isolation ● lack of quality support (National Heart Foundation 2003). These factors may influence other risk factors such as smoking, overeating and inactivity.
Obesity and inactivity	Cardiovascular disease. Reduced exercise tolerance.

mortality. Reducing the blood pressure below 90 mmHg significantly improves the outcome.

Subtle changes occur in the heart as a result of ischaemia-induced vascular remodelling and the effects of hyperglycaemia on the endothelium of large blood vessels that predispose the heart to failure (Standl & Schnell 2000). Heart muscle metabolism is critically dependent on glucose during periods of ischaemia but may not be able to utilise available glucose in the presence of insulin resistance or deficient insulin. Heart muscle performance is improved in the presence of insulin, which stimulates glucose uptake. Using an IV insulin infusion during the acute stages of an MI has been shown to improve outcomes because it normalises cardiac fuel substrates and protects cardiac muscle (Malmberg *et al.* 1995).

Table 5.2 Diabetes-specific abnormalities that predispose older people to cardiovascular disease, based on Dunning 2003

Abnormality	Cardiovascular effects
Metabolic	Relative or absolute insulin deficiency. Increase catecholamines. Reduced glucose utilisation. Increased free fatty acid production. Free radical damage. Reduced contractability. Increased O_2 consumption. Increased ischaemic injury.
Microvascular disease	Nephropathy, frequently in association with retinopathy and damage to the microvessels of the heart. Basement membrane thickening is the hallmark of diabetic microangiopathy. It affects various types of epithelium and several plasma proteins bind to the thickened epithelium.
Autonomic neuropathy	Postural hypotension. Abnormal cardiovascular reflexes. Loss of sinus arrhythmia. Resting sinus tachycardia. Painless myocardial ischaemia and infarction. Inability to increase heart rate or stroke volume to compensate for myocardial damage. Increased anaesthetic risk. Sudden death.
Endothelial damage in membranes or outer lining of large blood vessels.	Weak blood vessel walls. Impaired blood flow. Reduced tissue oxygenation and nourishment.
Hypertension	Thickened blood vessel walls. Increased strain on the heart.
Blood abnormalities	Platelet aggregation. Increased fibrinogen levels. Elevated PAI-1.

MI is 'silent' in 32% of people with diabetes, which leads to delay in seeking medical attention and may increase the mortality rate. 'Silent infarct' refers to the fact that the classic pain across the chest, down the arm and into the jaw associated with MI is not present or is not recognised. Only mild discomfort, which is mistaken for heartburn, may be present. The atypical nature of the chest pain may make it difficult for people to accept that they have had a heart attack and modifying risk factors may not be seen as essential. MI in older people may present as heart failure, cardiogenic shock, congestive cardiac failure (CCF), diabetic ketoacidosis, hyperosmolar coma or hypoglycaemia. These conditions put older people at risk of hypothermia, which further increases the mortality risk.

Diabetes is often diagnosed at the time of an infarct or during cardiac surgery. Emotional stress, and the associated catecholamine response, leads to increased blood glucose levels in 5% of patients admitted with coronary events. In some cases the blood glucose levels normalise during convalescence but need to be controlled in the acute stages. The person is at risk of diabetes and counselling about diabetes and its management is important.

Older people may be admitted with a cardiac event or develop cardiac problems while in hospital. A longer stay in hospital may be necessary for older people with diabetes and an MI and 35% die, often in the second week after the infarct (Karlson *et al.* 1993).

Short- and long-term morbidity and mortality of acute MI were shown to improve using IV insulin/glucose infusion followed by subcutaneous insulin injections for three months (DIGAMI) (Malmberg *et al.* 1995). However, not all experts agree with the DIGAMI approach. The suitability of subcutaneous insulin must be carefully considered, since it may lead to hypoglycaemia and falls. In addition, assistance may be required to help the person manage insulin. Reassessment of the need for insulin in previously undiagnosed people should occur after the acute episode resolves to rule out stress-induced hyperglycaemia.

Intravenous insulin targets the rapid increase in catecholamines, cortisol and glucagon that occurs in an acute MI. Insulin levels fall in the ischaemic myocardium and cardiac tissues are less sensitive to insulin. Glucose utilisation in cardiac muscle is impaired and free fatty acids (FFAs) are mobilised as fuel substrates. FFAs potentiate ischaemic injury, by direct toxicity, by increasing the demand for oxygen, or by inhibiting glucose oxidation. Using IV insulin during acute cardiac events followed by subcutaneous insulin for three months after the infarct has been shown to restore platelet function, correct lipoprotein imbalance, reduce plasminogen activator inhibitor (PAI-1) activity and improve metabolism in non-infarcted areas of the heart (Malmberg *et al.* 1995).

ACE inhibitors improve morbidity and mortality after an MI except where left ventricular function or heart failure is present. Aspirin, usually doses between 75 and 625 mg/day, is also frequently prescribed as a preventive measure to inhibit platelet aggregation and reduce inflammation and the formation of C-reactive protein (CRP), which is associated with insulin resistance (O'Brien 2003). Aspirin is contraindicated in some bowel conditions and where there is a possibility of haemorrhage. Care must be taken if the person uses some herbal medicines such as *Gingko biloba* and *Hypericum perforatum* (St John's wart).

People over 75 years with chronic angina may achieve equivalent outcomes to angioplasty or surgery with medicines, including symptom relief and quality of life (Pfisterer 2004).

5.2.1   Objectives of cardiovascular care

Preventing cardiovascular events is important in community and residential care settings and includes counselling about risk factor modification and providing appropriate diet and exercise opportunities as appropriate to the individual. Nursing care should be planned to allow adequate rest and sleep and reduce the possibilities of acute blood pressure elevations, such as those caused by stress and constipation. The objectives of care are to:

- Treat the acute cardiac event according to medical orders and the standard protocols in current use.
- Stabilise the cardiac status and relieve symptoms, such as pain, breathlessness and anxiety.
- Prevent extension of the presenting cardiac event and limit further cardiac events by controlling blood glucose levels.
- Provide psychological support to the individual and their family and carers.
- Prevent complications such as pressure areas, falls and confusion.
- Consider whether the person has made any advance directives concerning cardiac resuscitation.
- Plan appropriate post-discharge management, such as rehabilitation, medication and diabetes self-care management, and regular follow-up and assessment, including mental health and education needs.

5.2.2   Nursing responsibilities

Management in coronary care units is advisable for older people with dysrhythmias since there is an excess risk of heart failure beyond 2–4 days after the infarct and ~50% of deaths occur five or more days later. Diabetics are at risk of death at any cardiac enzyme level and cardiac enzymes are not a reliable indicator of infarct size, since more cardiac enzymes are released following reperfusion and pharmacological treatment.

Nursing responsibilities are to:

- Understand that the presentation of myocardial infarction can be atypical in people with diabetes. Presentation may be with CCF, syncope, vomiting, abdominal pain and fatigue that improves with rest. An ECG should be performed urgently if any of these symptoms are present.
- Provide psychological support and physical care, which includes monitoring blood glucose 2–4 hourly depending on the blood glucose level and route of insulin administration. If IV, monitor at least two hourly. If subcutaneous, four hourly is usually adequate.
- Provide adequate pain relief and control nausea and vomiting, which can contribute to hyperglycaemia. Sitting the patient upright, where possible, to aid breathing.
- Monitor cardiac status via continuous cardiac monitoring (EEG), cardiac enzymes, colour and respiratory rate.
- Administer medicines as prescribed and monitor the effect.

Often people on oral hypoglycaemic agents (OHAs) are changed to insulin during the acute stages of the MI to normalise cardiac fuel substrates and limit lipolysis and gluconeogenesis. Insulin is usually administered as an IV infusion, especially in the first 48 hours. Only clear, *short-acting insulin* is used via the IV route.

Practice point

Check the insulin carefully before preparing an insulin infusion. Note that insulin glargine (Lantus) and detemir are clear but *must not be given intravenously* (see Chapter 2).

The patient should be eating and drinking normally before the infusion is removed and a dose of subcutaneous insulin given to prevent hyperglycaemia developing, especially if the person has Type 1 diabetes. People need to be informed that insulin is being given to increase the glucose available to the myocardium and reduce free fatty acids in the blood. If subcutaneous insulin is required after discharge, early referral to a diabetes educator is recommended. The person should be encouraged to practise giving insulin under supervision.

- Be aware that non-cardiac selective beta-blocking agents can mask the signs of hypoglycaemia.
- Monitor physical status, which includes maintaining accurate fluid balance and renal output charts.
- Monitor blood pressure, lying and standing. Some antihypertensive medications can cause postural hypotension (see Table 5.3). Counsel the patient to change position gradually, especially on getting out of bed or out of a chair.
- Note any weakness, fatigue, CCF or unexplained hyperglycaemia, which may indicate an extension of the infarct or another infarct.
- Monitor serum electrolytes, blood gases and potassium levels. Report abnormalities to the doctor promptly because fluctuating potassium levels can cause or exacerbate cardiac arrhythmias.
- Monitor mental status. Confusion may indicate extension of the existing infarct, a second MI or stroke or be a side effect of drugs, hypoglycaemia or fluid overload.
- Prevent hypoglycaemia by carefully monitoring blood glucose levels and ensuring adequate carbohydrate intake to balance the insulin or OHAs.
- Take adequate steps to reduce falls risk.

Practice points

(1) The person may not recognise the signs of hypoglycaemia if:
   - they have autonomic neuropathy
   - non-cardioselective beta-blocking agents are used. Neuroglycopenic signs such as confusion, slurred speech or behaviour change may indicate hypoglycaemia and the blood glucose should be measured in these cases.
(2) The eyes should be assessed before thrombolytic medications are commenced. If proliferative retinopathy is present, bleeding into the back of the eye may occur and requires prompt treatment.

5.2.3 Preparing the patient for medical tests and procedures

Diagnostic procedures such as angiograms, which are often required when the person presents with a suspected MI, use radiocontrast dyes to define the blockage. These substances have been associated with renal complications. Adequate hydration before and after such procedures is essential. In addition, the urine output needs to be carefully monitored, especially if the person has renal disease. Some experts recommend stopping metformin 48 hours before angiograms and radiological investigations because of the risk of lactic acidosis.

Table 5.3 Indications for and potential adverse events associated with commonly prescribed antihypertensive agents.

Antihypertensive agent	Indications	Potential adverse effects
ACE inhibitors, e.g. Monopril, Coversyl, Accupril, Gopten. These drugs improve cardiac remodelling and stabilise the rate of progression of renal disease	Heart failure. Previous cardiac event. Microalbuminuria.	Hypotension with the first dose. Hyperkalaemia. Angioedema. Cough, which can become irritating to others. Renal impairment if renal disease is present.
Angiotensin receptor agonists	Albuminuria. Heart failure. Previous cardiac event. ACE inhibitor not tolerated.	Hypotension with first dose. Reduced glomerular filtration rate. Hyperkalaemia. Rarely angioedema and persistent cough. Renal impairment if renal disease is present. In combination with NSAIDs or COX-2 inhibitors can lead to fluid retention, oedema and kidney failure.
Beta-blocking agents (cardioselective agents preferred), e.g. atenolol, metroprolol	Heart failure. Previous cardiac event.	Hypo- or hyperglycaemia. Hypoglycaemic unawareness. Worse peripheral vascular disease. Erectile dysfunction. °†*Depression. †*Sleep disturbance.
Calcium channel blocking agents: a) centrally acting b) peripherally acting vasodilators		Gastrointestinal effects such as constipation, oesophageal reflux especially with centrally acting drugs. Flushing. Headache. Peripheral oedema.
Diuretics, e.g. low-dose thiazides such as Aprinox, Hygroton	Symptomatic heart failure.	Hyperglycaemia. Hyperkalaemia. Hyponatraemia. Dyslipidaemia. Hyperuraemia. Erectile dysfunction.
Sympatholytics, e.g. not with beta blocker. Aldomet, Hydopa, Catapres		°†Depression. †Postural hypotension.

* Already common in older people, † Increased risk of falls, ° Social isolation, inability to adequately self-care

People most at risk of renal damage are those who:

● Are older in age.
● Have established renal disease and/or proteinuria.
● Have hypertension.
● Have elevated serum creatinine.

5.2.4   Cardiac rehabilitation

Cardiac rehabilitation programmes may be very beneficial for older people and they should be encouraged to attend if they are physically capable of doing so (see Chapters 4 and 7).

- Encourage activity within tolerance limits. Physiotherapy, occupational therapy and exercise programmes confer cardiac benefits.
- Independence and autonomy should be encouraged.
- Inform the person about how and when to return to normal activity, including sexual intercourse.
- Ensure diabetes education is available. Refer to diabetes nurse specialist/diabetes educator and/or dietitian. Education should include the need to reduce cardiac risk factors as well as how to:
  (1)   recognise hypoglycaemia
  (2)   correctly administer insulin
  (3)   monitor blood glucose
  (4)   recognise further cardiac problems
  (5)   reduce cardiac risk factors
- Explain the reasons why several medicines are necessary.
- Encourage the person to have regular health checks.

5.2.5   Coaching

Coaching patients with coronary heart disease and suboptimal lipids has been shown to improve adherence to drug therapy and dietary advice. Coaching could be built into cardiac rehabilitation programmes (Vale *et al.* 2002) and could be particularly useful for older people with memory deficits. Coaching can help older people maintain independence and self-care by reminding them of important care strategies such as health-care appointments.

5.3   Hypertension

Key points

- Hypertension plays a key role in myocardial infarction and stroke.
- Controlling hypertension is an essential aspect of managing microvascular disease.
- More than one antihypertensive agent is often required.
- Hypertension and antihypertensive medicines significantly increase the risk of falls.
- Achieving blood pressure targets is dependent on compliance with medicines. Many people, especially older people, 'do not want to take more medicines'.

Controlling hypertension is difficult in older people, but is essential to reduce their risk of cardiac events and stroke. Hypertensive older people present with a range of clinical features that differ from those of younger hypertensive people and which influence management.

- Hypertension is common in older people and they tend to present with higher blood pressures than younger people. Hypertension may progress to cardiovascular disease, heart failure or renal impairment, all of which are common in older people. Hypertension is often overlooked and undertreated in older people (Duggan *et al.* 1997).
- Isolated systolic hypertension frequently occurs and has a greater influence on cardiovascular risk than diastolic blood pressure.
- Some antihypertensive agents cause significant side effects such as postural hypotension, which increases the risk of falls and other adverse events. Some people stop the medicines or reduce the dose without consultation with their doctors; therefore blood pressure control may be inadequate, wound healing impaired and peripheral blood flow to the feet compromised. For example, beta blockers may cause cold feet.
- The management regimen, including polypharmacy, makes the self-care more complex and older people may need assistance with their medicines.
- Older people benefit from effective antihypertensive therapy (Ramsay *et al.* 1999). However, blood pressure management guidelines are often complex and difficult for health professionals to follow so are not used (Ferrari *et al.* 2004).
- Systolic blood pressure is difficult to control. Daily medicine doses to achieve smooth blood pressure control can reduce the complexity of the regimen.
- Hypertension is a significant risk factor for stroke and ischaemic lesions in the white matter of the brain. These lesions increase as cognitive function declines (Skoog 1998). Hypertension is a significant risk factor for vascular dementia. The presence of cardiovascular disease and stroke increases the risk of dementia (Hansson 1999; Ivan *et al.* 2004). Stroke risk is significantly higher in people over 80.
- Older people are likely to have other diseases such as arthritis and be taking medications for these diseases.

5.3.1 Managing hypertension

A range of antihypertensive agents is used. These include:

- Angiotensin-converting enzyme (ACE) inhibitors.
- Angiotensin 2 receptor blockers if ACE inhibitors are not tolerated and there is no significant renal impairment. Research suggests that angiotensin 2 blockers slow the progression of renal disease in Type 2 diabetes when hypertension and microalbuminuria are present (Parving *et al.* 2001). In addition, the persistent cough associated with ACE inhibitors is less common with angiotensin 2 inhibitors, which improves compliance.
- Beta blockers and diuretics.
- Calcium channel blockers (Agarwal 2001).

The ACE inhibitors are usually the drugs of choice in people with diabetes. ACE inhibitors also have a renal protective effect by slowing the progression of micro-albuminuria. Therefore, these drugs may benefit older people by allowing fewer medicines to be used and reducing protein loss, which improves nutritional status, wound healing and immunity. However, the UKPDS (1998) showed that most people require two or more antihypertensive agents to adequately control their hyper-tensive risk factors. Therefore, polypharmacy is significant and makes adherence to the medication regimen more complex.

In addition, the risk of drug interactions increases with each medication added to the regimen; for example, combining an ACE inhibitor, diuretic and NSAID, which is common in older people with diabetes, can precipitate renal failure. Table 5.3 outlines the indications for and potential adverse events associated with commonly prescribed antihypertensive agents. Ideally these agents should be started at a low dose and titrated according to the blood pressure response. ACE doses require adjustment in older people with mild renal impairment. Hypotension on the initial dose is common and the person needs to be carefully counselled about preventive measures. Renal artery stenosis is relatively common and can lead to a significant fall in blood pressure, even at small doses (Howes 2001). Antihypertensive agents metabolised in the liver do not usually cause the same problems.

Non-drug measures used alone or to complement antihypertensive agents

Non-drug measures to manage hypertension should be instituted as part of the diabetes management plan and should continue even if antihypertensive agents are required. The measures include:

- Controlling weight by reducing the amount of fat and sweet foods in the diet and increasing the amount of fruit, vegetables and wholegrain cereals except where they are contraindicated, for example in enteral feeds and gastroparesis.
- Undertaking regular exercise where possible, for example tai chi, walking and swimming. At least 30 minutes per day is required. Exercise also helps control weight. Tai chi has been shown to improve balance, flexibility and cardiovascular health and reduce the risk of falls (Wang *et al.* 2004).
- Reducing salt intake.
- Limiting alcohol intake to two standard drinks per day for men and one for women and thin men.
- Stopping smoking. Referring the person to smoking cessation programmes such as the QUIT programme if they require assistance to stop.
- Controlling stress. Various methods, including tai chi, meditation and relaxation classes, are effective and should be chosen to suit the individual's preference and capability. In acute and residential care staff need to be alert to factors that increase stress in older people such as constipation, fear, inability to communicate and pain.

5.3.2 Blood pressure targets

The National Heart Foundation of Australia, the World Health Organization and the International Society for Hypertension Guidelines have defined blood pressure targets. The targets are shown in Table 5.4. Generally, a stepwise approach to reaching targets is adopted.

(1) Establishing baseline parameters such as blood pressure levels, risk factor profile and presence of other diabetes complications and comorbidities. Twenty-four-hour ambulatory blood pressure monitoring may be indicated in active, community-dwelling older people to distinguish between sustained hypertension and 'white coat' hypertension (Phillips *et al.* 2003).

Table 5.4 Blood pressure targets for people with diabetes and hypertension.

Medical status of the individual	Blood pressure target in mmHg
Over 65 years and established hypertension	<140/90
Diabetes	130/85
Diabetes and nephropathy	125/75

(2) Excluding secondary causes of hypertension such as endocrine diseases, e.g. hyperaldosteronism, Cushing's syndrome, renal artery stenosis or drug-induced hypertension.

(3) Determining baseline blood lipids, electrolytes, urea, creatinine, urinary albumin excretion rate, cardiac status, ECG or echocardiography.

(4) Modifying risky lifestyle behaviours that increase the hypertension risk, such as smoking.

(5) Introducing antihypertensive agents as indicated in Table 5.3.

Accurate blood pressure (BP) measurement

(1) Allow the person to rest for five minutes prior to measuring the BP.

(2) Ensure the person is seated with their back supported and their feet on the floor.

(3) Support the person's arm at the level of their heart (horizontal).

(4) Use an appropriate cuff size.

(5) Record the Korotkoff phase 1 sound for systolic measurements and the disappearance of sound for phase 2 or diastolic measurements.

(6) Perform two measurements and take the average.

(7) In many cases lying and standing measurements will be required.

5.4   Cerebrovascular disease

Stroke is a key consequence of hypertension, especially in older people, and is a major cause of morbidity and mortality. Many older people fear *having* a stroke and consider it almost worse than *dying from* a stroke. Almost every person who presents with a stroke has a history of hypertension.

The brain is supplied with blood by four main arteries: two carotids and two vertebral arteries. The clinical consequences of cerebrovascular disease depend on the vessels, or combination of vessels, involved. These consequences are transient ischaemic attacks (TIAs), cognitive dysfunction and confusion and stroke.

TIAs arise when the blood supply to a part of the brain is temporarily interrupted without permanent damage. Recovery from a TIA usually occurs within 24 hours. If TIAs occur frequently they can indicate impending stroke. Small repeated strokes that cause progressive brain damage can lead to multi-infarct dementia, which is common in people with diabetes. Signs that progressive damage is occurring include:

- Gradual memory loss.
- Diminished intellectual capacity.

- Loss of motor function.
- Incontinence.

Strokes are classified as thrombotic or haemorrhagic and occur when a major blood vessel in the brain becomes blocked. A great deal of the acute damage occurs as a consequence of postischaemic injury, but the causes are complex. Sustained ischaemia leads to changes in calcium homeostasis. Strokes frequently result in permanent damage and require prolonged rehabilitation. Self-care potential is often significantly reduced, as is quality of life, and depression is common. In these cases diabetes management should be discussed with the family or carers who will be responsible for assisting the person with diabetes at home or in residential care.

In addition to hypertension and hyperglycaemia, other predictors of stroke in older people with diabetes are diverse and include low level of wellbeing and high symptom burden (Araki *et al.* 2004).

5.4.1   Diagnosing stroke

Stroke may present acutely with paraesthesia and loss of consciousness, fainting or failing mental function. A careful history will elicit failing mental function. Improving the quality of life of stroke survivors is an important nursing function. Many instruments have been used to measure functional ability. These include:

- Barthel Index
- Functional Independence Measure (FIM)
- quality-of-life instruments such as the Sickness Impact Profile (SIP)
- SF-36.

Functional ability can often be improved by physiotherapy, occupational therapy and other rehabilitation procedures. However, functional ability is only one aspect of post-stroke life. 'Recovery from stroke' may not mean the same thing to stroke survivors, their family or health professionals (Doolittle 1991). Loss of bodily control in social situations often results in loss of meaning in life. The higher the functional ability after a stroke, the more likely the person is to engage in meaningful activities.

5.4.2   Managing stroke

The preventive measures needed to reduce the risk of stroke are the same as those needed to reduce the risk of cardiovascular disease.

- Carotid endarterectomy is indicated if the carotid arteries are significantly narrowed.
- Low-dose aspirin may be beneficial to limit platelet adhesiveness but doses used are often inadequate. The American Diabetes Association (2003) recommendations are 75–625 mg/day.
- Managing blood glucose levels. Research is under way in a number of centres into the efficacy of IV insulin infusions in the acute early stages of stroke. There are indications that outcomes improve.
- Anticoagulants may be required to manage TIAs and atrial fibrillation.
- Recent research suggests that caffeine reduces cerebral blood flow in people recovering from acute ischaemic stroke (Ragab *et al.* 2004). The study was small and further research is needed. However, encouraging people to reduce caffeine may

be warranted. In addition, limiting caffeine intake, especially at night, improves sleep and reduces bladder irritation and urinary incontinence (Fonda 2002).

- Nursing responsibilities include care during investigative procedures. Rehabilitation focuses on returning the person to optimal functioning and independence within their capabilities and supporting carers when necessary.

5.5 Intercurrent illness

Intercurrent illness such as influenza usually produces a rise in catecholamines, which cause hyperglycaemia and often lead to thirst, tiredness, polyuria and cognitive or behavioural changes. Reducing the blood glucose level is important to limit morbidity and make the person comfortable. Minor illness can often be treated in the community or residential care, provided the person is not cognitively impaired and the individual or their carer:

(1) Continues to take/administer their insulin, especially if they have Type 1 diabetes. Doses may need to be increased during illness to control the blood glucose and prevent metabolic abnormalities and ketones from developing.
(2) Tests the blood glucose every 2–4 hours and notifies the doctor if it remains elevated.
(3) Tests the urine or blood for ketones and consults the doctor if moderate to heavy ketones are detected. Ketone testing is essential in older people with Type 1 diabetes to prevent ketoacidosis (see Chapter 2).
(4) Continues to drink fluids and/or eat if possible. Recommended foods include:
    - sweetened jelly (not diet or low cal)
    - ice cream ($^1/_2$ cup)
    - custard with sugar ($^1/_2$ cup)
    - honey (3 teaspoons)
    - sugar (1 tablespoon)
    - sweetened ice block (one small or 90 mL)
    - egg flip, sweetened (8 oz)
    - tea or coffee + 4 teaspoons sugar
    - milk (10 oz)
    - Coca-Cola, lemonade or other sweetened soft drink ($^3/_4$ cup, not diet or low cal)
    - unsweetened tinned fruit ($^3/_4$ cup)
    - orange juice ($^3/_4$ cup)
    - apple juice ($^1/_2$ cup)
    - pineapple juice ($^1/_2$ cup)
    - orange (1 medium)
    - banana (1 small)
    - unflavoured yoghurt (100 g or $^1/_2$ carton)
    - flavoured (sweetened) yoghurt (200 g or 1 carton)
    - broth or soup.
(5) Carefully reads the labels on any medication taken or administered to treat the illness, to ascertain if it contains sugar, sugar substitutes or other ingredients such as adrenalin that cause hyperglycaemia.

(6) Rests.
(7) Keeps the phone number of the doctor, diabetes clinic or diabetes nurse specialist/diabetes educator beside the telephone and calls them if:
   ● they develop diarrhoea and/or vomiting
   ● they develop ketones in their urine or blood
   ● their blood glucose continues to rise
   ● they develop signs of dehydration (loss of skin tone, sunken eyes, dry mouth)
   ● the illness does not get better in 2–3 days or they develop fever or delirium
   ● they have trouble passing urine.

When notifying a doctor about a person living in a residential care facility, it is essential to provide the findings of an appropriate nursing assessment. The following information is required.

● Access to the person's medical notes and medication records. Have them available before telephoning.
● An indication of what changes have occurred since the doctor last reviewed the person. These include physical, psychological and social factors where relevant. For example, temperature, pulse and respiration, blood glucose level, blood pressure, pain (type and location and possible cause), nitrates in the urine, productive cough, reduced oxygen saturation and whether these parameters are increasing or falling, cognitive function and behaviour and mobility.

5.6   Diabetes and renal disease in older people

Key points

● Changes in renal function can affect fluid balance, drug reabsorption and excretion and increase the potential for adverse drug events.
● Renal disease is an important cause of drug toxicity necessitating a hospital admission.
● Diabetes may be the underlying cause of undiagnosed renal disease and incontinence.
● Regular screening for the presence of microalbuminuria is the most useful method of detecting early abnormal renal function.
● Hypertension may be an early indicator of renal disease.
● Hypoglycaemia may indicate an unexpected decline in renal function in people on OHAs or insulin.
● Serum creatinine is the most useful method of detecting abnormal renal function.
● Lower rates of creatinine are produced by older people and creatinine clearance rates can be misleading, especially in people with low muscle mass.

Diabetic nephropathy is a significant microvascular complication of diabetes. Diabetes is the second most common cause of end-stage renal disease in Australia and the UK (ANZDATA 2000: Department of Health 2001). Microalbuminuria is an early marker of renal function decline and occurs in up to 20% of people with diabetes. Over 40% eventually develop nephropathy. Some cultural groups are at significant risk of renal disease; these include Aboriginal and Torres Strait Island peoples, Pacific Islanders and Afro-Caribbeans. Diabetic vascular disease is both a macro- and microvascular disease process and there is a strong link with retinopathy. All of these processes are part of the generalised vascular disease that occurs in diabetes.

5.6.1   Risk factors for renal disease

The underlying nature of renal disease influences the rate at which renal function is lost. There is a strong link between hypertension and the progression to renal disease, because systemic blood pressure is transmitted through the renal circulation to the glomerular capillary loop. Elevated pressure in the loop accelerates damage to the remaining viable nephrons and hastens functional decline. The risk of end-stage renal failure increases as the diastolic blood pressure increases to >90–120 mmHg (Klag *et al.* 1996). Other risk factors include:

- Smoking, which hastens the decline in renal function.
- Hyperglycaemia. The Diabetes Control and Complications Trial (DCCT 1993) demonstrated that good control of blood glucose delayed the rate and progression of microvascular disease, including renal disease. Predialysis blood glucose control is an independent predictor of the outcome in people with Type 2 diabetes on haemodialysis (Wu *et al.* 1997).
- The presence of microalbuminuria and proteinuria, which are independent risk factors for the loss of renal function in people with diabetes (Keane 2001). Even moderate degrees of protein loss of 1 g/day indicate the person is likely to lose renal function quickly. Incipient renal disease is present when the albumin excretion rate reaches 20–200 µg/minute and becomes overt when it exceeds 200 µg/minute.

It is possible that proteinuria also plays a direct role in further injuring the kidney. Once overt proteinuria is present, the renal function decline is irreversible. Proteinuria is an important indicator of cardiovascular disease in Type 2 diabetes. Tests for microalbuminuria include:

- Timed urine collections either 12 or 24 hourly.
- Testing the first voided early morning specimen.

Microalbuminuria is due to:

- Increased permeability of glomerular capillaries.
- Raised glomerular capillary pressure.
- Loss of the negative charge in the capillary basement membrane.

It is accelerated by hypertension. The issues concerning hypertension discussed in the previous section apply equally to the management of renal disease. Clinical albuminuria follows microalbuminuria.

Often nephropathy coexists with retinopathy. These complications are often markers of each other and may be suggested by:

- Long duration of diabetes.
- Male sex.
- Increasing age.

Nephropathy has been divided into five basic stages.

(1) Early damage with increased glomerular filtration rate (GFR).
(2) Glomerular lesions and thickened basement membrane.
(3) Incipient nephropathy and microalbuminuria present denoted by an albumin excretion rate (AER) of 30–300 mg/day.
(4) Clinical nephropathy with overt proteinuria exceeding 500 mg/day and GFR <15 mL/minute.
(5) End-stage renal disease (ESRD). When the GFR is <10 mL/minute dialysis is required.

As the renal function declines symptoms and biochemical abnormalities such as uraemia develop.

Practice points

(1) People with diabetes develop other renal diseases besides diabetes nephropathy, including renal artery stenosis and chronic glomerulonephritis. Ischaemic nephropathy or renovascular disease is a common cause of renal failure in older people.
(2) Urinary tract infection may be symptomless or 'silent' in older people with diabetes. Many care facilities use cranberry juice or capsules as a preventive measure. In the past people were prescribed continuous low-dose antibiotics if urinary tract infections occurred frequently, but this practice is now less common.
(3) Intravaginal oestrogen significantly reduces recurrent urinary infections in menopausal women (Therapeutic Guidelines, Antibiotics 2003).

5.6.2 Delaying the progression of renal disease

Prevention

Early detection and treatment are essential so regular screening should be undertaken for the presence of microalbuminuria, while regular GFR, albumin excretion rate (AER) and urea (BUN) and creatinine measurements are also necessary. However, the creatinine does not rise until >50% of renal function has been lost. In addition, it is not an accurate indication of renal function in older people. BUN is a measure of protein catabolism and it is elevated by:

- Eating a high protein diet, which many people with diabetes are currently doing to reduce weight.
- Gastrointestinal bleeding.
- Infection.
- Metabolic stress such as hyperglycaemic states.
- Dehydration.
- Some drugs such as gluococorticoids and tetracycline.

Low BUN is often found in protein-malnourished people, those with liver disease and in the presence of polyuria.

An important aspect of prevention is adequate self-care. Education is essential and may need to include carers. Particular preventive measures nurses need to be aware of are as follows.

- Importance of performing routine urine tests in acute and residential care during illness. The presence of nitrates, blood or protein will require further investigation to determine the cause. This may include obtaining a specimen for culture and sensitivity to exclude urinary tract infection (UTI), especially in the presence of autonomic neuropathy.
- Need to manage blood glucose levels within safe acceptable limits for the individual, given that normoglycaemia and HbA_{1c} <7% may put older individuals at risk of hypoglycaemia and falls.
- Controlling lipids to help stabilise renal function. Lipid-lowering agents may be required (see Chapter 2).
- Controlling blood pressure (see section 5.2 and Chapter 2).
- Avoiding nephrotoxic agents. Nurses need to be aware of medications that have adverse effects on renal function, especially NSAIDS, which are often used by older people, complementary therapies (Chapter 11) and IV radiocontrast media.
- Nutritional management may help delay ESRD. In the later stages low-protein diets may ameliorate uraemic symptoms (Chan 2001). However, nutritional requirements differ according to the stage of renal disease. Nurses need to be aware that protein malnutrition is common in people with renal disease and may contribute to lethargy, skin problems and hypoglycaemia.

Managing blood glucose

Sulphonylureas may be contraindicated in older people with established renal disease. ESRD occurs in 25% of people diagnosed with diabetes before the age of 30 and dialysis is often needed. ACE inhibitors have been shown to delay or stabilise the rate of progression of renal disease and to decrease cardiac events (Keane 2001) (see Chapter 2) and are more effective than other anithypertensive agents in reducing the urinary albumin excretion rate and plasma creatinine in people with Type 2 diabetes who have other cardiovascular risk factors (Ravid *et al.* 1993). Likewise, ACE inhibitors reduce cardiovascular events and overt nephropathy, whether or not microalbuminuria is present (HOPE Study Investigators 2000).

People with significant renal disease require insulin therapy. However, lower doses of insulin are needed in people already on insulin because insulin, like many other drugs, is degraded and excreted by the kidney. Kidney damage delays degradation and excretion of many drugs and prolongs their half-life, which increases the risk of hypoglycaemia and drug interactions.

Anaemia appears to occur earlier in the decline of renal function than in non-diabetics and becomes more marked as the function declines. Renal anaemia is associated with fatigue, reduced quality of life, depression, left ventricular hypertrophy, reduced exercise capacity, malaise and malnutrition. Recombinant human erythropoietin (rhEPO) is the usual treatment, often in conjunction with intravenous iron if the ferritin is <300 μ/L. Cumming *et al.* (2004) found an association between anaemia and modest renal impairment in 3000 people over 65 and recommended considering diabetic renal disease when investigating anaemia in older people.

Dyslipidaemia is a feature of renal disease, usually hypertriglyceridaemia, and LDL and low HDL occur. Lipid-lowering agents, except the statins, are contraindicated. Thus, dietary measures become important.

5.6.3 Nutritional requirements

The nutritional needs of people with renal disease are individual and depend on the nephropathy stage and type of renal disease present. The aims of nutritional management are to maintain homeostasis and electrolyte balance, reduce uraemic symptoms and regularly reassess dietary requirements to ensure changing needs are addressed (National Kidney Foundation 2002). Nutritional goals before ESRD aim to retard the progression of renal damage by controlling blood pressure, lipids, glucose and electrolyte imbalance and reduce the accumulation of toxic substances. At the ESRD stage, dialysis losses need to be replaced and optimal nutrition achieved. Nutritional status in renal disease is affected by:

- Altered digestion metabolism and absorption of nutrients.
- Altered requirements.
- Altered taste and poor appetite.
- Blood loss due to sampling.
- Intercurrent illnesses.
- Psychosocial issues, including depression.

Protein and energy malnutrition are common and need to be corrected to prevent catabolism, lipid metabolism and anaemia. Low-protein diets are usually recommended for people with significant renal disease (0.6 g protein/kg/day) and adequate energy intake (35 kcal/kg/day). High biological quality protein is necessary to supply essential amino acids. Additional energy from carbohydrate and fat may be needed to spare body protein and maintain body weight.

Protein requirements usually increase once dialysis is commenced. Continuous ambulatory peritoneal dialysis causes higher losses than haemodialysis. Sodium restriction (80–100 mmol/day) is often recommended, but salt substitutes should not be used because they are usually high in potassium, which increases the serum potassium, which is usually already elevated in renal disease and haemodialysis. Water-soluble vitamin supplementation with Vitamins B and D group and Vitamin C may be required when dialysis commences. Fluid restriction is necessary when the renal output is low.

Anorexia is often a feature of renal disease and food smells can further reduce appetite and predispose the patient to nausea and vomiting and malnutrition. Small frequent meals may be more appealing. Malnutrition has implications for the individual's immune status and phagocyte function and increases the risk of infection (Churchill 1996). Referral to a dietitian is essential. The potassium, phosphate and fluid restrictions may conflict with the diabetes diet the person is accustomed to and a careful explanation about why the changes are necessary will be needed.

5.6.4 Medication management

Dose adjustments are needed for many medicines to avoid adverse events in older people, especially those with renal disease. Dose adjustments are especially necessary when drugs are initiated or added to existing drug regimes. A wide range of drugs is used in the elderly and dose adjustments are especially needed for drugs that are renally excreted, including digoxin, ACE inhibitors, narcotics, antimicrobials and OHAs (Howes 2001). Long-acting OHAs and long-acting insulin are usually contraindicated because of the risk of hypoglycaemia, as are drugs with a narrow therapeutic ratio and those where >50% of the drug is renally excreted.

Drug therapy needs to be closely monitored along with monitoring the renal function and nutritional status and non-drug alternatives used where possible. Body composition changes in older people can alter the volume of distribution of the drug and lead to a higher steady plasma state. Dose adjustments can be achieved by altering the dose interval or the amount of drug given. In general, it is preferable to reduce the dose to avoid unnecessary peak plasma levels and the associated toxicity.

5.6.5   Urinary continence

It is important to distinguish between continence changes associated with increasing age and those associated with illness. Uncontrolled diabetes is often a cause of frequent urination and nocturia, which make it difficult for many older people to remain continent. In addition, autonomic neuropathy can affect bladder function, lead to large residual urine volumes and predispose the person to UTIs, which in turn cause hyperglycaemia. Nurses can be aware of these changes and:

- Enable older people to access the toilet more frequently and be aware that going to the toilet at night is normal for older people.
- Provide extra fluids, especially during hot weather, unless fluid is restricted.

Some medicines cause frequent urination, e.g. diuretics. Hypnotics reduce awareness of the need to urinate. Immobility increases the risk of urinary incontinence (Fonda 2002).

Autonomic neuropathy poses particular problems with respect to managing continence. Catheterisation is no longer considered best practice. However, there are a number of continence strategies that can be implemented and referral to a continence nurse or continence clinic is recommended (see Chapters 2 and 7).

5.6.6   Renal dialysis

Most older people having dialysis live in the community but many live in residential aged care facilities. Dialysis is frequently required for ESRD. Dialysis is a filtering process that removes excess fluid and accumulated waste products from the blood. It may be required on a temporary basis during acute illness or for extended periods of time. Few older people receive a kidney transplant.

The presence of renal disease impacts on blood glucose control and other management strategies. Controlling blood glucose, managing comorbidities and diabetes complications and avoiding hypoglycaemia to achieve an acceptable quality of life may be the treatment goals. Co-ordinated care is essential since the person may be too ill or fatigued to make multiple visits to health services. The medication regimen should be reviewed and modified as necessary. Peritoneal dialysis and haemodialysis have different effects and self-management requirements.

Haemodialysis

Blood is pumped through an artificial membrane in the dialysis machine where it is filtered to remove metabolic waste before being returned to the circulation. Good venous access is required, usually in the arm or central venous access.

Haemodialysis is usually undertaken three times per week. Hypoglycaemia can occur as glucose is removed during dialysis. Insulin doses may need to be adjusted to include a lower dose or to omit the dose before dialysis and give a smaller dose after dialysis is complete. Hypotension is common when haemodialysis therapy is commenced for the first time. Hypotension often occurs if the person eats during dialysis because blood is diverted to the gastrointestinal tract for digestion. Not eating contributes to the fall in blood glucose.

Managing people undergoing haemodialysis consists of:

- Deciding an appropriate dialysis prescription.
- Minimising interdialytic fluid gains by deciding on appropriate amounts of fluid intake.
- Elevating the foot of the bed.
- Differentiating between disequilibrium syndrome, a set of neurological symptoms and characteristic EEG findings that occur during or after dialysis, and hypoglycaemia.
- Advising the patient to sit on the edge of the bed or chair to allow the blood pressure to stabilise before standing (Terrill 2002).
- Preventing coagulation after using anticoagulants. Many older people are already on these drugs and dose adjustment may be needed and the person monitored for bleeding.
- Strict aseptic technique and careful patient education, which are essential when managing dialysis therapies.
- Providing appropriate skin care to reduce uraemic itch.
- Providing diversional activities and ongoing psychological support

Peritoneal dialysis

In peritoneal dialysis the filtering occurs across the peritoneum and is an excellent method of managing kidney failure in people with and without diabetes. Uraemia, hypertension and blood glucose can be controlled without increasing the risk of infection if aseptic techniques are adhered to when changing bags.

Fewer problems occur with blood glucose control but some glucose is absorbed from the dialysate fluid, usually between 100 and 150 g/day depending on the glucose strength in the dialysate fluid. More glucose is absorbed from continuous automated overnight dialysing.

Continuous ambulatory peritoneal dialysis (CAPD)

CAPD is a form of peritoneal dialysis in which dialysate is continually present in the abdominal cavity. The fluid is drained and replaced 4–5 times each day or overnight if the patient is using automated peritoneal dialysis (APD). CAPD enables the person to be managed at home, which has psychological advantages. However, considerable education and support are needed to ensure the person knows how to care for the equipment and be metabolically stable.

Once insulin requirements are known, the doses can be divided between the bag exchanges, which achieves smoother blood glucose control because the insulin is delivered directly into the portal circulation and is absorbed in the dwell phase, which is closer to the way insulin is normally secreted after a glucose load. However, many modern insulin needles are not long enough to enable insulin to be added to the fluid and dose mistakes often occur. Therefore, some dialysis units continue to recommend subcutaneous insulin administration rather than adding the insulin to the bag.

The usual insulin dose may need to be increased if significant amounts of glucose are absorbed from dialysate fluids with a high glucose concentration and to account for insulin binding to the plastic of the dialysate bags and tubing. The continuous supplies of glucose and lactate in the dialysate fluid are calorie-rich energy sources and can lead to weight gain and contribute to hyperglycaemia. The availability of glucose-free solutions, such as Nutrimeal, and glucose polymers may help reduce complications associated with high insulin and glucose levels (Rutecki & Whittier 1993).

Practice point

Some blood glucose meters overestimate blood glucose levels (read higher than actual levels) in people being dialysed with Icodextrin dialysing fluids. Hypoglycaemia can be missed (Oyibo *et al.* 2002).

Objectives of care

The individual's ability to carry out the self-care tasks associated with diabetes and dialysis care needs to be assessed early when considering renal replacement therapy. Changed joint structure due to oedema and tissue glycolysation such as carpal tunnel syndrome and arthritis can limit the fine motor skills required to manage CAPD. Visual impairment due to retinopathy frequently accompanies renal disease and can limit self-care abilities, as can cognitive impairment and depression.

(1) Assessment includes:
   - knowledge of diabetes
   - ability to adopt preventive health-care practices
   - ability to use aseptic technique
   - usual diabetic control
   - presence of other diabetic complications such as autonomic neuropathy, cardiovascular disease and retinopathy that will impact on self-care
   - support available from family/carers and their ability
   - motivation for self-care
   - uraemic state.
(2) Thorough instruction about how to administer dialysate and any medications required, including how to recognise adverse drug-related events and the need to report illness or high temperatures immediately.
(3) Providing appropriate nutrition to meet protein energy needs and necessary supplements.
(4) Maintaining skin integrity by ensuring technique is aseptic, especially around the catheter exit site. Skin care is vital since people often develop uraemic itch and are likely to scratch, which represents a portal for infection.
(5) Monitoring metabolic parameters such as urea, creatinine and electrolytes carefully.
(6) Providing psychological support.
(7) Encouraging simple appropriate exercise.
(8) Ensuring adequate dental care and regular dental assessments.

(9) Managing pain and discomfort, especially associated with the weight of the dialysate.

(10) Regular foot care, especially if peripheral neuropathy is present because of the risk of infection.

Nursing management

Appropriate nursing care is essential and includes the following.

- Meticulous skin care.
- Regular daily inspection of the catheter exit site and early management of any redness, swelling, pain or discharge.
- Monitor fluid balance carefully:
  (1) measure all drainage
  (2) maintain progressive fluid balance to document input and output
  (3) report a positive balance of more than 1 litre. The aim of dialysis is usually to achieve a negative balance to maintain the dry weight.
- Monitor blood glucose.
- Perform regular medication reviews, which should include medication self-care practices.
- Monitor temperature, pulse and respiration and report abnormalities.
- Monitor nutritional status via intake and biochemistry results.
- Weigh daily to monitor fluid intake and nutritional status, when the patient is in acute or residential care.
- Ensure patency of tubes and monitor the colour of outflow:
  (1) cloudy
  (2) faecal contamination
  (3) very little outflow, which could indicate the tube is blocked, needs to be reported to the doctor for urgent management.
- Lethargy and malaise may be due to uraemia or high blood glucose levels; appropriate monitoring will help identify the cause.
- Warming the dialysate before adding prescribed drugs and before administration can reduce abdominal cramping.
- Ensure mouth care is carried out (see Chapter 2). Ice to suck may help relieve dry mouth discomfort.
- Assess self-care potential.
- Take appropriate steps to protect the kidney during routine tests and procedures by avoiding dehydration and infection.

Practice point

Ensure that appointments for multiple health services occur on the same day as much as possible.

Conducting a risk assessment prior to older people having IV contrast administered for radiographic investigative procedures is essential to avoid potential renal complications and allergies. Procedures include recent creatinine in patients on biguanides. Discontinue metformin for 48 hours before the procedure. Recheck creatinine (St. Vincent's Hospital 2004).

Table 5.5 Benefits and risks associated with using complementary therapies when renal disease is present.

Benefits	Risks
Reduce stress.	Contaminated products represent risk to kidneys.
Help the person cope with the demands of dialysis regimens.	Electrolyte imbalance, especially hypokalaemia.
Improve quality of life.	Tubular atrophy (aristolochic acid).
Maintain a positive attitude.	Haematuria.
Maintain mobility and dexterity.	Albuminuria, which may be difficult to distinguish from diabetic nephropathy.
Skin care.	Weight loss.
Meet spiritual needs.	Nephritis.
	Diuresis, yet sodium retention.
	Interaction with prescription drugs such as anticoagulants.
	Hypertension.

5.6.7 Complementary therapies and renal disease

Many people with chronic diseases use complementary therapies (see Chapter 11). The benefits and risks associated with using complementary therapies when renal disease is present are shown in Table 5.5. People with end-stage renal failure often try complementary therapies to alleviate the unpleasant symptoms of their disease. Some therapies, for example aromatherapy to reduce stress and maintain skin condition or counselling for depression, are beneficial and usually safe. Herbal medicines are popular with the general public but they may not be appropriate for people with renal disease (Myhre 2000).

The kidneys play a key role in eliminating drugs and herbal products from the system. Some of these drugs and herbs can cause kidney damage that may be irreversible and put already compromised renal function at great risk. In addition, some herbal products, particularly those used in traditional Chinese medicine (TCM), are often contaminated with drugs, heavy metals and other potentially nephrotoxic products (Ko 1998). Frequently these contaminants are not recorded in the list of ingredients for the product. As well as the direct effect of the herbs on the kidney, the intended action of particular herbs can complicate conventional treatment.

A herb used in TCM to treat diabetes, *Taxus celebica*, contains a potentially harmful flavonoid and has been associated with acute renal failure and other vascular and hepatic effects (Ernst 1998). Kidney damage can be present with few specific overt renal symptoms; therefore, it is vital that kidney and liver function is closely monitored in people taking herbs, especially if kidney function is already compromised by diabetes.

Practice point

Nurses must know when their renal patients are taking herbal medicines so that their kidney function can be closely monitored. Patients should be asked about the use of complementary therapies periodically and during medicine reviews and given appropriate non-judgemental advice about their use.

5.7   Eye disease and older people with diabetes

Keypoints

- Diabetes is not the only cause of visual loss in older people.
- Retinopathy is a significant complication of diabetes.
- People with visual loss are often able to care for themselves if they are provided with appropriate tools and information.
- Make sure the environment is safe and free of obstacles.
- Return belongings to the same place and explain things carefully before undertaking procedures.
- People with Type 2 diabetes often have signs of retinopathy at diagnosis.
- Prevention and early identification of visual deficits are essential. Visual loss or impairment has a large impact on the self-care and psychological wellbeing of people with diabetes.

Diabetic retinopathy is one of the microvascular complications of diabetes. It falls into two broad categories: non-proliferative (NPDR) and proliferative (PDR). The most common abnormalities are microaneurysms and dot and blot haemorrhages and exudates on the retina. New capillaries grow on the retina and are fragile and prone to sudden bleeding. Macular oedema also occurs in the region responsible for central vision, is the main cause of visual loss and occurs gradually. NPDR is the prominent type of diabetic retinopathy that occurs in older people. Visual loss is usually gradual, declines each year and is easily missed.

- Maculopathy.
- Retinopathy – stages of retinopathy have been described based on a system of photographic grading that requires comparison with a standard set of photographs showing different features and stages of retinopathy (DRS 1981).
- Generalised ocular oedema.
- Lens opacity or cataract, which makes it difficult to visualise or photograph the retina, which may need to be deferred until after the cataracts are removed or laser can be used. Cataract surgery may worsen retinopathy.
- Glaucoma is often also present in older people, as are a range of problems associated with long- and short-sightedness for which spectacles may be required.

Retinopathy is detected by examining the retina with an ophthalmoscope through dilated pupils or, more commonly, via retinal photography. Older people have small pupils and lens apertures that make retinal screening difficult.

Vision less than 6/24 is difficult to correct therefore regular screening is vital. In addition, managing hypertension, blood glucose control and stopping smoking are important preventive measures.

5.7.1   Risk factors for retinopathy

Factors that increase the risk of retinopathy include:

- Long duration of diabetes, the major risk factor for retinopathy which puts older people particularly at risk. After 20 years, 90% have some retinopathy.

- Poor blood glucose and lipid control, which over several years cause a variety of biochemical changes inside the endothelial cells of the retinal capillaries, which eventually leak and cause slow capillary death and retinal ischaemia.
- Atherosclerosis and renal disease.
- Smoking.
- Hypertension.
- Lipid abnormalities.

Hyperglycaemia can also distort the lens due to the accumulation of glucose, which causes blurred vision on a temporary basis that often takes some weeks to correct. This is very frightening and limits self-care and has safety implications. Visual changes can also accompany hypoglycaemia.

Most people with diabetes eventually develop some degree of retinopathy and are at increased risk of developing other diabetic complications if retinopathy occurs. Regular screening and appropriate preventive management needs to be commenced early to maintain older people in the community for as long as possible.

Visual impairment from non-diabetic causes often coexists with diabetes. People with diabetes also have an increased incidence of glaucoma and cataracts and there is an increasing correlation with age-related macular degeneration. This can be a significant disadvantage during diabetes education and general living because most diabetic and general health information contains essential visual components (IDF 2000).

Practice point

Vision can worsen in the short term when blood glucose control begins to improve such as when oral hypoglycaemic insulin agents are commenced.

5.7.2 Management and prevention

There is increasing evidence that ACE inhibitors can reduce the incidence of microvascular disease and may be the next preventive strategy. People can have severe retinopathy without being aware of it. Vision is not always affected and there is usually no pain or discomfort. Sudden loss of vision is normally an emergency. It may be due to:

- Vitreous haemorrhage.
- Retinal detachment.
- Retinal artery occlusion.

Reassurance, avoiding stress and sudden movement and urgent ophthalmological assessment are required. Laser treatment is very effective in preventing further visual loss. Once scar tissue forms in the retina or there is a dense vitreous haemorrhage, vitrectomy is necessary. Some exercises are contraindicated if retinopathy is present

5.7.3 Resources for people with visual impairment

People with significant loss of vision require assistance to perform blood glucose monitoring and to administer their own insulin. It is important to encourage independence as far as possible. Careful assessment is important and should include assessment of the home situation.

Vision Australia and the Royal National Institute for the Blind in the UK offer a variety of services for people who have degrees of visual loss. These services include:

- Assessing cognitive function.
- Assessing the person and the home situation and recommending modifications if necessary to improve safety, especially the risk of falls and other accidents such as burns.
- Low vision clinics.
- Education about how to cope in the community with deteriorating vision. This includes walking with a cane and in some cases guide dogs.
- A range of 'talking' equipment including watches, large print watches, clocks, books, liquid level indicator, key rings, signature templates, phones, magnifying glasses and calendars.

Other services include pensions, which may be available from the government.

5.7.4   Diabetes-specific aids for people with low vision

Various devices are available to help people continue to care for themselves. They can be obtained from diabetes associations and some pharmacies specialising in diabetic products.

(1) Insulin administration devices.
- Clicking syringes, Instaject devices, clicking insulin pens.
- Chest magnifying glass (available from some opticians).
- Magniguide, which fits both 50 and 100 unit syringes and enlarges the markings.
- Location tray for drawing up insulin if syringes are used.
(2) Blood glucose monitoring.
- Strip guides for accurate placement of the blood onto the strips.
- Talking blood glucose meters.
- Meters with large result display areas.
- Placing brightly coloured stickers to indicate the strip port.
(3) Medications.
- Dosette boxes that can be prefilled with the correct medications.
(4) Other self-care devices.
- Blood pressure monitors.
- Talking weight scales.
- Magnifying glass and lamps.

5.7.5   Nursing management of visually impaired patients

Aims of care

The aims of nursing care are to:

- Detect vision deficits early and institute appropriate screening and management.
- Encourage independence as far as possible.
- Ensure the environment is safe when the patient is mobile.

Nursing management of people confined to bed

- Introduce yourself and address the person by name, so they realise you are talking to them.
- Determine how much vision the person has. Assess if the blood glucose levels fluctuate at certain times of the day by undertaking regular blood glucose tests. High and low levels interfere with clear vision. If such a pattern emerges plan education and activities to avoid these times. Institute preventive measures to avoid such fluctuations such as mealtimes and medication doses.
- Visual impairment increases the risk of falls in older people. Help them recognise the route to the toilet and keep the passage clear.
- Some people prefer to be in a corner bed because it makes location easier, avoids confusion with equipment belonging to other patients and enables greater ease in setting up personal belongings.
- Introduce the person to other people in their ward or close by.
- If you move their belongings, return them to the same place.
- Explain all procedures carefully and fully before commencing.
- If eye bandages are required, make sure the ears and other sensory organs are not covered to improve communication.
- Consider having adjustable lighting for people with useful residual vision and make sure their vision aids do not get lost.
- Mark the person's medicines with large print labels or use a dose administration aid such as the Dosette.
- Indicate when you are leaving the room and concluding a conversation.

People who are mobile

- A central point, such as the bed, helps people orientate themselves to a room.
- When orientating a person to a new area, walk with them until they become familiar with the route.
- Keep pathways clear of obstacles where possible.

Mealtimes

- Describe the menu and let the person make a choice.
- Ensure the person knows their meal has been delivered.
- Offer assistance with the meal rather than help.
- Colour contrast is important for some patients. A white plate on a red tray-cloth may assist with location of place setting and plates with fitted guards and non-slip surfaces can help people feed themselves.
- Describe the location of the food on the plate; for example, 'The meat is at 2 o'clock'.

5.8   Diabetic neuropathy

Distal symmetric sensory polyneuropathy, usually referred to as diabetic neuropathy, affects 7% of people within the first year of diagnosis and 50% after 25 years.

Surprisingly, and significantly, screening for foot pathology, including neuropathy, is not undertaken in 50% of people with diabetes and many people are not taught foot self-care (Tapp 2004). This finding increases the likelihood that older people will have some form of foot pathology and be at risk of falls and foot ulcers.

Neuropathy affects the peripheral and autonomic nerves and can have devastating consequences such as foot amputation if appropriate preventive foot care is not undertaken. Peripheral sensory neuropathy is the most common form of neuropathy. The pathogenesis of neuropathy is poorly understood, but persistent hyperglycaemia plays a role. Degeneration of large and small myelinated nerve fibres occurs and nerve and blood supply to nerves is reduced.

Diabetic neuropathy is usually bilateral and symmetrical, which helps distinguish it from other common conditions in older people, such as arthritis which is usually asymmetrical. Peripheral sensory neuropathy presents in two forms that often overlap:

(1) Painful.
(2) Painless but with sensory loss.

Stages of peripheral neuropathy

- Chronic painful.
- Acute painful.
- Painless.
- Late complications (Vinik *et al.* 2000).

5.8.1 Presentation

People present with different symptoms, but commonly the symptoms of painful peripheral neuropathy are:

- Burning or short, sharp stabbing pain in the feet, especially at night.
- Pins and needles.
- Numbness.
- Hot, tight feet.
- Hyperalgesia.
- Allodynia.

When present, these symptoms can inhibit quality of life and sleep and may cause groaning in people unable to communicate pain. They also limit exercise and mobility. Regardless of whether the neuropathy is painful or painless, the loss of sensation puts the individual at significant risk of foot pathology, including pressure areas. From around the age of 60, people generally lose some of their peripheral sensation. Signs that indicate diabetes has a role are:

- Long duration of diabetes.
- Dry skin on the feet from anhidrosis.
- Clawed toes.
- Muscle stiffness.
- Unsteady gait with increased risk of falls.

5.8.2 Management

Management is difficult and depends on the symptoms present. No current treatment prevents or arrests the progression. However, spontaneous resolution often occurs when pain has only been present for a short time. It is important to:

- Exclude rest pain due to ischaemia.
- Improve blood glucose control in the acute situation, which might require medication and lifestyle review, but hypoglycaemia should be avoided.
- Manage pain where required. Strategies include simple analgesia and tricyclic antidepressants if sleep is disturbed. However, these agents may cause dry mouth, tachycardia and tiredness and aggravate urinary symptoms from prostate disease in men. Anticonvulsants such as gabapentin are effective for some people providing renal status is considered. People taking gabapentin should not drive until the dose is established because of the common side effects of drowsiness and fatigue. All these agents have dose-limiting side effects. Antiarrhythmic agents may help if burning pain is present but may cause bradycardia in older people with cardiac disease. Antiepileptic drugs also help in some circumstances. Topical capsaicin may benefit people if the pain is localised. Recently the opioid oxycodon has been used but morphine is ineffective. TENS, acupuncture and biofeedback may help.
- Provide education and regular foot inspection and care.
- Protect the feet.

Peripheral neuropathy must be distinguished from intermittent claudication, which can be achieved by taking a thorough history of the symptoms and brachial/ankle index measurements.

5.8.3 Foot care for older people with diabetes

Key points

- The presence of neuropathy represents significant physical, psychological, social and economic consequences for people with diabetes and for the health system.
- Foot complications are common in the elderly.
- Older people may have adequate knowledge about foot care but may not be able to care for their feet appropriately due to visual loss, limited mobility making it difficult to reach the feet, reduced manual dexterity and cognitive decline.
- Foot disease is a significant cause of hospital admissions.
- Fungal infections are often present and increase the risk of cellulitis and ulceration.

Diabetic foot pathology is multifactorial in nature due to micro- and macrovascular changes and neuropathy that predispose the person to trauma and infection, which are often not detected until significant pathology is present. The multifactorial nature of foot pathology in older people is shown in Figure 5.1. Foot care is often neglected in acute care settings but is often well catered for with podiatry services in residential care facilities. Early detection of foot problems is mandatory. Reduced vision, dexterity and cognitive function often preclude older people from caring for their own feet. These people need significant assistance and foot care.

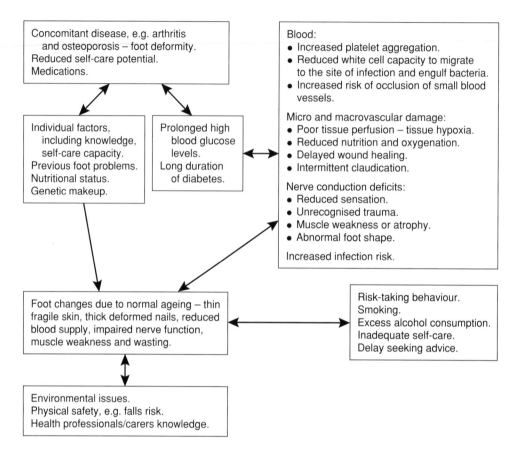

Figure 5.1 Schematic representation of the multifactorial nature of foot pathology in older people with diabetes. The Australian Pain Society recommends health professionals have a high level of suspicion that older people in residential care have unrecognised pain (~40%). The Society recommends the ten-minute Modified Residential Brief Pain Inventory be used and the Pain Assessment in Advanced Dementia Scale be used for people with severe dementia (Australian Pain Society 2004).

Managing foot infections

Foot infections are common serious problems. About 20% of admissions to hospital are for foot-related problems in people with diabetes. Infection can be present with few overt signs, which delays the diagnosis. Deep infections such as beneath a corn or callus can predispose the individual to septicaemia, osteomyelitis and Charcot's foot. Unrelieved pressure in bed- or chair-bound people can also cause foot ulcers.

Typically, a mixture of anaerobic, aerobic and Gram-negative organisms is present (Lipsky & Berendt 2000). Therefore, broad-spectrum antibiotics are needed and should be given IV if the infection is severe or the person has low resistance to infection. Antibiotics are often commenced on clinical grounds and modified on the basis of culture and sensitivity results from wound swabs.

Practice points

(1) Because foot infections are often deep-seated, superficial swabs are inadequate to detect causal organisms and decide treatment. In fact, they can delay appropriate treatment.
(2) Swabs should be taken from deep within the ulcer. Analgesics should be administered if pain develops.
(3) The healing rate, especially on plantar ulcers, is determined by the aetiology of the wound, not its size.

Management of foot infections includes the following.

- Antibiotics, IV if severe, which may be needed for up to six weeks if osteomyelitis is present.
- X-ray and MRI bone scans to detect bone deformity and foreign bodies.
- Surgical debridement and if necessary vascular surgery (femoral/popliteal bypass) to restore blood flow and prevent gangrene or amputation. Amputation may need to be reconsidered.
- Appropriate wound dressing depending on the type of wound present. The healing rate should be monitored and documented to determine progress and whether the antibiotic and/or dressing regimes need to be changed. Venous ulcers can be difficult to heal. They need to be treated quickly and aggressively to prevent further ulceration and decline.
- Rest and non-weight bearing is important. However, biomechanical measures such as contact casts that relieve pressure and allow the person to remain mobile improve mood and reduce isolation.
- Foot education for the individual, carers or health professionals.

Nursing care

Foot care is an essential aspect of caring for older people with diabetes. Provide care for *both feet* or remaining foot and the stump if the person has had an amputation.

- Appropriate assessment to identify people at risk of foot ulceration:
  (1) this includes testing sensation using 10 gram Semmes-Weinstein monofilaments, 128 H2 tuning forks and disposable neuropathy pins (Apelqvist *et al.* 2000)
  (2) ascertaining vascular status by checking capillary return and pedal, popliteal and groin pulses and performing Doppler studies to assess circulation
  (3) noting any foot deformity, areas of callus, colour and footwear
  (4) referral to a podiatrist may be necessary; also orthotics, specialist foot clinic and diabetes educator
  (5) knowledge of foot self-care
  (6) care potential of carers.
- Preventing trauma, including trauma from falls and unrelieved pressure. Use a bed cradle if the person is confined to bed. Elevate the feet when they sit out of bed.
- Pain management. Ill and cognitively impaired older people may not be able to communicate pain. The Australian Pain Society (2004) has developed specific pain

assessment tools to be used in these situations. The presence of pain can lead to behavioural problems and further complicate cognitive deficits as well as reducing the quality of life. Appropriate language should be used when asking about pain, for example 'soreness' or 'discomfort'.

- Achieve an appropriate level of glycaemic control by appropriate medication and nutrition management and activity where possible.
- Monitor blood glucose.
- Maximise arterial blood flow by keeping the foot down and venous return by elevating the feet. Review the need for beta blockers (see Chapter 2), reducing caffeine consumption and wearing non-restrictive footwear.
- Attend to appropriate foot hygiene:
  (1) wash in lukewarm water using pH-neutral products that do not dry the skin, especially in malnourished older people and those on steroid medications
  (2) check water temperature is not too hot before people enter a bath, to prevent burns
  (3) dry feet carefully, especially between the toes to prevent maceration and portals for infection
  (4) apply urea cream or Eulactol to prevent dry skin and cracks. Sometimes these products cause stinging if deep cracks are present
  (5) if bandages are required, ensure they do not encircle the toes or foot and reduce the circulation, which could result in gangrene.
- Ensure shoes are worn when ambulating. Slippers should only be worn for short periods because they are associated with an increased risk of falling. High heels, loafers and sandals also increase falls risk (Koepsall *et al.* 2004).
- Control odour when infection and gangrene are present. Some wound dressings eliminate odour by absorbing bacteria. Aromatherapy essential oils placed on the surface of secondary dressings can help eliminate odour.
- Nutritional review if foot ulcers are present to maximise healing potential.
- Bed rest is important if foot ulcers are present. If bed rest is necessary it is important to ensure that:
  (1) regular toileting is attended to and hand-washing facilities are provided afterwards
  (2) meals are placed where the person can reach them and assistance given if necessary
  (3) pressure care is attended to.

5.8.4 Autonomic neuropathy

The autonomic nervous system controls the automatic functions of the body. There are three main divisions of the autonomic nervous system:

- Sympathetic nervous system.
- Parasympathetic nervous system.
- Enteric nervous system.

Autonomic neuropathy is a group of symptoms caused by damage to the autonomic nerves which affects approximately 30% of people with diabetes (Aly & Weston 2002). Symptoms develop slowly and are rare, therefore the prevalence of autonomic neuropathy in older people is difficult to assess. Other conditions common in older people also cause autonomic neuropathy, for example Parkinson's disease. Autonomic neuropathy is more common in people over 55 years with diabetes than in non-diabetics.

Common features of autonomic neuropathy are:

- Postural hypotension and syncope.
- Dysphagia due to reflux oesophagitis, gastroparesis, feeling of fullness often associated with flushing, and constipation and intermittent diarrhoea.
- Hypoglycaemic unawareness.
- Bladder atony and asymptomatic urinary tract infection.
- Erectile dysfunction.

The functions and manifestations depend on which nerves and organs are involved. Autonomic neuropathic changes often occur concomitantly with age-related changes (see Chapter 1). Many of these changes affect the gastrointestinal tract; they include reduced peristalsis, gastric motility and emptying and reduced acidity of gastric juices (Aly & Weston 2002; Durrance 2003). Intestinal absorption and blood flow are diminished, which has nutritional, blood glucose and drug implications. Delayed gastric emptying can cause oesophageal reflux and dysphagia.

When the vagal nerve is involved, gastroparesis often occurs, resulting in bloating, diarrhoea, often at night, and vomiting after food. Sitting up after meals and eating small meals may relieve these symptoms. Gastrointestinal infections occur and antibiotics may be needed to combat bacterial overgrowth. Medicines such as domperidone and cisapride may stimulate gastric emptying. Cisapride is associated with cardiac arrhythmias and an ECG should be performed and serum potassium and magnesium levels measured before commencing the drug. Adverse drug interactions increase the likelihood of cardiac abnormalities.

If the cardiovascular nerves are affected, the tone in the sympathetic arterioles is lost, causing postural hypotension. Postural hypotension is more common in older people and is further aggravated by autonomic neuropathy. Antihypertensive and antianginal agents often precipitate postural hypotension and a medication review should be undertaken.

Postural hypotension complicates the management of hypertension and increases the risk of falls. Cardiovascular status is disrupted by reduced beta receptor responsiveness and baroreflex function. Resting tachycardia, loss of diurnal variation in blood pressure, blurred vision, cognitive impairment, weakness and reduced exercise tolerance may be present. Fludrocortisone is sometimes used in severe postural hypotension but it is associated with fluid retention, hypertension and hypokalaemia. Less frequently, midorine is used.

Erectile dysfunction can be extremely distressing for men (see Chapter 10). An autonomic bladder predisposes the person to incomplete bladder emptying, leaving significant volumes of residual urine which may lead to urinary tract infection, incontinence or acute metabolic disturbances such as DKA and HONK (see Chapter 4).

Other signs of autonomic neuropathy include hyperhidrosis, gustatory sweating, anhidrosis and redness of the feet, all of which contribute to foot pathology.

Hypoglycaemic unawareness is a common feature and occurs due to the blunted counterregulatory response to falling blood glucose levels and is exacerbated by the gastrointestinal manifestations and reduced appetite.

Managing autonomic neuropathy

Management is difficult and often aims at symptom management. The main management strategies are shown in Table 5.6 according to the type of neuropathy present. Unpredictable swings in blood glucose are difficult to manage and make it difficult to tailor the medication regimes. Rapid-acting insulin may be a viable alternative. The

Table 5.6 Management of autonomic neuropathy according to the system affected. Regular blood glucose monitoring is recommended to reduce the risk of hypoglycaemia. Education is essential. Psychological support is imperative.

System affected	Management strategies
Gastrointestinal	Smaller, more frequent meals that are easily digested. Low in fat. Gluten free.
	Monitor food intake to determine foods most likely to cause symptoms.
	Metoclopramide, cisapride, erythromycin.
	Cholestyramine chelate. Bile salts.
	Elevate the head of the bed to reduce oesophageal reflux.
	Review medicines to reduce the risk of adverse events. Short-acting preparations may be preferred.
	Prophylactic antibiotics may be needed to reduce bacterial overgrowth. Consider the need for drugs such as narcotics that slow intestinal contractions.
	Parenteral nutrition may be needed in severe cases.
	Surgery to remove bezoars.
	Gentle abdominal massages and/or compresses.
Cardiovascular and postural hypotension	Elevate the head of the bed.
	Elastic stockings.
	Medicines such as fludrocortisone or midodrine.
	Moving from lying or sitting to standing positions slowly to reduce likelihood of falls.
Urinary tract	Encourage regular bladder emptying.
	Consider prophylactic preventive measures such as daily cranberry juice or low-dose antibiotics to prevent urinary infections or intravaginal oestrogen for recurrent urinary infections in postmenopausal women.
	Reduce alcohol intake if relevant.
Skin	Good hygiene and skin care.
	Good foot care.
Erectile dysfunction	See Chapter 11.
Counterregulatory response to low blood glucose	Regular blood glucose monitoring to detect patterns and plan activity and food to reduce the risk of hypoglycaemia.
	Hypoglycaemia management education.
	Review of medicines. Long-acting agents may not be the best choice.

psychological impact can be profound due to the unpredictability of symptoms and cause embarrassment and withdrawal from social functions, isolation and depression. In the future, high-frequency gastric simulation, which electrically stimulates the stomach to empty, may be more readily available and affordable.

Nursing management

Prepare people appropriately for diagnostic procedures depending on the particular system involved, for example:

- Gastric emptying times.
- Voiding cystourethrogram.
- Valsalva manoeuvre to assess cardiovascular neuropathic involvement.

Adopt preventive strategies such as:

- Regular blood glucose monitoring to detect increases and falls and an overall pattern.
- Improving blood and lipid control by detecting and managing abnormalities early.
- Through regular monitoring, notifying doctors of persistent abnormalities.
- Appropriate medication administration and monitoring of outcomes.
- Ensuring the diet and fluid intake are adequate and monitoring intake and output. Small frequent light meals. In some cases a fluid balance chart will be necessary.
- Correctly applying graduated compression stockings to reduce venous pooling.
- Encouraging activity.
- Taking note of signs and symptoms that indicate neuropathy may be present.
- Providing psychological support.
- Assisting with diabetes education.

Provide palliative and supportive care:

- Ensure the environment is safe to minimise the risk of falls.
- Take care when moving the person from lying to sitting or to standing and in the bath or shower to account for postural hypotension.
- Maintain blood glucose at an optimal level to prevent hypo- or hyperglycaemia and the consequent risks, including falls.
- Ensure feet are protected from bedclothes and other risk factors for ulcers.
- Use aseptic technique for procedures.
- Identify whether enteral feeds are required and if so, the most suitable feeds and feeding regimen. Revise medicines to ensure they can be administered via an enteral tube (see Chapter 2).

5.8.5 Restless legs syndrome

Some older people have restless legs syndrome, a chronic disabling condition that affects 5–10% of the population with a preponderance in women. It is often undiagnosed and untreated. It is different from peripheral neuropathy and needs to be distinguished from it in order to offer appropriate treatment. The criteria for diagnosis are:

- Desire to move legs with a sensory discomfort.
- Motor restlessness.

- Leg discomfort at rest relieved by movement.
- Discomfort worse in the evening and at night (Medical Medscape News 2004).

Periodic limb movements occur in 80% of people with the syndrome and disrupt sleep and daily functions and can exacerbate behavioural problems. Continuous treatment is required, especially for older and severely affected individuals. Dopaminergic drugs have been the treatment of choice. Recently, pergolide as a single evening dose has been shown to reduce arousal and increase subjective improvement (Wetter *et al.* 1999; Trenkwalder *et al.* 2004).

5.8.6 Pressure ulcers

Pressure ulcers are significant, common and costly medical problems in older people. They are rare in residential aged care in Australia but are more likely to occur when the person is in acute care facilities. Pressure ulcers reduce quality of life and increase morbidity and mortality. Having specific pressure ulcer protocols in place can reduce the prevalence of pressure ulcers and therefore costs.

Healing can be delayed in the presence of malnutrition, cardiovascular disease and deformities that cause pressure. Treatment needs to be instituted early and focus on prevention. Common factors associated with pressure ulcer development are:

- Immobility.
- Incontinence, using catheters and mechanical urine collection devices.
- Altered mental status, which might be permanent or occur as a result of DKA, HONK or hypo- or hyperglycaemia.
- Poor nutritional status.
- Antidepressant and sedative medications.
- Inadequate blood glucose control.
- Previous pressure ulcers, including at-risk feet.
- Severe illness, especially requiring enteral feeding.
- Peripheral neuropathy

The Braden Scale can be used to predict risk and plan care (Horn *et al.* 2004). Management strategies include relieving the pressure, managing any infection present, appropriate dressings and topical antiseptics or debridement when indicated (see also p. 177). A new platelet-derived growth factor, Regranox, is being trialled in Europe and the USA that may prove useful in the future.

5.9 Diabetes and osteoporosis

Recent research suggests osteoporosis is an important public health problem, which is predicted to increase due to the ageing population (Therapeutic Guidelines: Endocrinology 2004). Thirty to fifty per cent of women can expect to sustain fractures and 30% of older women have hip fractures. Diabetes significantly increases the risk of falls and fractures (see Chapter 5). Thirty per cent of older men have hip fractures due to osteoporosis. The presence of diabetes is an independent risk factor for the development of osteoporosis (Chau & Edelman 2002). The intrinsic characteristics of Type 1 diabetes mellitus and lifestyle factors seen in Type 2 diabetes may partly explain this phenomenon.

Osteoporosis is characterised by a decrease in bone mass and bone quality, encompassing low bone mass and deterioration in the microstructure of the bone, which increases the risk for fracture (WHO 1994). Importantly, osteoporosis can be diagnosed before fractures occur and risk reduction strategies implemented. One in two women and one in three men over 65 are likely to develop osteoporosis. The presence of Type 1 diabetes is associated with lower bone mineral density (BMD) (Brown & Sharpless 2004). Several researchers have shown that older people with diabetes are at a higher risk of hip fracture but the association needs to be considered in context. All older people with diabetes are at a higher risk of falling (see Chapter 5). Fractures in older people with diabetes are not confined to hips. Foot fractures frequently occur and are probably partly due to obesity and/or neuropathy (Schwarz *et al.* 2001).

There appears to be no relationship between duration of diabetes, current HbA_{1c} and BMD (Brown & Sharpless 2004). However, an association between BMD and the presence of diabetes complications may exist, in particular peripheral neuropathy (Rix *et al.* 1999), where mobility and walking, i.e. weight-bearing activity, are reduced, often as a consequence of numbness due to peripheral neuropathy.

However, other risk factors include family history of osteoporosis, other disease processes such as endocrine diseases, malabsorption syndromes, which may occur as a consequence of diabetic gastroparesis, renal disease, connective tissue disease such as arthritis and some medications that cause bone loss, for example glucocorticoids. In older people any disorder that increases falls risk also increases risk of trauma and fractures.

Lifestyle factors and nutritional deficiencies also influence BMD; for example, many older people do not get enough Vitamin D because they do not have enough exposure to sunlight. Fracture risk can be assessed by dual energy X-ray absorptiometry (DEXA). In addition, the risk of osteoporotic fractures is raised even with only moderate bone loss. Significantly, <40–50% of women and <20% of men at risk of osteoporosis receive treatment.

Practice points

(1) Trauma plays a role in most fractures but bone fragility alone is often enough to precipitate vertebral fractures.
(2) Any older person with diabetes who sustains a fracture should be investigated for osteoporosis.
(3) Systemic illness, weight loss, metabolic abnormalities, hyperglycaemia and pain may indicate osteoporosis or fracture.

5.9.1   Management

Prevention strategies

- Regular monitoring, including fracture risk.
- Dietary review and supplementation, Vitamin D, calcium, e.g. 600 mg elemental calcium.

- Medication review, using medicines that cause osteopenia at the lowest possible effective dose.
- Encourage physical activity to improve muscle strength, mobility and balance. Exercise can increase BMD. However, if osteoporosis is present the risk of high-impact exercise and falls needs to be considered.
- Review environment.

Management

- Manage presenting fracture and institute falls prevention strategies such as modifying the environment. Hip protectors, vision checks.
- Relieve pain.
- BMD to estimate initial bone loss or ongoing bone loss.
- Spinal radiographs to detect any unrecognised compression fractures.

Medications

- Medications are prescribed to prevent bone loss and/or increase bone mass.
- Dietary calcium and Vitamin D supplementation.
- Bisphosphonates such as alendronate and risedronate raloxifene, low-dose calcitriol, with regular monitoring of serum calcium and creatinine to prevent hypercalcaemia. If calcitriol is used, oral calcium supplements should be avoided to reduce the risk of hypercalcaemia. Dietary revision and advice may be needed. Teriparatide.

Diabetes

- Improve blood glucose control.
- Manage complications such as peripheral neuropathy, that increases the risk of falls, and gastroparesis that causes malabsorption.

5.10   Falls

Key points

- Falls are common in older people.
- Diabetes complications represent considerable falls risk, over and above the usual falls risk factors.
- Diabetes-specific contribution to falls risk is underrecognised in most currently used falls risk assessment tools.

Many factors contribute to falls. Falls are included with long-term diabetes complications because the complications significantly contribute to the falls risk. In addition, the contribution of diabetes, its treatment and complications was not included on any of the current falls risk tools identified.

   In 1998 in Australia, 1014 older people died as a direct consequence of falls and 45 069 were hospitalised because of falls (AIHW 2001). One in three people over

65 years fall at least once in a 12-month period (Sturmberg 2001; Hill *et al.* 2003). The falls rate in residential facilities is up to 50% and serious injuries occur in 9% of people who fall, in particular hip fractures, other fractures, lacerations and loss of confidence, which is not surprising given the incidence of chronic illnesses in older people (Krueger *et al.* 2001). People sustaining hip fractures are ten times more likely to live in care facilities than in the community. People who fall often do so repeatedly.

There is a great deal of research and literature relating to developing falls risk profiles, falls assessment tools and falls incident report tools, environmental falls hazard assessment tools and falls risk assessment and management tools (Commonwealth Department of Health and Aged Care 2000; Day *et al.* 2002). While many of these cite chronic medical conditions, foot problems, visual impairment and postural hypotension (Hill *et al.* 2003), consideration of other diabetes-specific contribution to falls is not generally included. Commonly, there is more than one reason for the fall and sometimes the cause of the fall is not immediately apparent.

Falls are the sixth leading cause of death in older people. Falls are multifactorial and can occur through the direct effect of the disease or indirect effects such as weakness, visual problems and poor balance. Table 5.7 outlines the diabetes-specific direct and indirect contribution to falls. These factors should be considered in addition to the falls risk factors usually documented. Only diabetes-specific information is addressed here.

5.10.1 Management

Management consists of:

(1) Prevention.
(2) Managing the consequences of the fall such as fractures, bruises, haematomas and lacerations.
(3) Managing the psychological and social consequences of falls.

Management strategies include the following.

- Appropriate risk assessment.
- Provide appropriate diabetes foot care. Comorbidities and insensate feet increase the falls risk (Wallace *et al.* 2002). Ensure appropriate footwear is worn, e.g. shoes with laces or buckles rather than slippers or slip-on shoes.
- Nutritional care is important. Falls risk increases with obesity. People with BMI >30 kg/m^2 are at increased risk of falls (Wallace *et al.* 2002). Vitamin D supplements improve the risk of osteoporosis (Bischoff-Ferrari *et al.* 2004).
- Manage blood glucose levels to prevent hypoglycaemia or hyperglycaemia and other short- and long-term complications that significantly increase the likelihood of falls.
- Ensure complication status is documented and assessed regularly to identify changing falls risk, including depression.
- Undertake regular medication review to ensure medicines, doses and dose intervals are appropriate. Try to prevent adverse drug-related events that might precipitate falls.
- Eliminate long-acting medicines, anticonvulsants, narcotics, OHAs and insulin, antihypertensives and some classes of antidepressants where possible or use at the lowest possible dose.
- Encourage mobility or exercise. Weekly regular exercise reduces falls (Barnett *et al.* 2003). The optimal type of physical activity depends on the individual, but

Table 5.7 The contribution diabetes makes to falls in older people. These factors should be considered in addition to existing falls risk assessment processes.

Diabetes-specific risk factor	Signs and symptoms	Consequences
Skin – dry, fragile skin	Skin tears and pressure ulcers. Bruises and haematoma. Fever may or may not be present.	
Infection – urinary tract, URTI, foot ulcers	Fever may or may not be present. Polyuria, nocturia, often 'silent'. May be offensive-smelling urine. Anorexia, breathing difficulties, confusion, behavioural change. Pain may or may not be present. Unstable gait.	Getting out of bed at night. Disturbed sleep. Impaired cognition. Impaired gait.
Dehydration – electrolyte imbalance, HONK, DKA	Hyperglycaemia. Dry skin and poor tissue turgor, dry mucous membranes. Lethargy. Altered consciousness. Polyuria, polydipsia, incontinence. Deterioration in functional status. Cardiac arrhythmias. Hyperglycaemia.	
Long-term complications Peripheral neuropathy	Pain may or may not be present. Tingling, burning, paraesthesia. Disturbed sleep. Changed foot structure.	Unsteady gait. Inability to sense how high they lift their feet and misgauging heights. Reduced mobility.
Autonomic neuropathy	Delayed food absorption/gastric emptying. Anorexia. Postural hypotension leading to dizziness. Constipation/diarrhoea.	Hypoglycaemia. Unsteady gait. Syncope.
Retinopathy	Visual loss.	
Nephropathy	Fatigue malaise. Hypertension. Oedema. Confusion.	Hypoglycaemia.
Cardiovascular disease, thrombosis	Hypertension. Confusion.	Stroke/MI. Syncope. Unsteady gait. Confusion.

Medicines
  Blood glucose lowering agents (OHA/insulin)
  Antihypertensives
  Diuretics
		Hypoglycaemia
		Postural hypotension
		Polyuria

strength and resistance training, balance re-education, tai chi, walking programmes and functional activity programmes have all been shown to reduce falls risk (Day *et al.* 2002). Agility training reduces the falls risk if it is maintained for at least six months. The possible need to adjust medicines and food intake should be considered when recommending exercise activity programmes to older people. Tai chi under appropriately qualified supervision is a useful exercise strategy to assist with improving balance, socialisation and physical and mental wellbeing (Schneider & Morgan 2004).

- Recognise and manage acute illness promptly.

5.11   Diabetes and wound management

Key points

- Diabetes affects all facets of wound healing and wound management.
- Assessment must include objective and subjective information pertaining to the wound and to the host.
- Wound healing is more difficult in older people with diabetes.
- Treat the cause and take a multidisciplinary approach.
- Treatment must include strategies other than wound products.
- Wounds must be regularly evaluated and documented with defined goals of treatment.

The existence of diabetes directly affects all facets of wound management in the older person with diabetes. In fact, diabetes itself can contribute to the development of a wound, for example diabetic foot wounds.

5.11.1   Normal ageing and wound healing

Initially, ageing can contribute to the development of a wound due to changes in skin structure, which increase the likelihood of injury. In addition, normal ageing affects the way wounds heal (Desai 1997). Ageing effects include:

- Changes in vascular function and thermoregulation.
- Reduced inflammatory response, thereby reducing the number of lymphocytes transported to the site.
- Reduced mast cells that are necessary for angiogenesis.
- Reduced number of growth factors released.
- Reduced quality in collagen formation, thereby reducing tensile strength and increasing the risk of dehiscence.

5.11.2   Effects of diabetes on wound healing

Diabetes affects all aspects of wound healing (Silhi 1998).

- Thirty to forty per cent of wound healing can be attributed to contraction, compared to 80–90% in people who do not have diabetes.

- Hyperglycaemia affects collagen synthesis and the capacity of phagocytes to travel to the wound site and engulf bacteria.
- Very poor glycaemic control results in dehydration that in turn affects the transport of waste products and healing mediators.
- Long-term poor glycaemic control (indicated by an HbA_{1c} >7%) causes red blood cells to become larger because of excessive glycosylation. As a result they have difficulty moving through the microcirculation, which reduces oxygen levels in the wound.
- Blood vessels are more rigid and therefore do not dilate in response to the initial inflammatory phase required for normal wound healing, thus oxygen exchange and white blood cell transport to the infected site are reduced.
- Increased fibrinogen levels thicken the blood, which slows transport.
- People with diabetes have increased circulating free radicals, which in turn allows macrophages to destroy a larger area of the wound during the reconstructive phase.

Diabetes can also make it difficult to assess a wound because:

- Blood vessels supplying the lower limbs are often calcified, which makes it difficult to obtain a correct Ankle Brachial Index (ABI) because the blood vessels around the calf cannot be compressed. The ABI is used to determine the presence of arterial disease in lower limbs and to diagnose whether the ulcer is arterial or venous.
- The absence or muting of the inflammatory response (redness, heat, swelling and pain) makes it difficult to identify whether infection is present.
- Absent or reduced sensation in the feet and lower limbs due to peripheral neuropathy can significantly reduce pain generated by wounds to those areas.

5.11.3   Wound assessment

Wound assessment in people with diabetes is the same as in non-diabetics. The most important aspect of wound management is performing a detailed wound assessment as well as determining the person's physical, mental and social history, nutritional status, medications and allergies, biochemistry and imaging results. The assessment enables the cause of the wound to be diagnosed and an appropriate management plan formulated. The plan should include using non-product strategies and appropriate wound product(s) that maximise wound healing. The wound should be reassessed at regular intervals to determine progress. As the wound changes, different combinations of wound products and non-product strategies will be required. Optimising diabetes control is an important consideration.

Wound healing may not be achievable in all older people with diabetes. Therefore, quality-of-life issues need to be incorporated in the wound management care plan. Wound management requires a team approach that includes the person with the wound and/or their carers. The following factors should be assessed.

History of the wound

Compile a detailed history of the wound.

- What caused it?
- Is it an acute or chronic wound? This may directly influence realistic healing targets; for example, a wound that has been present for two years is unlikely to heal in two weeks.

- What products have been used, for what length of time, how long were they kept *in situ* and were they evaluated (problems still exist in acute hospital units when nurses change wound product types from day to day)?
- What investigations were performed?
- Were antibiotics prescribed? If so, which ones? Were they effective?
- Who has been involved in treating the wound, for example the GP, naturopath, home visiting nursing service, self-management?
- Have other adjunct therapies been used such as hyperbaric oxygen, maggots?
- Have other therapies been used such as medical honey, vitamins, supplements or other complementary products? (Refer to Chapter 11.)
- Has the person applied their own home remedies to the wound?
- Did any allergies or painful reactions to treatments occur? If so, indicate what they were and how they were managed.

Skin

- Is the skin healthy and nourished or dry, thin and malnourished in appearance? Has the skin been badly damaged by sun? An increasing number of leg ulcers are skin cancer lesions.
- Is the surrounding skin inflamed, swollen and hot to touch? If any of these factors are present, they may indicate infection.
- Bruising.
- Old scars or signs of other pathologies such as venous eczema on the lower limbs in the presence of leg ulcers, allergies to medications or wound products, psoriasis.
- Injury to skin caused by tapes or other wound products.

Wound colour

The colour of the wound indicates the stage of healing and can denote the presence of infection. The common colours that differentiate stages are as follows.

- Pink – epithelisation.
- Red – healthy granulation.
- Yellow – slough.
- Green – infection. However, some zinc wound products will cause a greening of the wound exudate.
- Black – eschar.

Size of the wound

The size of the wound should be assessed at presentation and then on a regular basis.

- Measure the wound opening and always check for undermining by using a probe. If undermining is present outline the actual size of the wound by using a permanent marker on the skin.
- Measure the depth and use a probe to identify if sinuses are present.
- Use measuring tapes, measure grids and photographs, especially digital photographs that can be printed or downloaded onto electronic patient files, to record the healing process. They should be dated and a Bradma patient label attached.

Odour

The smell of the wound can be a clue to the presence of infection.

- An offensive odour could indicate infection. Some hydrocolloid dressings can leave a 'stale' odour and yellow exudate.
- Note whether the odour changes.

Exudate

Assess the presence or absence of any exudate.

- 'Relative' measurements of small, moderate and large.
- Note the colour of any exudate and the consistence and presence of bleeding or clots.
- Note whether the exudate changes.
- A green exudate invariably means infection. However, if a zinc-based dressing is used, wound exudate can turn green in the presence of zinc wound products and may not be indicative of infection.

Pain

The presence of pain may indicate infection, mechanical discomfort due to dressing or be unrelated to the wound. Note the type, site and degree of pain.

- Constant or intermittent.
- Sharp or dull.
- Relieved by analgesia.
- In the case of leg ulcers, is it relieved by raising or lowering the leg (very important when determining if a leg ulcer is arterial or venous in nature)?
- Pain may be absent due to reduced sensation caused by peripheral neuropathy. Consider referred pain, for example from changed gait due to peripheral neuropathy.

Other observations/investigations

- Wound swabs taken from clean wounds where pus has been expressed and not from old wound and dressing debris present when the dressing is initially removed.
- Biopsy is a more accurate method of assessing the bacterial burden in chronic wounds. All wounds are colonised by a variety of bacteria. When host resistance is compromised, for example where diabetes is combined with chronological age and comorbidities, the host is often overcome by the number or virulence of micro-organisms (Carville 1998).
- Blood tests that include haemoglobin to identify anaemia, albumin to identify protein status, a raised white cell count which may indicate infection, HbA_{1c} to determine glycaemic control, zinc and Vitamin C levels, which are important nutrients and supplements in wound healing.
- X-rays of diabetic foot ulcers often fail to identify osteomyelitis.
- Bone scans are useful to identify osteomyelitis.
- Sinusgram to determine extent of wound sinuses.

Diabetes

The degree of blood glucose control can affect wound healing. Note the:

- Type of diabetes: Type 1 or Type 2, steroid-induced diabetes.
- Duration of diabetes and treatment.
- Glycaemic control (HbA$_{1c}$ and capillary blood glucose testing). Poor control (HbA$_{1c}$ >7%), even short term, may require substantial management changes. The full diabetes team needs to be involved to deal with dietary needs, blood glucose monitoring, medication changes and, for example, commencing insulin. The podiatrist must be involved with all foot ulcers and in the modification of footwear.

Nutritional status

Nutritional status is an important determinant of wound healing. A significant number of older people are malnourished despite the appearance of being overweight, which is attributed to reduced activity rather than excessive calorie intake. Wounds require an increased intake of protein, calories and vitamins, which may need to be in the form of supplements. Perform a mini nutritional assessment or other similar tests (see Chapter 2), to identify clients over the age of 65 who are at risk or who are malnourished. Blood albumin levels are a useful indicator of nutritional status (normal >35 mmol/L). Identify the barriers to good nutrition (see Chapter 2). Coexisting autoimmune disorders, such as rheumatoid arthritis, in addition to affecting joints, can also be a causative factor for leg ulcers, vasculitis and vascular disease.

Medications

Many older people are on several medications in addition to their diabetic medications.

- Corticosteroids, which suppress the body's inflammatory response, reduce collagen synthesis and the number of available growth factors, cause hyperglycaemia, fluid retention, hypertension, muscle wasting and thinning of the skin.
- NSAIDS (including aspirin and paracetamol) suppress the inflammatory response and alter the availability of growth factors.
- Anticoagulants increase the risk of bleeding and affect angiogenesis.
- Beta blockers reduce circulation to lower limbs and the feet, often causing cold feet.
- Diuretics can affect angiogenesis
- ACE inhibitors can affect angiogenesis

Consider the possibility of adverse drug events that might have contributed to the wound in the first place such as trauma from a hypoglycaemic episode.

Reduced oxygen supply

This delays healing and can be caused by:

- Smoking.
- Respiratory disease.
- Vascular insufficiency.
- Anaemia.

Other factors to consider

- Abuse is common in older people and can lead to clotting dysfunction and Vitamin B deficiency that causes nerve damage. In addition, it causes brain and liver damage and clouds judgement and recognition of hypoglycaemia, putting the person at risk of trauma.
- Available financial resources to purchase wound products and treatments.
- Physical and cognitive ability to comply with the wound regimen.
- Level of social support available to assist with wound management at home and to attend assessment appointments.
- Degree of mobility.
- Continence.
- Consider whether quality of life can be obtained without the wound healing if a better management regimen cannot be attained.
- Are there wound 'ownership issues'? Are different health professionals and carers using a variety of wound products without a plan or detailed evaluation?
- Is the environment contributing to trauma, such as spills, handrails?

5.11.4   Wound treatment strategies

Wound products should be selected according to the type of wound, as in any person without diabetes. Commonly used wound dressings generally include film dressings, which have been shown to reduce the discomfort of painful peripheral neuropathy, hydrogels, foams, alginates, hydrocolloids, hydroactive, hydrofibre and silver-impregnated dressings.

Cadexomer iodine products are now used widely in diabetes wounds. Unlike other iodine products, they are not toxic to fibroblasts and reduce bacterial loads. The product can be applied to a wound as a powder (which can sometimes be initially uncomfortable as it has a 'drawing' effect on the wound bed), paste sheet or gel. The product is used widely within the community setting as it needs to remain *in situ* for three days. Over this time, iodine is slowly leaked into the wound bed and the polymers absorb the exudate. After three days the dark brown product is a white bulking paste. A secondary dressing such as foam is required. Cadexomer iodine may not be suitable for people with thyroid dysfunction and for large wounds over prolonged periods of time.

Medical honey contains antibacterial properties that appear effective against *Pseudomonas* and some antibiotic-resistant strains such as MRSA. Supermarket table honey does not contain the properties required to treat wounds. Medical honey requires a daily regimen and a secondary dressing and can be expensive to purchase, unlike the ineffective table honey.

Practice point

As a wound changes, so too must the product. Different stages of healing require different wound products.

Non-product wound-healing strategies

These include nutrition (see Chapter 2). Exudate contains protein; therefore highly exudating wounds lose a significant amount of protein. Protein supplements are often required as part of the total wound management plan. Protein drinks can be used or protein powders, which can be added to food and fluids without producing a detectible taste. Zinc and Vitamin C are required for wound healing. Some practitioners advocate zinc and Vitamin C supplements to assist with wound healing. Multivitamins are often used.

All pressure wounds require pressure to be relieved. Most neuropathic foot ulcers are in fact pressure ulcers, usually caused by footwear. Therefore, treatment includes modifying existing footwear or the purchase of new footwear. Putting the person with a neuropathic foot ulcer back into the offending shoe, the cause of their ulcer, will not promote healing (Mulder & Armstrong 2003; Maciejewski *et al.* 2004).

Some patients require total casting in order to completely relieve pressure on the ulcer, which may be required for many weeks and may impact on their mobility. Spencer (2000) identified the need for more investigation into the effectiveness of the wide range of pressure-relieving products and interventions when treating diabetic foot ulcers.

Improving glycaemic control assists overall wound management. Poor diabetes control over a prolonged period saturates red blood cells with glucose, reducing their ability to enter the microcirculation, especially to a wound bed. Hyperglycaemia increases the risk of infection and the likelihood of dehydration, which further reduces circulation effectiveness. Older people with a chronic wound may require insulin therapy to improve diabetes control and enhance wound healing.

Hyperbaric oxygen may enhance wound healing. When an individual breathes 100% oxygen during a 'dive' in a hyperbaric chamber, plasma oxygen increases and easily diffuses into tissues (Rowe 2001), including tissues that are often hypoxic in older people with multiple chronic conditions such as diabetes, hypertension and peripheral vascular disease. Diabetic wounds are considered more likely to have a deficient oxygen supply, which directly impacts on fibroblast proliferation and collagen synthesis. Hyperbaric oxygen often improves healing rates of diabetic foot ulcers and may even prevent lower limb amputations in some cases. Barriers to this therapy include:

- Availability of dive chambers.
- The intensive and long-term commitment required to attend a hyperbaric centre for half a day, five days each week for up to 20 weeks consecutively.
- Wounds still require dressings.
- Older people may have physical or cognitive conditions preventing them from accessing the service.

Surgical intervention may be required to enable healing to occur. Surgical interventions include insertion of a balloon or bypassing blocked leg arteries to improve arterial flow to the lower leg and to the foot. More recently, bypassing the smaller vessels in the foot has been pioneered with promising results.

5.11.5   Quality-of-life issues

People with chronic wounds are more likely to become depressed. Changes to body image, reduced mobility and a direct and very real impact on their financial resources to pay for wound treatments all affect a person's emotional capacity to deal with a chronic wound. The person may become increasingly isolated if their mobility is limited, the wound is odorous and causes embarrassment and when the wound is managed at home. Support groups for people with leg ulcers are being developed to provide social interaction and emotional support.

Practice point

Effective wound management requires a multidisciplinary approach.

References

Agarwal, R. (2001) Treatment of hypertension in patients with diabetes. Lessons from recent trials. *Cardiology Review*, **9**, 36–44.

Aly, N. & Weston, P. (2002) Autonomic neuropathy in older people with diabetes mellitus. *Journal of Diabetic Nursing*, **6**(1), 10–15.

American Diabetes Association (2003) *Clinical Management Guidelines.* http://care.dia-betesjnls.org/content/vol28/supp_1#POSITION STATEMENTS (accessed 20.2.04).

ANZDATA Registry (2000) *Australian and New Zealand Dialysis Transplant Registry.* Adelaide, South Australia.

Apelqvist, J., Bakker, K., Van Houtum, W., Nabuurs-Franssen, M. & Schaper, N. (2000) The international consensus and practical guidelines on the management and prevention of the diabetic foot. *Diabetes/Metabolism Research and Review*, **16**(suppl 1), s84–s92.

Araki, A., Murotani, Y., Kamimiya, F. & Ito, N. (2004) Low well-being is an independent predictor for stroke in elderly patients with diabetes mellitus. *JAGS*, **52**, 205–10.

Australian Institute for Health and Welfare (AIHW) (2001) *Falls by the Elderly in Australia. Trends and Data for 1998.* AIHW, Canberra.

Australian Pain Society (2004) www.aspc.org.au (accessed 2004).

Barclay, L. (2004) *Poor oral health linked to coronary heart disease.* http://medscape.com/viewarticle/469444?mpid=25173 (accessed 26.2.04).

Barnett, A., Smith, B., Lord, S., Williams, M. & Baumand, A. (2003) Community-based group exercise improves balance and reduces falls in at-risk older people: a randomised controlled trial. *Age and Ageing*, **32**(4), 407–14.

Bischoff-Ferrari, H., Dawson-Hughes, B. & Willett, W. *et al.* (2004) Effect of Vitamin D on falls: a meta-analysis. *Journal of the American Medical Association*, **291**(16), 1999–2006.

Brown, S. and Sharpless, J. (2004) Osteoporosis: an under-appreciated complication of diabetes. *Clinical Diabetes*, **22**(1), 10–20.

Bush, T. (1991) Epidemiology of cardiovascular disease in older persons. *Ageing*, **3**(1), 3–8.

Carville, K. (1998) *Wound Care Manual*, 3rd edn. Silver Chain Foundation, Perth.

Chan, M. (2001) Nutritional management in progressive renal failure *Current Therapeutics*, **42**(7), 23–7.

Chau, D. & Edelman, S. (2002) Osteoporosis and diabetes. *Clinical Diabetes*, **20**(3), 153–7.

Churchill, D. (1996) Indications for long-term results and limitations of peritoneal dialysis. In: *Replacement of Renal Function by Dialysis* (eds C. Jacobs, C. Kjellstrand, K. Koch & F. Winchester). Kluwer Academic Publishers, Boston.

Commonwealth Department of Health and Aged Care Injury Prevention Section by The National Aging Research Institute (2000) *An Analysis of Research on Preventing Falls Injury in Older People: Community, Residential Aged Care and Acute Care Settings.* Commonwealth Department of Health and Aged Care, Canberra.

Cumming, R., Mitchell, P., Craig, J. & Knight, J. (2004) Renal impairment and anaemia in a population-based study of older people. *Internal Medicine Journal*, **34**, 20–3.

Day, L., Fildes, B., Gordon, I., Fitzharris, M., Flamer, H. & Lord, S. (2002) Randomised factorial trial of falls prevention among older people living in their homes. *British Medical Journal*, **325**, 129–33.

DCCT (1993) The effect of intensive treatment of diabetes on the development and progression of long-term complications in insulin-dependent diabetes mellitus. *New England Journal of Medicine*, **329**, 977–87.

Department of Health (2001) *Diabetes National Service Framework: Standards for Diabetes Services.* Department of Health, London.

Desai, H. (1997) Ageing and wounds part 2: healing in older age. *Journal of Wound Care*, **6**(5), 237–9.

Doolittle, N. (1991) Clinical ethnography of lacunar stroke. *Journal of Neuroscienctific Nursing*, **20**, 169–73.

DRS (1981) Photocoagulation treatment of proliferative diabetic retinopathy: clinical implications of DRS findings. *Ophthalmology*, **88**, 583–600.

Duggan, S., Aylett, M., Eccles, M. & Ford, G. (1997) Defining hypertension in older people from primary care case notes review. *Journal of Human Hypertension*, **11**(3), 193–9.

Dunning, T. (2003) *Care of People With Diabetes*, 2nd edn. Blackwell Publishing, Oxford.

Durrance, S. (2003) Older adults and NSAIDs: avoiding adverse reactions. *Geriatric Nursing*, **24**(6), 348–52.

Ernst, E. (1998) Harmless herbs? A review of the recent literature. *American Journal of Medicine*, **104**(2), 170–8.

Ferrari, P., Hess, L., Pechere-Bertschi, A., Muggli, F. & Burnier, M. (2004) Reasons for not intensifying antihypertensive treatment (RIAT): a primary care antihypertensive intervention study. *Journal of Hypertension*, **22**(6), 1221–9.

Fonda, D. (2002) Urinary incontinence and bladder dysfunction in older persons. In: *Second International Consultation on Incontinence*, Paris, July 1–3 (eds P. Abrams *et al.*). Health Publications, Plymouth, UK.

Hansson, L. (1998) Hypertension in the elderly: state-of-the-art treatment. *British Journal of Urology*, **81**(1), 17–20.

Hansson, L. (1999) Recent intervention trials in hypertension initiated in Sweden – HOT, CAPPP and others. *Clinical and Experimental Hypertension*, **21**(5–6), 507–15.

Hansson, L., Petitet, A. & Safar, M. (1995) Blood pressure and serum lipids in hypertensive men and women aged 60–97 years. *Blood Pressure Supplement*, **3**, 26–30.

Hill, K., Barrett, C., Smith, R. & Lindeman, M. (2003) Falls. In: *Aged Care Nursing. A Guide to Practice* (eds S. Carmody & S. Forster). Ausmed Publications. Melbourne.

HOPE Study Investigators (2000) Effects of ramipril on cardiovascular and microvascular outcomes in people with diabetes mellitus: results of the HOPE study and MICRO-HOPE substudy. *Lancet*, **355**, 253–9.

Horn, S., Bender, S. & Ferguson, M. *et al.* (2004) The national pressure ulcer long term care study. *Journal of the American Geriatrics Society*, **52**(3), 359–67.

Howes, L. (2001) Dosage alterations in the elderly: importance of mild renal impairment. *Current Therapeutics*, **42**(7), 33–5.

Huang, E., Meigs, J. & Singer, D. (2001) The effect of interventions to prevent cardiovascular disease in patients with type 2 diabetes. *American Medical Journal*, **11**(8), 663–42.

International Diabetes Federation Consultative Section on Diabetes (2000) *Position Statement on Diabetes Education for People who are Blind or Visually Impaired.* International Diabetes Federation, Brussels.

Ivan, C., Seshadri, S. & Beiser, A. *et al.* (2004) Dementia after stroke: the Framingham Study. *Stroke*, **35**(6), 1264–8.

Karlson, B., Herlitz, J. & Hjalmarson, A. (1993) Prognosis of acute myocardial infarction in diabetic and non-diabetic patients. *Diabetic Medicine*, **10**, 449–54.

Keane, W. (2001) Metabolic pathogenesis of cardiorenal disease. *American Journal of Kidney Disease*, **38**(6), 1372–5.

Klag, M., Whelton, P. & Randau, B. *et al.* (1996) Blood pressure and end-stage renal disease in men. *New England Journal of Medicine*, **334**(1), 13–18.

Ko, R. (1998) Adulterants in Asian patent medicines. *New England Journal of Medicine*, **339**, 847.

Koepsall, T., Wolf, M., Buchner, D. *et al.* (2004) Footwear style and risk of falls in older adults. *Journal of the American Geriatrics Society*, **52**, 1495–501.

Krueger, P., Brazil, K. & Lohfeld, L. (2001) Risk factors for falls and injuries in a long-term care facility in Ontario. *Canadian Journal of Public Health*, **92**(2), 117–20.

Lipsky, B. & Berendt, A. (2000) Principles and practice of antibiotic therapy of diabetic foot infections. *Diabetes/Metabolism Research and Reviews*, **16**(suppl 1), s42–s46.

Maciejewski, M., Wallace, C., Reiber, G., Hayes, S., Smith, D. & Boyko, E. (2004) Effectiveness of diabetes therapeutic footwear in preventing reulceration. *Diabetes Care*, **27**(7), 1774–82.

Malmberg, K., Ryden, L., Efendic, S., Herlitz, J., Nicol, P. & Waldenstrom, A. (1995) Randomised trial of insulin-glucose infusion followed by subcutaneous insulin treatment in diabetic patients with acute myocardial infarction (DIGAMI study) effects on mortality at 1 year. *Journal of the American College of Cardiology*, **26**, 57–65.

Medical Medscape News (2004) *Pergolide helpful for restless legs syndrome.* http://www.medscape.com (accessed May 2004).

Merritt, S. (2004) Sleep-disordered breathing and the association with cardiovascular risk. *Cardiovascular Nurse*, **19**(1), 19–27.

Mulder, G. & Armstrong, D. (2003) Management of the diabetic foot ulcer in the elderly population. *Clinical Geriatrics*, **11**(4), 46–53.

Myhre, M. (2000) Herbal remedies, nephropathies and renal disease. *Nephrology Nursing Journal*, **27**(5), 473–80.

National Heart Foundation (2003) *Medical Journal of Australia*, **178**, 272–6.

National Kidney Foundation (2002) Clinical practice guidelines for nutrition in chronic renal failure. Kidney outcome quality initiative. *American Journal of Kidney Disease*, **35**(96), suppl 2.

O'Brien, R. (2003) Aspirin use in diabetes Part 2: dosage and treatment recommendations. *International Journal of Metabolism by Fax*, **VI**(19), I.

Oyibo, S., Richard, B. & McLay, L. *et al.* (2002) Blood glucose overestimation in diabetic patients on continuous ambulatory peritoneal dialysis for end-stage renal disease. *Diabetic Medicine*, **19**, 693–6.

Parving, H., Lehnert, N., Brochner-Mortensen, J., Gomis, R., Anderson, S. & Arner, P. (2001) The effect if Ibesartan on the development of diabetic nephropathy in patients with type 2 diabetes. *New England Journal of Medicine*, **345**, 870–8.

Pfisterer, M. (2004) Long-term outcome in elderly patients with chronic angina managed invasively versus by optimized medical therapy: four year follow-up of the randomized Trial of Invasive versus Medical therapy in Elderly patients (TIME). *Circulation*, **110**(10), 1213–18.

Phillips, P., Popplewell, P. & Wing, L. (2003) Diabetes and hypertension – double trouble. *Medicine Today*, 1–9.

Ragab, S., Lunt, M., Birch, A., Thomas, P. & Jenkinson, D. (2004) Caffeine reduces cerebral blood flow in patients recovering from an ischaemic stroke. *Age and Ageing*, **33**(3), 299–303.

Ramsay, L., Williams, B. & Johnston, G. *et al.* (1999) Guidelines for management of hypertension. *Journal of Human Hypertension*, **13**(9), 569–92.

Ravid, M., Savin, H. & Jutrin, I. (1993) Long-term stabilising effect of angiotensin-convertin enzyme on plasma creatinine and on proteinuria in normotensive Type II diabetic patients. *Annals of Internal Medicine*, **118**, 577–81.

Ritz, E. (2001) Advances in nephrology: success and lessons learnt from diabetes. *Nephrology Dialysis Transplant*, **16**(suppl 7), 46–50.

Rix, M., Andreassen, H. & Eskildsen, P. (1999) Impact of peripheral neuropathy on bone density in patients with Type 1 diabetes. *Diabetes Care*, **22**, 827–31.

Ronaldson, S. (2000) *Spirituality. The Heart of Nursing*. Ausmed, Melbourne.

Rowe, K. (2001) Hyperbaric oxygen therapy: what is the case for its use? *Journal of Wound Care*, **10**(4), 117–21.

Ruskin, P. & Rosenstock, J. (1992) The genetics of diabetes complications. Blood glucose and genetic susceptibility. In: *International Textbook of Diabetes Mellitus* (eds K. Albert, R. DeFronzo, H. Keen & P. Zimmet). John Wiley, Chichester.

Rutecki, G. & Whittier, F. (1993) Intraperitoneal insulin in diabetic patients on peritoneal dialysis. In: *Dialysis Therapy* (eds A. Nissenson & R. Fine). Hanley & Belfus, Philadelphia.

Schneider, C. & Morgan, S. (2004) Tai Chi and fall prevention in the elderly. *Alternative Medicine Alert*, **7**(1), 1–4.

Schwarz, A., Sellmeyer, D. & Ensrud, K. *et al.* (2001) Older women with diabetes have an increased risk of fracture: a perspective study. *Journal of Clinical Endocrinology and Metabolism*, **86**, 32–8.

Silhi, N. (1998) Diabetes and wound healing. *Journal of Wound Care*, **7**(1), 47–51.

Simons, L., Simons, J., Freedlander, Y., McCallum, J. & Palanioppan, L. (2003) Risk functions for prediction of cardiovascular disease in elderly Australians: Dubbo study. *Medical Journal of Australia*, **178**, 113–6.

Skoog, L. (1998) Status of risk factors for vascular dementia. *Neuroepidemiology*, **17**, 2–9.

Spencer, S. (2000) Pressure relieving intervention for preventing and treating diabetic foot ulcers. In: *Cochrane Database of Systematic Reviews*, Issue 3. Cochrane Library, Oxford.

St. Vincents Hospital (2004) *Departmental Policy for Managing People with Diabetes Having Procedures in Radiology*. St. Vincent's Hospital, Melbourne.

Standl, E. & Schnell, O. (2000) A new look at the heart in diabetes: from ailing to failing. *Diabetalogia*, **43**, 1455–69.

Stranders, I., Diamant, M. & Gelder, R. (2004) Admission blood glucose levels as risk indicator of death after myocardial infarction in patients with and without diabetes mellitus. *Archives of Internal Medicine*, **164**, 982–8.

Sturmberg, J. (2001) Falls in the elderly. *Australian Family Physician*, **30**(6), 583–6.

Tapp, R. (2004) Diabetes care in an Australian population: frequency screening examinations for eye and foot complications of diabetes. *Diabetes Care*, **27**, 688–93.

Terrill, B. (2002) *Renal Nursing: A Practical Approach*. Ausmed Publications, Melbourne.

Therapeutic Guidelines: Antibiotics (2003) Therapeutic Guidelines Ltd, Melbourne.

Therapeutic Guidelines: Endocrinology (2004) Therapeutic Guidelines Ltd, Melbourne.

Trenkwalder, C., Hundemer, H. & Lledo, A. *et al.*, the PEARLS Study Group (2004) Efficacy of pergolide in treatment of restless legs syndrome: the PEARLS Study. *Neurology*, **62**(8), 1391–7.

UKPDS Group (1998) Intensive blood glucose control with sulphonylureas or insulin compared with conventional treatment and risk of complications in patients with Type 2 diabetes (UKPDS 33). *Lancet*, **352**, 837–53.

Vale, J., Jelinek, M., Best, J. & Santamaria, J. (2002) Coaching patients with coronary heart disease to achieve cholesterol targets: a method to bridge the gap between evidence-based medicine and the 'real world' – randomised controlled trial. *Journal of Clinical Epidemiology*, **55**, 245–52.

Vinik, A., Park, T., Stansberry, K. & Henger, P. (2000) Diabetic neuropathy. *Diabetologia*, **43**, 957–73.

Wallace, C., Ruber, B. & LeMaster, J. *et al.* (2002) Incidence of falls, risk factors for falls, and fall-related fractures in individuals with diabetes and a prior foot ulcer. *Diabetes Care*, **25**(11), 1983–6.

Wang, C., Collet, J. & Lau, J. (2004) The effect of tai chi on health outcomes in patients with chronic conditions: a systematic review. *Archives of Internal Medicine*, **164**(5), 493–501.

Wetter, T., Stiasny, K. & Winkelmann, J. *et al.* (1999) A randomized controlled study of pergolide in patients with restless legs syndrome. *Neurology*, **52**(5), 944–50.

World Health Organization (1994) *Assessment of Fracture Risk and Its Application to Screening for Postmenopausal Osteoporosis*. Report of a WHO Study Group, Geneva.

Wu, M., Yu, C. & Yang, C. (1997) Poor pre-dialysis glycaemic control is a predictor of mortality in Type II diabetic patients on maintenance haemodialysis. *Nephrology Dialysis Transplant*, **12**, 2105–10.

Chapter 6
Educating and Communicating with Older People

Trisha Dunning

Key points

- Older people often do not receive adequate diabetes education.
- Education needs to be tailored for older people and aim to foster self-efficacy and self-esteem.
- Older people like to have advice in writing.
- Older people are individuals and 33% were born overseas, therefore information should be culturally relevant and supplied according to individual needs.
- Regular knowledge assessment is important.
- Information must be consistent between all health professionals caring for older people with diabetes.
- Carers and significant others should be included in the education programme.

6.1   Introduction

Diabetes education is an integral part of the management of diabetes and is an ongoing process. However, diabetes education programmes often do not meet the needs or learning styles of older people (Bruce *et al.* 2003). The goal of diabetes education programmes is to assist people to accept their diabetes and integrate the diabetes management tasks into their lifestyle to achieve and maintain a balanced lifestyle and optimum metabolic control. Some older people are unable to perform some self-care tasks and require assistance. In these cases their carers also need education. However, in 1999, 69% of older people lived in family households, mostly with their partners. Only 8% lived in residential aged care facilities (AIHW 2002).

Standardised diabetes education guidelines exist, but most are not developed for older people. In addition, each person should be assessed and a teaching plan developed to ensure individual learning needs are addressed. As with younger people with diabetes, the education requirement consists of survival and ongoing education. Survival skills, which refer to the minimum information required for the person to be safe at home, enable the person to understand what diabetes is and how to care for themselves. Ongoing education consists of continuing to provide information as required.

The psychological and intellectual changes that accompany normal ageing can affect how education is provided and the outcome of education sessions. These changes include:

- Decline in short-term memory.
- Small decline in both simple and complex motor performance.
- Reduction in reaction time by approximately 20%, usually affecting information processing such as decision making. The reaction time declines further when:
  (1) complex decisions are required
  (2) the stimulus or cue to action is weak or not relevant to the individual
  (3) the motor sequence needed to complete the task is complex.
- Reduced ability to understand concepts.
- Increased cautiousness and unwillingness to change or take risks.
- Low self-image and self-efficacy, which may inhibit the person from participating in group programmes (Crandall 1980; Pitt 1986).
- Sensory loss.

However, despite these changes healthy older people retain their verbal ability, long-term memory, judgement and creativity unless they have cognitive impairment, dementia or depression. Major depression is closely associated with inadequate self-care in people with diabetes, including compliance with medicines, blood glucose monitoring, exercise and diet, and the use of more medical services (Lin *et al.* 2004).

6.2   Characteristics of older learners

Older learners are, by definition, adults. Therefore the principles of adult learning apply to older people. Essentially adults:

- Have established beliefs, attitudes, problem-solving and decision-making processes, behaviours and habits.
- Have a great deal of life experience. They learn best when the information is relevant to their everyday lives and they can put new information into the context of what they already know.
- Like to have an overview of what the education session will involve. The education is more likely to be effective if the person:
  (1) believes they need information about diabetes
  (2) believes their lives will be affected if they do not know about diabetes and how to manage it
  (3) has confidence in their ability to manage
  (4) expects and actually has positive benefits from the education.
- Learn by sharing their experiences with other people and bring a variety of experiences and knowledge to any learning encounter; therefore, they respond to interactive teaching styles.

However, as people grow older some of these factors change and older people may:

- Have poor self-esteem and hearing and vision problems that make it difficult for them to participate in education sessions.
- Be reluctant to ask questions and become passive learners.
- Have fixed beliefs and behaviours, which may be at odds with those needed for appropriate diabetes care.

- Have cognitive, sensory or physical deficits that impact on their ability to learn or perform tasks.
- Be isolated, have financial burdens or depression, all of which inhibit learning.
- Not regard diabetes as serious or a priority in their lives. Many of these factors also apply to younger people with diabetes.

Health professionals often have specific ideas about what could/should be taught and what older people are capable of learning and doing, especially in residential aged care where learned helplessness develops (Weinberg & Chappell 1996). Learned helplessness refers to the feeling of not being in control of one situation and transferring the feeling to other situations. Effective education for older people should be based on providing simple, concise, relevant information delivered at a pace to suit the individual, and maintaining autonomy as far as possible is essential. An empowering education framework allows the individual's needs to be clarified and opportunities for negotiation to take place to ensure essential issues are not overlooked.

Education encounters evoke emotional as well as cognitive and rational feelings. The following issues need to be assessed when designing an empowering education encounter for older people.

- How to encourage older people to identify and express what they wish to know about diabetes management.
- The individual's feelings and beliefs.
- Psychosocial situation (see the ecomap in Chapter 2).
- Education level.
- Coping style
- Learning style. Enquiries about what worked in the past can help identify the best way to structure the education session.
- Goals for the session and future education sessions.
- Ability to carry out self-care behaviours.

The learning process for older people is much more effective if a partnership based on mutual respect can be established (Coulter 1997). Health professionals can have a powerful influence on the beliefs and attitudes of their patients and must use the relationship with integrity (Dunning & Martin 1998).

6.3 Survival skills

Survival skills are taught at diagnosis. The specific information needed depends on the type of diabetes the person has and the treatment. Where relevant, the family or carers should be involved. Minimal information for safety is given and written information to aid memory and act as a cue to action should be supplied. However, specific concerns/questions need to be addressed even when written information is supplied.

Some relevant survival skills are the ability to:

- Know the effect of medicines and food on blood glucose levels.
- Name their insulin or medicines or carry a list in their health record.
- Demonstrate correct care and administration of insulin.
- Correctly monitor their blood or urine glucose and ketones and appropriately document the results.
- Realise the significance of ketones in the urine and the appropriate response.

- Recognise the signs and symptoms, causes and appropriate treatment of hypoglycaemia.
- Know why it is important to have regular meals containing an appropriate amount of carbohydrate and low fat.
- Know who and how to contact if help is required.
- Demonstrate safe disposal of sharps.
- Care for their feet.

A sample diabetes education record of survival information and a plan for further teaching is shown in Table 6.1.

Table 6.1 Sample diabetes survival information record.

DIABETES EDUCATION RECORD

Patient details/Bradma

Name: ....

Address:

....

....

D.O.B.: ....

Language spoken: ....

Understanding of primary language/English: good ☐   fair ☐   poor ☐
Other communication issues, e.g.
  Cognitive deficit:
  Hearing ☐ with hearing aid
  Vision   ☐ with glasses

How assessed? ....

Indicate perceived level of skill and understanding attained:

....

....

Information covered:

  1. What is diabetes? ....

  2. Management:

  - diet ....

  - exercise ....

Table 6.1 (*cont'd*)

• tablets ....

• insulin ....

3. Blood glucose monitoring □ Method ....

4. Urine blood ketone testing ....

5. Urine glucose testing □ Method ....

6. Insulin administration □ Method ....

7. When to take medications ....

8. Possible adverse effects of medications ....

9. Sharps disposal ....

10. Hypos .... 11. Sick days ....

12. Foot care .... 13. Exercise ....

14. Dentist .... 15. Travel & driving ....

Other information discussed:

....

....

Family/carer support:

....

....

Education material supplied (list):

....

....

Blood glucose record book ....

Further education required: Yes □   No □

MedicAlert:

Enrolment in Diabetic Association: ....

6.4   Ongoing education

Education can be continued on an individual basis or in group programmes. Education is a lifelong process. Both individual and group sessions are usually employed. Group programmes can be effectively carried out in retirement settings (Wendel et al. 2003). The same may be true of low-level care and can address transport difficulties, costs, reduced mobility and social isolation.

Groups have been shown to improve satisfaction with care and lead to better health outcomes and uptake of preventive care such as immunisation (Beck et al. 1997). In addition, attendances at emergency departments and hospital admissions were reduced. Evaluation from older participants in group programmes indicates that weekly sessions over one to one and a half hours aid information retention and enhance socialisation (Wendel et al. 2003).

Over time, the individual should gradually learn how to:

- Cope in special situations, such as eating out, managing during travel and exercise/activity, in terms of medication and food intake.
- Undertake or seek appropriate foot care to prevent foot problems and hospital admissions.
- Maintain acceptable blood glucose control.
- Ensure they have regular examination of the eyes, feet, blood pressure, cardiovascular system and kidney function to prevent or delay the development of long-term diabetic complications.

6.5   Useful teaching strategies for educating older people

It is essential to carry out a physical and mental and education assessment to identify knowledge deficits and facilitators of and barriers to learning. Assessment tools such as ADLs and mini-mental examinations might be useful and the learning goals of the individual need to be defined. Strategies include the following.

- Give people the option of having relatives or carers present.
- Pace the teaching according to the needs of the individual or group. Allow time.
- Proceed from the simplest information to more complex concepts/tasks.
- Break each topic into smaller chunks and use illustrations and practical examples to explain the information.
- Allow people to practise skills or solve problems.
- Use a variety of teaching methods to cater for individual learning styles.
- Seek feedback, ask questions and involve people in the teaching encounter.
- Allow time, but do not have sessions too long because it is difficult for older people to concentrate for long periods and sitting may become uncomfortable.
- Use clear concise handouts to complement and reinforce the information provided. Researchers have shown that older people find handouts valuable (McKenna et al. 2003). Older people indicate that they refer to and follow written health information. Conversely, in the same study, GPs only issued written material if the person asked for it or thought the person was interested. They were mostly likely to hand out information provided by self-help organisations, specialist clinics,

government health departments or pharmaceutical companies. They were least likely to use Internet or other electronic material. Participants in Wendel *et al.*'s (2003) study also indicated that they welcomed written information and that large-print, easy-to-see information helped them remember what they had been taught.

These findings suggest that an important aspect of diabetes education is alerting people to the need to ask for written information. Using non-glossy paper and having a clear contrast between the background and the print can enhance readability. For example, black print on a red background is difficult to read and pastel colours often look alike to older people.

In general, font size should be at least 14–16 and in sentence case. All upper case letters (capitals) are difficult to read. Sans serif fonts are also preferable. Spacing the information and using short, simple sentences in active language make it easier for older people to absorb the information. If necessary, SMOG, FLESCH or CLOZE readability tests can be performed.

- Plan to deliver the education at an appropriate time and in a suitable quiet, well-lit environment.
- When using empty food packages as examples, provide 'no name' brands as well as brand names to cater for people on a limited budget.
- Use food models to demonstrate serving sizes of relevant foods on a standard plate.
- Supermarket tours, modifying recipes and exercise programmes promote learning, socialisation and support.
- Consider referring the person to other non-diabetes education programmes such as arthritis management.

6.6   The learning environment

Having an appropriate learning environment is as important as the teaching strategy. Important environmental aspects to consider are:

- A quiet environment without distractions such as busy posters, music, passers-by.
- Adequate lighting.
- Comfortable temperature.
- A clean uncluttered teaching space.
- Adequate contrast between the background and teaching material, which applies to equipment as well as written material.
- Ensuring the older person has their hearing aid switched on and appropriate glasses.
- Ensuring the individual is comfortably seated and free of pain.
- Planning the education session so that it does not conflict with another important activity such as a meal or outing.
- Ensuring access is easy for people in wheel chairs or on walking frames or using walking sticks.

Practice points

Education methods that incorporate behavioural strategies and experiential learning and are offered in small chunks, are more likely to be effective.

6.7 Empowerment

Diabetes education is appropriate and essential for older people but knowledge alone will not necessarily result in appropriate health behaviours or self-care. Beliefs, attitudes, satisfaction and disease status are some of the factors that affect knowledge and behaviour. These factors are not constant and they need to be assessed on a regular basis, for example deciding what is happening at the particular time, what could/will change and how the changes will affect the individual and their relatives or their care needs.

Empowerment models of diabetes education are based on shared governance and consideration of the whole person. Empowerment models emerged when health professionals realised that people with diabetes must be, and mostly want to be, responsible for their own care. Empowerment arises from three basic characteristics.

(1) The person with diabetes makes choices that affect their health care.
(2) The individual is in control of what they learn and the self-care practices they adopt.
(3) The consequences of their choices affect their diabetes outcomes.

Therefore, empowerment is a collaborative approach to care where management is designed to help the individual make informed choices and maximise their knowledge, skills and self-awareness. Empowering education strategies requires health professionals to accept the legitimacy of an individual's goals, even if they result in suboptimal control (Anderson *et al.* 1996). An essential aspect of empowerment is that the individual is responsible for their decisions. However, some people require specific instructions. In addition, stress and anxiety at specific times can impair an individual's ability to take control in acute situations, as can cognitive and physical deficits.

Practice point

Health professionals must provide consistent information to avoid confusing the individual.

6.8 The role of the nurse in educating older people

Education is an independent nursing function and is a vital part of the diabetic treatment plan. Therefore, teaching older people in acute, community and residential care facilities is well within the scope of professional nursing practice. Some key points should be kept in mind when educating older people with diabetes.

● The aim of diabetes education is to achieve autonomy and empowerment within the limits and capacity of the individual.
● Consider the psychological and social impact of diabetes on the individual and their carers.
● Encourage questions and discussion.
● Ask open questions, allow people time to respond and use active listening.

Table 6.2 Factors that influence teaching and learning. Reproduced with permission from Dunning 2003.

Factor	Patient	Nurse
Health beliefs	✓	✓
Social support	✓	
Wellbeing/illness	✓	✓
Environment	✓	✓
Knowledge	✓	✓
Skills	✓	✓
Time	✓	✓
Perceived responsibility	✓	✓
Work priority		✓
Perception of teaching role		✓

- Teach specific skills and allow the person time to practise new skills, such as administering insulin.
- Encourage people to discuss their difficulties and concerns about diabetes.
- Relate new information to the person's experience.
- Provide written information in an appropriate format.

In acute care settings, learning is facilitated when the need/readiness to learn is perceived and immediately applied in a given situation; that is, 'teaching at a teachable moment'. Teachable moments often occur when the ward staff are performing routine nursing care such as blood glucose tests or giving injections.

Teaching is non-verbal as well as verbal. In fact, >60% of communication is non-verbal. People learn by observation so the nurse can be a role model and care should be taken to perform procedures correctly and to refer questions to another person if the answer is not known. In this way, formal and informal ongoing education in the ward is possible and desirable.

Many factors can influence teaching and learning. Some of these are shown in Table 6.2. It is the responsibility of the teacher to ensure that the environment is not distracting. Noise in a busy ward can make conversation difficult and hinder learning. The patient should be as comfortable as possible and free from pain.

6.8.1 Encouraging self-management

People learn about their individual responses to illness through trial and error (Kralik *et al.* 2004). Therefore, education programmes where the individual plays a passive role may not be successful. Learning diabetes self-management can be a dynamic, interactive process that enables the individual to actively self-care despite physical and mental limitations. Manias *et al.* (2004) identified several issues that need to be addressed in acute care settings to promote self-care.

- Being willing to encourage people to monitor their own blood glucose and administer insulin.
- If possible, adjusting medicine administration times to be consistent with home times.

- Carefully explaining any new medicines and what they are for.
- Allowing the person to use their familiar medicine systems such as Dosette boxes and insulin administration devices.
- Appropriately tailoring structured learning opportunities for people with poor cognition can enable older people to administer insulin and monitor their blood glucose levels (Braun *et al.* 2004).

References

Anderson, R., Funnel, M. & Arnold, M. (1996) Using the empowerment approach to help patients change behaviour. In: *Practical Psychology for Clinicians* (eds B. Anderson & R. Rubin). American Diabetes Association, Alexandria.

Australian Institute of Health and Welfare (AIHW) (2002) *Australia's Health No. 8*. AIHW, Canberra.

Beck, A., Scott, J., Williams, P. *et al.* (1997) A randomised trial of group outpatient visits for chronically ill older HMO members. The Cooperative Health Care Clinic. *Journal of the American Geriatrics Society*, **45**, 543–9.

Braun, A., Miller, A., Miller, R., Leppertt, K. & Schiel, R. (2004) Structured treatment and teaching of patients with type 2 diabetes mellitus and impaired cognition function – the DICOF trial. *Diabetic Medicine*, **21**, 999–1006.

Bruce, D., Davis, W., Cull, C. & Davis, T. (2003) Diabetes education and knowledge in patients with type 2 diabetes from the community: the Fremantle Diabetes Study. *Journal of Diabetes and Its Complications*, **17**, 82–9.

Coulter, A. (1997) Partnerships with patients: the pros and cons of shared clinical decision making. *Journal of Health Service Policy*, **2**, 112–21.

Crandall, R. (1980) *Gerontology: A Behavioural Science Approach*. Addison-Wesley, London.

Dunning, T. (2003) *Care of People with Diabetes*, 2nd edn. Blackwell Publishing, Oxford.

Dunning, P. & Martin, M. (1998) Type 2 diabetes: is it serious? *Journal of Diabetes Nursing*, **2**, 70–6.

Kralik, D., Koch, T., Price, K. & Howard, N. (2004) Chronic illness self-management: taking action to create order. *Journal of Clinical Nursing*, **13**, 259–67.

Lin, E., Katon, W. & Von Kroff, M. (2004) Relationship of depression and diabetes self-care, medication adherence, and preventative care. *Diabetes Care*, **27**, 2154–60.

Manias, E., Beanland, C., Riley, R. & Baker, L. (2004) Self-administration of medication in hospital: patient's perspectives. *Journal of Advanced Nursing*, **42**(2), 194–203.

McKenna, K., Tooth, L., King, D. *et al.* (2003) Older patients request more information: a survey of use of written patient education materials in general practice. *Australasian Journal on Ageing*, **22**(1), 15–19.

Pitt, M. (1986) *Psycho-Geriatrics*. Churchill Livingstone, London.

Weinberg, L. & Chappell, N. (1996) *Perceived Control and Learned Helplessness in Older People: Choice and Powerful Others*. Centre on Ageing, University of Melbourne, Melbourne.

Wendel, I., Duros, S., Zable, B., Loman, K. & Remsburg, R. (2003) Group diabetes patient education. A model for use in a continuing care retirement community. *Diabetes Educator*, **28**(1), 37–44.

Chapter 7
Rehabilitation, Respite and Palliative Care

Trisha Dunning

Key points

- Older people account for the majority of participants in general rehabilitation programmes.
- Older people's premorbid functional and cognitive statuses are strong determinants of the outcome of rehabilitation.
- Older people benefit from rehabilitation programmes, especially when the disability is recent.
- Rehabilitation should start as soon as possible.
- Rehabilitation may be a direct consequence of having diabetes.
- The rehabilitation process may take longer in the older person with diabetes.
- Rehabilitation is an opportunity to address diabetes self-care deficits and implement and evaluate new management strategies to reduce risks.
- Disability can impact on the individual's sense of control and motivation to maintain their diabetes management.
- Caring for older people with diabetes can be a significant burden on family caregivers especially if they are also old.

7.1 Rehabilitation

Older people with diabetes may require rehabilitation after an acute short-term complication, such as ketoacidosis or hyperosmolar coma, or as a consequence of long-term complications such as retinopathy or amputation, or because of general disability as a consequence of age or comorbidities (see Chapters 4 and 5). In general terms, rehabilitation aims to restore function in disabled people or limit the amount of assistance they require (Cameron & Kurrle 2002). For older people, rehabilitation is often required to help them manage the usual activities of daily living (ADLs), including diabetes self-care tasks.

Older people need to be assessed initially to ensure they are referred to the most appropriate programme. People with cognitive impairment or who were not independently self-caring before the need for rehabilitation arose are likely to have different outcomes from those who were fully independent. The Barthel Index can be used to establish the degree of assistance needed to perform ADLs; however, it may not adequately reflect ability to manage diabetes self-care tasks such as blood glucose testing or medication management.

Rehabilitation occurs in acute, subacute and residential aged care settings and in the person's home. Goals should be specific and the outcomes monitored according to the presenting problem. For example, grooming and feeding ability usually precede climbing stairs after a stroke (Cameron & Kurrle 2002). Amputee programmes should focus on stump as well as foot care. In addition to impaired function, the social and psychological consequences and risk of depression need to be assessed. The presence of depression is likely to affect the rehabilitation process and outcomes. A number of factors affect the extent of impairment.

- The disease process/cause of the impairment, including duration, severity, type of disability and the extent to which it can be corrected.
- Individual patient factors such as physical status, presence of comorbidities, psychological outlook, coping strategies, willpower.
- Degree of support available, resources including finances, the services available in the health sector and community (Sinclair & Finucane 2001).

Rehabilitation should commence as soon as possible to limit the functional decline that comes from immobility and the associated risk of further comorbidities such as pneumonia, weakness and loss of muscle bulk and strength, pressure areas and apathy and social isolation. There are many well-described rehabilitation programmes for amputees, people who have had a stroke or myocardial infarction and vision loss and older people should be encouraged to attend. The education and self-care plan as well as medication regimen may need to be adjusted.

Rehabilitation has been defined as the processes involved in restoring and maximising an individual's physical, mental and social level of functioning (Gray et al. 2002). Older people with diabetes are often over-represented in both inpatient and outpatient rehabilitation services and programmes, probably due to the long-term health problems associated with having diabetes, such as stroke, myocardial infarction, falls and lower limb amputation. According to Sinclair & Finucane (2001), 'the elderly diabetic patient tends to have the worst of both worlds, with multiple impairments both related and unrelated to diabetes'. These impairments include:

- Visual impairment caused by retinopathy and/or a higher incidence of glaucoma and cataracts.
- Peripheral neuropathy resulting in a higher risk of falls and foot ulceration, which may lead to lower digit or limb amputation.
- Mononeuropathies such as Bell's palsy.
- Autonomic neuropathy leading to postural hypotension, hypoglycaemic unawareness, falls and other debilitating conditions.
- Tissue glycolysation causing conditions such as carpal tunnel syndrome.
- Higher rate of cognitive impairment from Alzheimer's disease or vascular dementia.

Therefore, older people with diabetes may not fit into typical clinical pathways and short-term rehabilitation programmes. If their degree of disability is significant, the risk of depression increases. The rehabilitation process also directly impacts on family members, many of whom may have had little input into the individual's diabetes management prior to the occurrence of a critical incident, such as stroke.

According to Gray *et al.* (2002), several factors can be responsible for poor rehabilitation outcomes:

- Severe and incapacitating illness.
- Poor endurance levels.
- Altered cognition.
- Persistent urinary or faecal incontinence.
- Depression or poor motivation.
- Poor social support.
- Barriers in hospital or at home.
- Financial constraints.

The older person with diabetes or their family may feel guilty about their poor compliance with diabetes management prior to a critical health incident that requires rehabilitation services. Others exhibit self-blame or blame health professionals. For example, a smoker with diabetes who has undergone a lower limb amputation may blame himself or herself for being in such a predicament, be blamed by their family and/or be blamed by health professionals. Yet with a compliant older person with diabetes, health professionals may be at a loss to explain why seemingly good diabetes control and adherence to management regimens resulted in the same outcome as for the non-compliant individual. The person with diabetes and their family may mourn not only the loss of physical independence, but independence and a sense of control associated with diabetes self-management.

7.1.1 Cardiac rehabilitation

The majority of people who present with an acute cardiac event are over 65 and have reduced capacity to exercise and a great chance of having other comorbidities that reduce mobility and contribute to depression (Ades 1999). Nevertheless, older people are likely to attend rehabilitation programmes if they are referred by a medical specialist (Ades *et al.* 1992). Cardiac rehabilitation programmes provide the opportunity for older people to participate in aerobic and resistance training activities that improve cardiovascular fitness, mobility and flexibility and mood (see Chapter 5). In addition, they often provide diabetes education and strategies to support behaviour modification such as diet, smoking cessation and relaxation training. Importantly, they provide information about when it is safe to resume sexual activities.

7.1.2 Neurological rehabilitation

All people with diabetes, including older people, are at a higher risk of having a stroke. A stroke occurs due to a blockage (clot or embolus) in an artery supplying the brain or haemorrhage within the brain. If hyperglycaemia is not controlled in the initial stages of a stroke, the degree of ischaemia and tissue reperfusion is reduced, which in turn can lead to damage in a greater area of the brain (Kawai *et al.* 1997). The disabilities resulting from stroke can have a profound effect on the individual's ability to manage their diabetes. Depending on the areas of the brain affected, there may be paresis, dysphasia or aphasia, changes in mobility, behaviour and cognition, which include:

- Impaired swallow reflex, requiring vitamised meals and thickened fluids or even long-term or permanent enteral therapy, which impacts on how and by whom medicines are administered.
- Reduced mobility, which affects a significant component of normal diabetes management. It also directly affects the person's ability to attend health appointments, shop and remain an active contributor to their community. It may increase the person's risk for developing foot ulceration and increases the falls risk.
- Hemiplegia, which impacts on an individual's ability to perform blood glucose monitoring, administer insulin and prepare food.
- Cognitive changes increase the risk of vascular dementia occurring.
- Reduced ability to detect hypoglycaemia symptoms due to altered neurological pathways, which affects the person's ability to recognise falling blood glucose levels and increases the risk of falls. There is a greater reliance on others to detect and treat hypoglycaemia; for example, impaired speech may prevent the individual from verbally notifying carers if they do recognise hypoglycaemic symptoms or impaired mobility may mean they cannot access treatment.

Practice point

Early education, intervention and innovative education strategies are required to assist the person who has had a stroke to adjust to their new reality (Hernandez 1994). The person who has had a stroke may find their previous diabetes medicines are no longer adequate to maintain good glycaemic control. For example, a normally very active person treated with oral hypoglycaemic agents who becomes immobile, and therefore unable to utilise glucose to the same degree, may require insulin to achieve stable blood glucose levels. Starting insulin is a daunting prospect at the best of times. It can be overwhelming for the individual and their family after a stroke. They often fear that eventual discharge home will be jeopardised because of the need to have insulin injections. Compassion and understanding by health professionals and sound and open communication are essential during this period.

7.1.3 Transient ischaemic attacks (TIA)

TIAs often precede carotid artery thrombotic strokes (Gray et al. 2002). TIAs occur when the supply of blood to the brain is temporarily interrupted (Dunning 2003). Until a few years ago, some health professionals held the view that people with diabetes did not experience TIAs, progressing to a stroke, which is incorrect. People with diabetes do experience TIAs; however, the symptoms of TIA can last for a few seconds or minutes and often mimic hypoglycaemia. Signs and symptoms of TIAs in people with diabetes may include:

- Dizziness.
- Visual disturbances.
- Sudden loss of hearing.
- Difficulties speaking.

It is imperative that the person with diabetes checks their blood glucose level when symptoms are present to differentiate between TIAs and hypoglycaemia. If blood glucose levels are above 4 mmol/L and there has not been a sudden drop in blood glucose levels, such as a sudden reduction from 20 mmol/L to 5 mmol/L, a TIA should be considered, especially if the person can report hypoglycaemic-like symptoms and is not at risk of hypoglycaemia, for example someone controlled on diet. TIAs result from blockages to the carotid arteries. Health professionals may be able to hear carotid bruits through a stethoscope. Otherwise, Doppler, ultrasound and/or an angiogram may be required. Significant carotid artery blockage requires a carotid endarterectomy to reduce it. Daily aspirin may also be prescribed.

7.1.4 Lower limb amputation

The amputation of a limb is a traumatic time for the person with diabetes and their family. Their lives will be changed forever. In addition, the person's life expectancy will also be reduced. Often they have undergone months of foot ulcer treatment, including extensive and expensive wound dressings, hyperbaric oxygen therapy and surgery to either improve arterial blood supply or to amputate a toe or part of a foot. Where the blood supply is adequate, the surgeon performing a lower limb amputation always tries to preserve part of the leg below the knee to make it easier to fit a prosthesis and allow a greater level of independence.

Blood glucose control leading up to an amputation is often labile due to recurrent, hard-to-treat infections, enforced immobility, pain and stress. The source of the infection is removed along with the amputated foot, pain is usually markedly reduced, mobility is encouraged and surprisingly, stress often subsides. Therefore, diabetes medication requirements may need to be reduced in order to prevent hypoglycaemia from occurring. Wound management continues to be a primary focus of care (see Chapter 5). Stumps are at a higher risk of poor healing and/or wound breakdown, especially if the person has profound peripheral neuropathy and has sensory loss as far as the knee or poor arterial circulation.

7.1.5 Issues relating to blood glucose monitoring

Prior to a critical incident requiring hospitalisation and rehabilitation services, the individual may not have performed home blood glucose monitoring. Therefore, the activity may be new to the person and its relevance to their ongoing care not fully understood by the individual or their family. A disability in the short term or permanently can have a profound effect on an individual's sense of self-control over diabetes if they were previously performing home blood glucose monitoring independently.

Blood glucose meters are small and compact and relatively easy to use – if you can see and have the functional use of both hands. However, the digital graphics displayed on blood glucose meters are often quite small and opening blood glucose strip containers or removing blood glucose electrodes from prepacked foil containers can be very difficult for many older people with diabetes, even those who have not had a stroke. Assembling the lancet device and removing the used lancet can also be difficult, as can the calibration process required each time a new container of blood glucose strips or electrodes is opened. Blood glucose strips and electrodes should only be removed from their packages when a test is performed because normal moisture in the air can affect the accuracy of the strips.

Some strategies that can assist the person with diabetes to gain or retain independence in self-blood glucose monitoring include using:

- A magnified fluorescent lamp to perform the test if visual acuity is poor. The intense light and the magnified image can make a difference.
- Brightly coloured stickers to indicate where to insert the blood glucose strip or electrodes. Some 'discreet' blood glucose meters are so small it is difficult to see where the strip insertion site is located.
- Hospital or health institution blood glucose lancets that require only minimal twisting of a plastic cap to activate the mechanism. Although the lancet is single use only, it is still cost-effective.
- Velcro to ensure that blood glucose meters adhere to the surface and do not slip as the strip is inserted or blood applied.
- Computer software programs that can be downloaded so health professionals have access to blood glucose readings if manually recording results is too difficult for the individual. The meters should be properly set up to ensure the correct date and time are activated on the screen.
- Talking blood glucose meters or interfacing devices that fit onto existing meters that verbally instruct the person what to do and what the blood glucose level is.

7.1.6   Administering medicines

Several products now exist to assist the person who is unable to open tablet containers or cannot remember to take the right tablets at the right time. These include Dosette boxes and Webster packs, which are examples of dose administration aids that assist the person to take their medicines correctly at the designated time. However, simplifying medicine regimens, reducing the number of medicines and dose frequency and changing the format to small tablets or liquids may achieve greater compliance. Supervision by family members or carers may also be beneficial or necessary if the person frequently forgets to take their medicine or requires assistance.

Insulin administration is fraught with difficulty in terms of client self-management and administration in residential aged care facilities. The introduction of insulin pens several years ago revolutionised the way insulin was administered. Most people changed from using syringes to using insulin pens. Insulin pens can be disposable or non-disposable. They are relatively cheap to buy and convenient to use, especially when insulin needs to be administered outside the home environment. However, nearly all insulin pens currently available require full functioning, including dexterity and strength, of both hands in order to safely administer insulin. The individual who has suffered a stroke and remains hemiplegic or a person with severe arthritis who has very limited movement in their hands can be at a disadvantage if insulin pens are the only option considered for insulin administration.

Insulin syringes are an alternative and although it may still be too difficult for the individual to safely draw up an insulin dose unassisted, up to seven days supply of insulin can be predrawn by a family member or health professional and left in the refrigerator for the person to self-administer at the required time. If the person requires more than one injection each day, two different coloured containers can be placed inside the refrigerator containing the breakfast dose and evening meal dose. The person with diabetes removes the relevant syringe and administers the insulin unassisted. Insulin

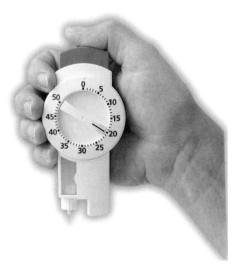

Figure 7.1 Innolet™ Novo Nordisk insulin device. Note the large clock-like face that makes the device familiar to people and the large size of the numbers that make dialling up an insulin dose easy to accomplish. The large size of the device makes it easy for people with limited manual dexterity to manage.

can be administered from predrawn syringes using only one functional hand and minimal dexterity or strength. If the person drawing up the insulin does not refit the syringe caps to the syringe too tightly, the person with diabetes can easily remove it to give their dose. People can use disposable pens that are preset at the required dose and have the pen needle already in place even if they have limited manual dexterity.

One disposable insulin pen currently on the market (see Figure 7.1) partly addresses the challenges for older people administering their own insulin. The Innolet™ device was designed for older people and enables those with disabilities to be more independent in terms of their insulin administration. The clock face makes it easy to see to dial up the insulin dosage and there is large writing and clearly audible clicks can be heard as each unit is dialled. In addition, minimal strength and dexterity are required when pushing the plunger downwards. Currently, the Innolet™ is only available with two insulin types, Mixtard 30/70™ and Protaphane™.

Insulin regimens for older people requiring insulin may now be reviewed due to the release of 24-hour-acting insulins. Lantus™ (glargine) has a flat action profile; that is, it has no onset of action time or peak action time and the action remains constant over the entire day (see Chapter 2). The role of Lantus™ in the care of older people, especially those with disabilities, has not been fully explored but the possibilities are encouraging. For example, instead of the homebound person with diabetes being dependent on home visiting nurses coming twice a day to administer insulin, Lantus™ could be administered once a day. A daily Lantus™ injection, with its flat profile of action, means that, provided the injection is given at roughly the same time each day, a visiting nurse could in fact administer this insulin at two o'clock in the afternoon. The flexibility could have a tremendous effect on the very finite resources currently available to visiting home nurses, by allowing the peak insulin admin-istration times, early morning and late afternoon, to be rationalised.

7.1.7 Diabetes self-management in rehabilitation and residential facilities

Older people with diabetes, people residing in residential care or currently admitted to inpatient or rehabilitation services should carry out as much of their own diabetes management as possible to maximise their independence and self-esteem. Self-participation reduces the risk of depression and may relieve some anxiety associated with changes made to diabetes management, as a result of changes in physical and mental functioning. Self-participation should be documented as part of the care plan and management goals (see Chapter 3). If insulin is required and is either a new man-agement strategy or the insulin administration device needs to be changed to meet the changing functional needs of the individual, self-insulin administration can be taught in reverse. That is, start with the person actually administering their insulin dose using the device already loaded by nursing staff. Once the person is confident and com-petent giving the injection, work backwards and have the individual attach or remove the needle, if they are using an insulin pen. Then have them perform the two unit air shot (an action required with all pen devices). Actually assembling the device could be the last skill to master.

This process may take some time to complete, but it does allow the individual the opportunity to develop skills and, more importantly, to build confidence and a sense of achievement. In the inpatient rehabilitation environment it may also allow overnight or weekend leave to occur more easily, which also assists the individual to meet their goals.

7.1.8 Hypoglycaemia and rehabilitation

As previously mentioned, symptoms of hypoglycaemia may change or be completely absent once an individual experiences a critical health incident requiring rehabilita-tion or restorative services. The treatment of hypoglycaemia may also need to change. For example, after a stroke or Bell's palsy, the person may be required to eat only a vitamised diet and thickened fluids because of an impaired swallowing reflex.

Hypoglycaemia management traditionally focuses on thin fluids such as Lucozade™, glucose tablets or glucose jellybeans. Providing these treatments for a person with an impaired swallowing reflex could put them at a very high risk of aspiration and chok-ing. Placing glucose powder into thickened fluids or vitamised foods quickly reverses the hypoglycaemia initially and also reduces the possibility it will recur because the fluids and foods usually have a lower Glycemic Index™ (see Chapter 4). Prepacked 15-gram tubes of glucose paste or gel are available and are an ideal treatment for hypoglycaemia when swallow reflex is impaired. The paste or gel can be squeezed onto a spoon and safely swallowed. If the tube has a soft plastic opening, the open-ing can be inserted directly in the mouth and contents squeezed into the mouth. This practice is sometimes used for reversing hypoglycaemia in very young children.

When older people with diabetes require enteral therapy, hypoglycaemia can be effectively and safely treated by mixing 10 grams of glucose powder in water and inserting the resultant fluid directly in the feed tube. Please refer to Chapter 2.

Hypoglycaemia may be more likely to occur in people with diabetes undergoing rehabilitation. For example, during an acute admission, the person may have been bedbound, being treated for an acute infection, experiencing higher levels of stress and a greater degree of pain. These issues are usually less acute in a rehabilitation or restorative environment. Often people in rehabilitation settings are given frequent physiotherapy or occupational therapy activities to perform out of hours which constitutes extra physical activity and increases the hypoglycaemic risks. When there is a prolonged gap between mealtimes, for example between the evening meal which is served around 5 pm to when breakfast is served the following morning, activity and prolonged fasting increase the risk of hypoglycaemia. Providing late night suppers is an important part of preventing overnight hypoglycaemia in rehabilitation settings.

If limited food resources are available out of hours, effective suppers can include a hot chocolate drink made with full milk, not half milk and half boiling water, a bowl of ice cream or a similar dairy dessert or a piece of fruit. The traditional sandwiches or biscuits and cheese that are often distributed with the evening meal, to be eaten by the patient later for supper, often have a high Glycemic Index™ and may not last long enough to prevent the blood glucose levels falling overnight. Likewise, confused people often consume the supper at the same time as their meal.

Overnight blood glucose measurement should be part of the care plan to identify whether overnight hypoglycaemia occurs, because hypoglycaemic symptoms may not be present or the symptoms may have changed significantly as a result of other disease processes.

7.2   Residential care

The proportion of older people per population living in residential aged care facilities varies. The leading causes of admission to a residential care facility are cognitive deficits, falls and incontinence. Twenty five per cent of older people are cared for in residential aged care settings in the UK (Croxon 2000) and 8% in Australia where the majority of older people are cared for in the community (AIHW 2002). Various levels of care are provided in these facilities, from supervision only through to high levels of dependency where qualified nursing care is necessary 24 hours a day.

Older people living in residential care facilities are a vulnerable population, with chronic diseases, increasing frailty and age. Diabetes management is often less than optimal, care is fragmented and staff often have insufficient knowledge about diabetes (Benbow *et al.* 1997) which leads to increased rates of hospitalisation (Wolffenbuttel *et al.*1991; Sinclair *et al.*1997). Comorbidities and cognitive decline often complicate management. In particular,

- Individual treatment targets and complication reviews are often not undertaken. In Australia care plans for residents in aged care facilities have been required under legislation since 1997.
- Specialist contribution in a timely manner to prevent comorbidities may not occur.
- There is inadequate blood glucose monitoring and metabolic review, including HbA_{1c} and lipids.

7.2.1   Aims of diabetes management in residential care

Individual aims, depending on a complete assessment, will need to be developed to maintain optimal function and wellbeing within the individual's functional and cognitive capabilities, enabling the person to manage their diabetes wherever possible (see Chapter 3). In order to achieve these goals, the following issues need to be considered.

- Provide a safe environment to enable residents to function to the best of their ability.
- Achieve an optimum level of metabolic control that reduces excursions in blood glucose levels and prevents the consequences of hyperglycaemia (see Chapters 2 and 4) and hypoglycaemia and the attendant risk of falls and injury.
- Ensure that regular appropriate screening of complications, including renal, and HbA_{1c}, foot care, dental health, vision, self-care potential and mood is carried out to reduce the risk of intercurrent infections, morbidities, the need for assistance and falls.
- Monitor blood glucose levels at appropriate intervals to detect deviations from the target range so that strategies can be put into place quickly to manage the situation and reduce the physical and cognitive effects of the abnormalities and deterioration that could require hospital admission.
- Manage coexisting disease, such as urinary tract and respiratory infections, appropriately and quickly.
- Provide a balanced diet that contains essential nutrients and supplements as required according to the individual nutritional assessment, disease status and medication regimen.
- Plan medication interventions according to the principles of quality use of medicines (see Chapter 9) and administer considering mealtimes and activity levels. Observe for adverse events.
- Increase the frequency of blood glucose monitoring and assessment of vital signs if intercurrent illness is present, a fall occurs or physical or mental changes such as confusion develop.
- Develop strategies to communicate with the individual.

7.3   Respite care – caring for family caregivers

Respite care is vital for older people living in the community and being cared for by family or carers. Many family carers are also elderly and their health and wellbeing are put at significant risk by the burden of care. Often they have reduced immunity and sleep deprivation and worry about what will happen to their relative if they become ill or incapacitated. Respite care should be available on a regular basis to support the significant role these carers perform. Negative health outcomes such as depression, psychosocial impairment, concerns about managing symptoms and deficits and providing physical and emotional care, managing a family and providing transportation are especially difficult (Bakas et al. 2004). These issues are exacerbated by short length of stay in hospital following an acute event.

The overall aim of respite care is that the older person will return home. However, the change in routine and the connotations of being 'put away' or 'dumped' that are common reactions of older people need to be sensitively and patiently dealt with, offering reassurance. Planning respite should occur in advance and informing the older person allows them time to adjust to the situation. Planning the care also enables the carer to have a break before they reach the burnout point.

Nurses in respite care need to be tolerant of the carers, who often feel guilty and find fault with the nursing care. Often, skilled nursing care improves the older person's health status and represents an opportunity for diabetes assessment to take place. Preparing the room with familiar objects from home before the person arrives and explaining usual routines when they arrive can help orient the person to the new environment.

7.4   Palliative care

Many older people will require palliative care, as a consequence of either diabetes complications or other disease, including cancer. There is very little evidence on the frequency of blood glucose monitoring and diabetes medicines at the end of life. However, in keeping with the philosophy of keeping the person comfortable, avoiding pain, hyper- or hypoglycaemia symptoms, dehydration and incontinence to maintain dignity and quality of life, allows them to complete unfinished business and move on. Monitoring and some medicines may be needed.

7.5   Spiritual care for older people with diabetes

Spiritual needs often become apparent through particular situations, often as physical health declines. People often need support to review the situation and decide how spiritual needs can be met, for example being able to spend time in a sensory garden, chapel or alone. Importantly, spiritual care is not separate from other necessary care; it is part of holistic practice. Nurses can provide spiritual care for older people by affirming their current circumstances, beliefs and relationships and helping them to identify their needs.

Reviewing their life journey is a naturally occurring phenomenon in older people (Ronaldson 2000, p. 113). Nurses can help older people travel their spiritual journey by listening, affirming and questioning to help the individual find meaning and worth in their new situation. Spiritual isolation is often a consequence of social isolation, especially for frail older people, and can be difficult to address. Social isolation and spiritual deprivation may well hasten cognitive and functional decline. Certainly depression is common in older people and significantly affects their self-efficacy and self-care and leads to further decline (see Chapter 8). Home visiting nurses often provide a vital link for housebound older people. Referring people for spiritual care should be considered.

In some cases, meditation and walking a labyrinth or finger labyrinth can help people focus on their spiritual journey. Prayer, purifying rituals, meditation and reflection are particularly important to some religions. Ensuring optional functioning and comfort to help the person complete unfinished business is an important aspect of spiritual and palliative care. Over one-third of adult Americans pray as well as using conventional and complementary therapies to address their health concerns; 75% pray to stay well and 22% pray for specific medical conditions. Most people in this study were older than 30, well educated and suffered from chronic conditions such as pain, depression and allergies. Most did not discuss the role of prayer in their self-health management with their doctors (McCaffrey *et al.* 2004).

References

Ades, P.A. (1999) Cardiac rehabilitation in older coronary patients. *Journal of the American Geriatrics Society*, **47**(1), 98–105.
Ades, P.A., Waldmann, M.L., Polk, D.M. & Coflesky, J.T. (1992) Referral patterns and exercise response in the rehabilitation of female coronary patients aged greater than or equal to 62 years. *American Journal of Cardiology*, **69**(17), 1422–5.
Australian Institute of Health and Welfare (AIHW) (2002) *Older Australia at a Glance 2002*. AIHW, Canberra.
Bakas, T., Austin, J., Jessup, S., Williams, L. & Oberst, M. (2004) Time and difficulty of tasks provided by family care givers of stroke survivors. *Journal of Neuroscience Nursing*, **36**(2), 95–106.
Benbow, S., Walsh, A. & Gill, G. (1997) Diabetes in institutionalised elderly people: a forgotten population. *British Medical Journal*, **314**, 1868–9.
Cameron, I. & Kurrle, S. (2002) Rehabilitation and older people. *Medical Journal of Australia*, **177**, 387–91.
Croxon, S. (2000) Diabetes in United Kingdom care homes. *Practical Diabetes International*, **17**(3), 70–1.
Dunning, T. (2003) *Care of People with Diabetes: A Manual of Nursing Practice*. Blackwell Publishing, Oxford.
Gray, L., Woodward, M., Scholes, R., Busby, W. & Fonda, D. (2002) *Geriatric Medicine*, 2nd edn. Ausmed Publications, Melbourne.
Hernandez, C. (1994) The challenges of teaching clients with cerebrovascular accidents to manage their diabetes. *Diabetes Educator*, **20**(4), 311–16.
Kawai, N., Keep, R. & Betz, L. (1997) Hyperglcyaemia and the vascular effects of cerebral ischaemia. *Stroke*, **28**(1), 149–54.
McCaffrey, A., Eisenberg, D., Legedza, A., Davis, R. & Phillips, R. (2004) Prayer for health concerns: results of a national survey on prevalence and patterns of use. *Archives of Internal Medicine*, **164**, 858–62.
Ronaldson, S. (2000) *Spirituality. The Heart of Nursing*. Ausmed, Melbourne.
Sinclair, A.J. & Finucane, P. (2001) *Diabetes in Old Age*. Wiley, Chichester.
Sinclair, A., Allard, I. & Bayer, A. (1997) Observations of diabetes care in long-term institutional settings with measures of cognitive function and dependency. *Diabetes Care*, **20**, 778–84.
Wolffenbuttel, B., Van Viet, S., Knols, A., Slits, W. & Sels, J. (1991) Clinical characteristics and management of diabetes patients residing in a nursing home. *Diabetes Research and Clinical Practice*, **13**, 199–206.

Chapter 8
Mental Health, Depression, Dementia and Diabetes

Trisha Dunning and Michelle Robins

8.1   Mental health and depression

Key points

- Psychiatric conditions are more common in people with diabetes compared to the non-diabetic population.
- Depression is common in older people, especially those living in residential care.
- Anxiety and depression can coexist.
- There is a higher prevalence of mental health problems in older people with reduced physical or cognitive functioning.
- Depression in older people can be recurrent in nature.
- Depression directly affects glycaemic control and diabetes management.

8.1.1   Introduction

A diagnosis of diabetes is associated with increased levels of anxiety, fear and depression (Beeney *et al.* 1996; Goldney *et al.* 2004). In fact, anxiety and depression have been identified as part of the adaptation to coping with diabetes (Lo & MacLean 2001). Depression is a debilitating condition that affects a significant number of older people and their carers (Goldney *et al.* 2004) (see Chapter 2) and is costly in terms of human suffering and resources.

Chronological age is not a specific risk factor for the development of depression (Bird & Parslow 2002), but up to 15% of older people living in the community experience depressive symptoms. A recent Australian study indicates that at least 24% of people with diabetes of all ages are depressed (Goldney *et al.* 2004) and the incidence rises sharply in older people living in residential facilities. Up to one in four residents has depression and 20% of newly admitted residents develop a depressive episode within their first year living in a facility (Gray *et al.* 2002). The incidence of major depression is as high as 25% in older people with chronic illnesses (Reynolds 1999). In addition, late-onset depression identified in older people is more likely to be recurrent in nature (Cluning 2001).

Depression often remains undiagnosed in older people. Many health professionals and family members often consider depression to be part of normal ageing yet in Australia, the second highest suicide rate occurs in men over 85 (Bishop 2000). Despite the well-documented association between depression and diabetes, most well-established long-term complication screening procedures do not include screening for depression. For example, depression screening was only included on the Australian National Complication Screening and Benchmarking Tool, ANDIAB, in 2003.

The incidence of depression is higher for people with diabetes regardless of their age. A growing body of knowledge is emerging that indicates that the prevalence of depression in older people with diabetes is significant and impacts directly on their ability to manage their diabetes. Some studies indicate that the rate of depression in older people with diabetes is double the rate in non-diabetics (Anderson *et al.* 2001) and represents higher health costs through increased service utilisation (Ciechanowski *et al.* 2000).

8.1.2   *Identifying depression*

According to Gray *et al.* (2002), a depressive episode is defined as the presence of the following three features:

(1)   A depressed mood not influenced by circumstances, which is present for the entire duration of most days, for at least two weeks.
(2)   Loss of interest or pleasure in activities or interests normally enjoyed.
(3)   Reduced energy.

In addition, at least four of the following symptoms are usually present:

- Loss of self-esteem or confidence.
- Inappropriate or excessive guilt and, sometimes, false beliefs or delusions.
- Recurrent thoughts of worthlessness and despair leading to thoughts of death or suicide.
- Poor concentration span and indecisiveness.
- Agitation or significant reduction in activity levels.
- Sleep disturbances.
- Changes in weight influenced by alterations in dietary intake.

Depression often presents differently in older people (Miller 1999) (see Table 8.1). As a result, validated screening tests to identify depression or threats to the wellbeing of older people were developed and include the following:

- Geriatric Depression Score.
- Diabetes Quality of Life Measure (DQOL).
- Cornell Depression Rating Scale.
- Medical Outcome Study Health Survey 36-item Short Form (SF-36).
- Health-Related Quality of Life Survey (HRQoL).
- Elderly Diabetes Impact Scales (EDIS) – Japan.
- Elderly Diabetes Burden Scale (EDBS) – Japan (replaced EDIS).
- Hospital Anxiety and Depression Scale (HADS).
- Audit of Diabetes Dependent Quality of Life (ADDQoL).

Table 8.1 Comparison of presenting symptoms of depression in younger and older adults with diabetes. Reproduced with permission from Miller 1999.

Depressed younger adults	*Depressed older adults*
More likely to report emotional symptoms.	Report more cognitive and physical symptoms.
Sense of hopelessness, uselessness and helplessness.	Apathy, exaggeration of personal helplessness.
Negative feelings towards self.	Sense of emptiness, loss of interest, withdrawal from social activities.
Insomnia.	Hypersomnia, early waking.
Eating disorders.	Anorexia, weight loss.
More verbal expression of suicidal ideation than successful attempts, more passive means of suicide.	Less talk about suicide, but more successful attempts and more violent means of suicide.

8.1.3 Factors associated with depression in residential aged care facilities

People who are depressed rarely state 'I feel depressed'. Some clues to the presence of depression are:

- Talking about the physical symptoms and believing they have a serious 'physical' illness (Cluning 2001).
- Grief over lost opportunities and abilities leading to a sense of powerlessness and learned helplessness, which impacts on other aspects of life, including self-care.
- Withdrawing from communal activities or attending activities but remaining aloof or being overly critical.
- Difficulty establishing relationships with staff and other residents in the first four weeks after admission.
- Experiencing chronic pain.
- Having had a stroke.
- Not receiving any visitors at least once a week.

8.1.4 Differentiating depression from dementia

Miller (1999) provided a useful summary to assist with the very difficult task of distinguishing between depression and dementia. However, a significant number of people in the early stages of dementia who retain some insight often have depressive moods when they realise 'things are slipping away' from them. Table 8.2 outlines the difference between depression and dementia. If depression is treated, behaviours associated with dementia improve.

Table 8.2 Identifying different signs and symptoms of depression and dementia. Reproduced with permission from Miller (1999).

Parameter	Depression	Dementia
Onset of symptoms	Abrupt onset, possibly involving a triggering event.	Gradual onset, recognised only in hindsight.
Presentation of symptoms	Exaggeration of memory problems and other cognitive deficits.	Unawareness of symptoms.
Memory and attention	Memory and attention deficits attributable to lack of motivation and inability to concentrate.	Impaired memory, especially for recent events, poor attention, strong attempts to perform well.
Emotions	Consistent feelings of sadness and being 'down in the dumps', unresponsive to suggestions.	Labile affect that changes in response to suggestions, possible apathy owing to cognitive impairments.
Response to questions	Slowed, apathetic, frequent response of 'I don't know' with no effort expended.	Evasive, angry, sarcastic, use of humour, confabulation or social skills to cover up deficits.
Personal appearance	Little or nor concern about appearance because of lack of motivation or diminished self-esteem.	Inappropriate dress and action owing to impaired perceptions and thought processes.
Physical complaints	Anorexia, weight loss, constipation, insomnia, decreased energy.	Vague fatigue and weakness, complaints are inconsistent and easily forgotten.
Neurologic features	Complaints of dysphagia without physical basis.	Aphasia, agnosia, agraphia, apraxia, preservation.
Contact with reality	Exaggerated sense of gloom, possible auditory hallucinations or self-derogatory delusions.	Denial of reality, illusion more predominant than hallucinations; if present, delusions are aimed at explaining deficits.

8.1.5   Causes of depression

The causes of depression are multifaceted and include:

- A triggering event such as the death of a spouse.
- Loneliness or isolation.
- Recurrent or almost constant presence of pain, for example painful diabetic peripheral neuropathy.
- Urinary and/or faecal incontinence.
- Inability to perform activities of daily living (ADLs).
- Weight gain as a result of diabetes drug therapy, such as sulphonylureas and insulin (see Chapter 2).
- Loss of independence, for example poor diabetes control, which can be a reason for cancelling a driver's licence.
- Financial concerns and difficulties.
- Level of education.
- Sense of loss of control.
- Impaired cognition.
- Reduced physical functioning due to chronic illness, for example diabetes, stroke, Parkinson's disease, rheumatoid arthritis, dependence on oxygen therapy.
- Adverse reactions to medicines such as antihypertensives, which are commonly used in people with diabetes, steroids and non-steroidal agents, anti-Parkinson disease drugs and analgesics.
- Alcohol.
- Diabetes-related complications such as impaired vision, need for enteral feeds and renal failure requiring renal dialysis.
- Duration of diabetes.

8.1.6   How does depression impact on diabetes?

Researchers suggest there are two pathways by which depression occurs in older people with diabetes. One explanation is that when motivation to adhere to diabetes management plans and strategies is reduced, worsening diabetes control and adverse outcomes result. However, interestingly, there may be a common pathogenesis, involving the autonomic and sympathetic nerves, shared by both diabetes and depression, which may account for the association between the two conditions (Black *et al.* 2003).

When depression is present, it directly impacts on all aspects of diabetes management and includes:

- Poor adherence to dietary guidelines.
- Reduced dietary intake, even anorexia.
- Poor compliance with medication regimens.
- Reduction or cessation of home blood glucose monitoring.
- Reduced compliance with health appointments and complication screening.

Depression increases the risk for adverse diabetes-related outcomes. Black *et al.* (2003) found that when diabetes and depression were both present in older Mexican Americans with Type 2 diabetes, they had a greater incidence of macro- and microvascular complications and disability. Treating depression improves mood and functioning and exercise to some extent but not other aspects of self-care, such as diet and metabolic control (Williams *et al.* 2004).

8.1.7 Strategies to improve self-worth for older people living in the community

One of the greatest challenges facing diabetes health professionals, and in fact all health professionals, is that diabetes is often not 'the' priority for the person with diabetes. For example, the person nursing their spouse through illness often neglects their own health and wellbeing, because their main priority is completely directed toward their partner's needs. Therefore, diabetes control often falters during such periods, often causing significant health problems for the person with diabetes who makes a conscious decision to ignore such problems.

'Giving permission' to an individual to reduce the level of their diabetes self-management may allow them to deal with other concerns and come back to day-to-day diabetes management at a later time. Setting a time frame for the temporary reprioritising of diabetes self-management tasks is as important as determining which tasks can be put aside for a time. For example, blood glucose testing could be reduced to minimal testing for a period of one month when a person temporarily has difficulty incorporating all aspects of diabetes management into their lives. As part of such an agreement, a contract of sorts might be drawn up stipulating that the person will eat three meals each day and take their diabetes medications as prescribed.

8.1.8 Strategies to improve self-worth for residents with diabetes

The entire diabetes management is often taken away from residents with diabetes in residential aged care facilities, even in low-care facilities, which are not obliged to provide medical equipment. Where possible, even in the presence of impaired cognition, enabling the individual to have more input into their diabetes management improves their self-esteem.

In order to include people with diabetes in self-care in residential facilities, it is often necessary to change existing thinking and staff practices. Depression needs to be considered and discussed at care planning meetings and with the managing doctor. Some strategies include:

- Encouraging the person to choose what food they eat, the snacks they keep in their room and the type and time of their supper.
- Recognising the individual needs to have treats and enjoy special occasion foods the same as everyone else in the facility.
- Encouraging the person to administer their insulin where possible under supervision.
- Allowing the person to perform their own blood glucose tests if possible.
- Encouraging the person to participate in exercise and community activities.
- Avoiding labelling the person as 'the diabetic' or having a separate 'diabetic table' in the dining room or 'diabetic meals', thus stigmatising residents.
- Avoiding blaming residents for labile blood glucose levels and accusing them of eating foods they should not eat.

- Using complementary therapies such as St John's wort, massage, acupuncture and tai chi to improve wellbeing and reduce stress (see Chapter 11).

8.1.9 Useful counselling skills

Ongoing support and creating and maintaining a therapeutic relationship between health professionals and the older person with diabetes suffering from depression, although resources intensive, may prove to be one of the most effective treatments. Useful tools to achieve such a therapeutic relationship include:

- Being empathetic – when the, person says 'I feel terrible', respond by acknowledging their feelings, 'Yes, that makes sense'.
- Active listening – clarifying by repeating phrases.
- Observing non-verbal cues, which make up most of what we communicate.
- Validating how the person feels – 'I understand how you must feel'.
- Setting realistic goals.
- Providing encouragement and acknowledging when gains, however small, have been made.
- Antidepressant agents, which should be used in conjunction with counselling and/or cognitive behaviour therapy. However, they should be chosen appropriately and used at the lowest possible dose for the shortest possible time. It should be noted that some antidepressant medicines contribute to hyperglycaemia. Unfortunately, there are insufficient low-cost counselling services for older people in many countries.

8.1.10 Anxiety

Anxiety and depression can coexist and may be sequential. Often both need to be treated simultaneously. Some medicines can cause anxiety, including some antidepressants, antihypertensives, steroids, non-steroidal anti-inflammatory agents and bronchodilators (Jeffreys 2004). It is important to distinguish anxiety attacks from hypoglycaemic episodes, especially if impaired cognitive functioning is also present.

8.1.11 Quality of life

Quality of life (QOL) is an important determinant of how an individual, regardless of their age, accepts and lives with their diabetes. Compared to younger people, older people identify QOL as being more important than length of life (Medical Research Council 1993). Dunning (2003) identified four categories of factors that can affect QOL.

(1) Medical – diabetes type, treatment regimen, level of metabolic control and presence of complications. The greater the severity and effects of diabetes-related complications, the poorer the QOL reported by clients.
(2) Cognitive – acute and chronic blood glucose control and neuropsychological changes can reduce QOL for the person with diabetes and their family.
(3) Attitudinal – self-efficacy, locus of control and social support. Individuals with good support will have a better QOL and reduced risk of depression. Strategies

that focus on empowerment or enablement can improve an individual's sense of wellbeing.

(4) Demographic – gender, education level, ethnicity and age. Men report better QOL than women and young people better than older people. Higher education is associated with a higher QOL.

Interestingly, the level of glycaemic control rarely relates to the level of wellbeing (Testa *et al.* 1998). However, the presence of diabetes symptoms is more directly related to QOL measurements. Maaravi *et al.* (2000) identified nutritional status as a major determinant of QOL in a population aged over 70 years living in the community. There are conflicting views about the effects of the different types of diabetes treatment on the QOL of older people. For example, Petterson *et al.* (1998) found QOL was lower in people treated with insulin. In contrast, Reza *et al.* (2002) observed improvements in SF-36 scores in mental health, social functioning and vitality. Reza *et al.* also noted that carer strain was lower in situations where people were treated with insulin.

8.2   Dementia and diabetes

Key points

- Impaired cognition may be present at the time of diagnosis due to hyperglycaemia and the associated dehydration and electrolyte imbalances.
- Acute impaired cognition may be a symptom of hypoglycaemia.
- There is a higher incidence of Alzheimer's disease in older people with diabetes.
- Vascular dementia (VaD) is a complication of diabetes.
- Impaired cognition can result from other diabetes-related complications, such as transient ischaemic attacks (TIAs) and stroke.
- Specific and unique strategies are required to safely manage older people with diabetes and impaired cognition.

8.2.1   Introduction

Dementia is a progressive deteriorating neurogenerative disease that results in generalised impairment of intellectual functioning and interferes with social and occupational functioning. Cognitive function deteriorates and leads to a decline in the ability to perform basic activities of daily living. There may be memory loss, impaired visual spatial skills, behaviour and personality changes and a decline in thinking ability (Moss *et al.* 2002). Unlike delirium, dementia is characterised by gradual, progressive, irreversible cerebral dysfunction. Delirium and dementia resemble each other and delirium must be ruled out whenever dementia is suspected.

Changes in personality and behaviour are seen as non-cognitive manifestations of dementia. Dementia may be overlooked as a barrier to providing diabetes education and care for older people. It is becoming evident that identifying early cognitive impairment should be a routine part of the assessment process before providing diabetes education and care for older people (see Chapter 6).

8.2.2 Scope of the issue

Prevalence rates for dementia increase with age. In Australia, approximately one in four people over the age of 85 years has dementia (Gray *et al.* 2002). The two main forms of dementia are Alzheimer's disease (AD), accounting for 70% of known dementias, and vascular dementia (VaD), representing 20%. In up to 20% of people both dementias are present. Some researchers have proposed changing the current classification structure for dementia when people also have diabetes because mixed pathologies of AD and VaD often coexist (Stewart & Liolitsa 1999). Yaffe *et al.* (2004) suggested women with impaired fasting glucose have worse baseline cognitive scores than non-diabetic women although their scores were better than women with diabetes. The risk of cognitive impairment in women with impaired glucose tolerance (IGT) and diabetes increases twofold. Therefore, women may have cognitive impairment at diagnosis since IGT usually precedes the onset of diabetes.

Three pathways of association between diabetes and the development of dementia have been identified (Phillips & Popplewell 2002).

(1) Cardiovascular disease causing TIAs and stroke can result in multifocal damage to the brain, thus contributing to dementia.
(2) Hypoglycaemia, especially if recurrent and frequent in nature, may lead to permanent neuronal destruction, causing damage similar to infarcts.
(3) Persistent hyperglycaemia increases protein glycosylation and contributes to the development of advanced glycosylated end-products (AGE). AGE are found in the plaques and tangles seen in Alzheimer's disease.

Some authors suggest hyperinsulinaemia is associated with insulin resistance and may contribute to the neurofibrillary lesions seen in the brains of people with Alzheimer's disease (Gasparini *et al.* 2002). Hypertension is also cited as being associated with the development of Alzheimer's disease and VaD, partly due to the resultant reduced elasticity of blood vessel walls, which increases vascular resistance and reduces the ability to respond to changing circulation demands. However, some authors disagree with Gasparini *et al.*'s hypothesis (Posner *et al.* 2002).

Stroke is a well-known complication of diabetes and it is possible for people to have cerebral infarcts without suffering a clinical stroke. Arvanitakis *et al.* (2004) conducted detailed neuropsychological tests in four domains of cognitive function – episodic memory, semantic memory, working memory and visuospatial ability – in 824 older women with diabetes and dementia. They found these functions were lower at baseline in diabetics than non-diabetics but declined at the same rate. However, perceptual speed was lower at baseline and declined faster in women with diabetes. A history of stroke did not change any of the relationships that were identified.

Arvanitakis *et al.* (2004) postulated that possible links between diabetes and cognitive function included:

- A direct effect of insulin on memory and plasma amyloid levels.
- A genetic link between diabetes and Alzheimer's disease.
- The effects of AGE on the neurological structure and function.

Other researchers also indicate that older people with diabetes have poorer cognition and hyperglycaemia reduces cognitive functioning (Morley & Flood 1990). Grodstein *et al.* (2001) found that women with diabetes aged between 70 and 78 years of age performed worse than those without diabetes on tests measuring general cognitive function, immediate and delayed verbal recall and verbal fluency and suggested that longer duration of diabetes and lack of pharmacological treatment of diabetes appeared to be associated with poorer cognition performance. Data presented at the American Diabetes Association Meeting in 2004 suggested that oral hypoglycaemic agents may reduce the risk of dementia in Type 2 diabetes by reducing hyperglycaemia and they improved memory within four months but not learning ability (Rouse 2004).

Logroscino et al. (2004) found women with Type 2 diabetes have about 30% greater chance of poor cognitive function than women without diabetes, increasing to 50% after 15 years' duration of diabetes. A earlier study (Kalmijn et al. 1995) found older men with impaired glucose tolerance (or prediabetes) had reduced cognitive function similar to men with diabetes. High-level care residents with diabetes have significantly higher levels of both cognitive and physical disability than non-diabetic residents and these disabilities cannot be accounted for by other comorbidities (Sinclair et al. 1997).

8.2.3   Identifying dementia

The initial indication of dementia can be made using Folstein's Mini-Mental State Examination (MMSE). Out of a possible score of 30, measurements between 18 and 26 may suggest mild dementia, 10 and 17 suggest a moderate form of dementia, whilst scores under 10 indicate severe dementia. However, it is important to realise that issues such as impaired hearing or vision and cultural and education background can influence the results (Phillips & Popplewell 2002). Diabetes treatment may also play a role. For example, older insulin-treated people have been shown to have higher rates of brain atrophy compared to similar cohorts treated with oral hypoglycaemic agents and those without diabetes (Ushida et al. 2001).

With the advent of expensive drugs to treat Alzheimer's disease, CT and MRI imaging are increasingly incorporated into the diagnostic assessment (Gray et al. 2002). Other diagnostic tests of cognitive function include digit symbol tests, clock drawing test and the trials B tests. However, taking a detailed history is important to gather all available information to assist with a diagnosis.

Practice points

(1)   Different stages or levels of dementia are identified by a person's functioning level; therefore, regular reassessment and review of diabetes-related management strategies are required.
(2)   The presence of dementia makes managing diabetes complex and challenging but should not be seen as a legitimate reason to deny or reduce access to diabetes services.

While there are still many unanswered questions about the relationship between diabetes and dementia, the literature suggests that the people with diabetes and mental symptoms have 'accelerated brain ageing' (Bent et al. 2000; Biessels et al. 2002). These symptoms are seen as diabetic encephalopathy and reduced spatial learning. A person with dementia usually presents with a history of changes in their everyday behaviour (Cluning 2001), including forgetfulness, confusion and reduced cognition and level of understanding.

8.2.4   Stages of progression in dementia

Nay & Garratt (1999) outline three main stages of AD. The first stage is char-acterised by absent-mindedness, emotional instability and poor concentration, which are often overlooked. These symptoms can worsen to include spatial disorientation, perception disturbances, changes in personal appearance and hygiene and a tendency to blame others and an inability to successfully perform daily tasks. Depression is often present at this time, because the person is aware that something is 'not quite right' (Katona 1994).

During stage two, the person may withdraw and demonstrate variable behaviour including anger, transient crying, poor sleep patterns, disorientation and profound short-term memory loss. Stage two may last up to 12 years, which is important to remember when planning diabetes management and care. At this stage, a person usually cannot live safely by themselves in the community. Their gait often changes, they cannot recognise their own face in a mirror and issues with continence emerge, as might other behaviours such as exhibitionism.

Stage three is often the shortest in duration, lasting up to two years. Profound decline in physical and cognitive functioning occurs, finally resulting in stupor and coma.

As a result of these changes people with dementia have difficulty receiving, pro-cessing and responding to environmental stimuli. Stress negatively affects individuals with dementia and may precipitate anxiety and dysfunctional behaviour. Six main groups of stressor have been identified (McCloskey 2004):

- Fatigue.
- Changes in usual routines, environment or caregiver. For example, acute care envir-onments fluctuate from understimulation to overstimulation from movement and noise, which can be overwhelming.
- Demands that exceed functional capacity.
- Multiple competing stimuli.
- Affective responses to perceptions of loss, including anger.
- Physical stressors such as pain and poor metabolic control.

Managing these factors can be difficult but reducing stress where possible by provid-ing a calm, stable environment is likely to be beneficial for the individual.

8.2.5   Impact on diabetes education

An individual's mental status directly affects their ability to learn, retain, recall and problem solve, which has a direct impact on diabetes education for the older person with diabetes who also has impaired cognition. Older people with Type 2 diabetes have greater deficits in their ability to process verbal and non-verbal material compared to matched non-diabetic subjects (Reaven *et al.* 1990). Reaven *et al.* also indicated that the higher the HbA_{1c}, the poorer the learning, reasoning and complex psycho-motor functioning. Croxson & Jagger (1995) identified lower MMSE results in older people with diabetes, even newly diagnosed people, compared to non-diabetic subjects. There appears to be an even stronger association between diabetes and Alzheimer's disease if the individual is treated with insulin (Ott *et al.* 1996).

The presence of impaired cognition may be short term; that is, when glycaemic control is significantly improved, cognition may also improve (Meneilly et al. 1993). Hyperglycaemia can impair cognition in a variety of ways including:

- Dehydration, causing electrolyte imbalance.
- Polyuria, especially nocturia whereby sleep is interrupted by the need to go to the toilet frequently overnight.
- Lethargy, impacting on a person's ability to care for themselves and be involved or interested in the world around them.
- Severe presentation of hyperglycaemia in the form of hyperosmolar non-ketonic coma (HONK), often requiring admission to an intensive care unit.

Educating a person with short-term impaired cognition needs to be conducted very differently from that of younger people with diabetes. For example, a longer-term approach to education is required. Group education will not be appropriate at this stage. Individual education strategies will need to focus on the person's partner/carer or other family members who should have a more active role in the management of the individual's diabetes. For example, a person with impaired cognition may need to rely on family to perform home blood glucose monitoring or administer insulin. Home nursing services may need to be initiated as a front-line strategy. Education in the home, a familiar and non-threatening environment, may prove to be more conducive to learning for the patient and family. Home education sessions also allow more immediate assessment of knowledge.

Other benefits to home education include the ability to:

- Develop rapport with the patient and family.
- Check the contents of the fridge and cupboards to assess how much food is in the house, which denotes probable food intake.
- Identify if food is out of date or of a type or quality that should not be consumed.
- Measure how activities of daily living (ADLs) are being achieved in terms of cooking, shopping, hygiene and home maintenance.
- Identify the type of footwear worn every day at home.
- Check blood glucose meter memory function to determine if home testing is being achieved.
- Monitor, to a degree, medication compliance by checking Webster packs and other medication in the house.

Education materials may need to be low literacy and large print. Videos may prove useful as a teaching tool. However, by assessing the individual within their home, it may be possible to organise small changes in usual routines to fit into diabetes management strategies, which may therefore have a minimum impact on the individual's day-to-day life. Identifying goals and time frames is vital. Goals may include blood glucose levels in a higher range if hypoglycaemia is occurring or less frequent blood glucose monitoring and a greater reliance on behaviour assessment and three-monthly HbA_{1c} levels.

Although those with dementia forget people's names, incidents in their lives and words, they can retain many of their long-practised skills (Cluning 2001). For example, they may still be able to cook some particularly useful meals that fit within diabetes eating guidelines. Continuing such activities can assist the person with diabetes and dementia to feel that they are contributing to their management, even though they are unable to learn newer skills such as blood glucose monitoring.

Practice points

(1) Never assume that a person with dementia is unaware of what is going on around them and what people are saying, even if they appear not to be actively participating (Cluning 2001). Always include the person with diabetes and dementia in the teaching session with family members where possible, talking to them directly, rather than ignoring them and talking only to family members.

(2) Do not talk to the person with dementia in a demeaning manner, for example using 'baby talk'; however, do try to use simpler words and break down complex concepts into small, simple chunks.

(3) Try to maintain eye contact and positive facial expressions. More information about educating older people can be found in Chapter 6.

8.2.6 Impact of dementia on treatment and management strategies

Management may vary for individuals living alone. For example, greater focus will need to be placed on activities of daily living rather than simply diabetes management and include the following:

- Support services at home such as Meals-on-Wheels and home help.
- Surveillance services, especially in terms of supervision of medication administration and meals.
- Day-care services.
- Supermarket pick-up and drop-off services from local councils.
- Hygiene needs with particular emphasis on toileting, hand washing and good foot care.
- Setting up shared management plans with general practitioners, for example agreed glycaemic control levels, medication management, frequency of review and evaluation of care plans.

Nutrition

Labile eating patterns are common in people with dementia. Due to poor short-term memory, some people with dementia cannot remember when they last ate, which can result in a person eating several meals each day.

More commonly, people with dementia are anorexic. Poor appetite, reduced taste sensation, increasing difficulty eating and a reduced concentration span to sit and eat a meal all contribute to a poor and reduced dietary intake. Several strategies can be employed to maximise dietary intake:

- Serving one course at a time, rather than three, which minimises confusion and mixing foods together.
- If at all possible serving food on a resident's own crockery from home in a residential facility, thus allowing them to recognise something familiar which may help create a sense of calmness.
- Putting foiled meals from home meal delivery services onto plates to maximise their appearance.
- Serving favourite foods or meals.
- Allowing grazing instead of serving three main meals. For example, leaving fruit on a platter and allowing the person to return to the plate as often as they wish

could be encouraged. Note that this practice may not be approved by some residential facilities on the grounds of hygiene.

- Encouraging low Glycemic Index™ dairy products such as ice cream, milk shakes, custard and hot chocolate drinks when food is refused. Such products provide one to two serves of carbohydrate and reduce the risk of hypoglycaemia in residents on oral hypoglycaemic agents or insulin.
- Encouraging the person to participate in meal preparation or at least be close to the kitchen so that they can smell food cooking, which may increase the sense of appetite and awareness that mealtime is approaching.
- Reducing environmental stimuli if aggressive or negative behaviours occur during mealtimes. For example, turn off the television and play soft music instead.
- Using food cues such as warm face cloths before the meal (see Chapter 11).

Practice point

If the person with dementia is able to make decisions, offer simple choices such as 'Do you want chicken or steak?' rather than 'What do you want to eat?' (Miller 1999).

Nutritional status should be monitored to ensure that malnourishment does not occur. Weight should be measured regularly as well as other parameters including serum albumin, especially if the person has a current wound. Regardless of whether or not cognitive impairment is present, older people often require protein and vitamin supplements. Encourage adequate fluid intake because dehydration causes lethargy and confusion (see Chapter 4).

Medication

Impaired cognition has a direct impact on compliance with medicines. The person with dementia often does not take medicines correctly or at all. Some oral diabetes agents are now manufactured in higher dosages or slow-release forms that reduce the need to take several tablets to achieve effective doses. For example, glimepiride has four different dosages but they are all formulated in sizes of one tablet and all have duration of action of 24 hours. According to company product information, glimepiride should be taken once a day in the morning.

No studies were identified that examined whether people with dementia could take their daily sulphonylurea at another time of the day, particularly if they are behaviourally more compliant and likely to take their tablets later in the day rather than in the morning. Metformin, although contraindicated in frail elderly people with diabetes and renal disease, now comes in 1 g tablets, which allow people on a 1 g dose to take one tablet rather than taking two 500 mg tablets.

Repaglinide, though currently not available on the Australian Pharmaceutical Benefits Scheme (PBS), may be an ideal oral agent for people with diabetes and impaired cognition. The tablet is only taken when a meal is eaten. Thus, if a meal is omitted, repaglinide is not administered. It is much faster acting and has a shorter half-life than other sulphonylurea agents. Thus, it is less likely to produce severe hypoglycaemia so may be an ideal agent for a person who often refuses to eat a meal, which puts them at risk of hypoglycaemia.

A range of new insulin pens and devices make insulin administration easier and more aesthetically pleasing. One device, the Innolet™ (see Figure 7.1), was developed largely for the elderly population requiring insulin therapy. The device resembles an egg timer. It is easy to dial up the dose and requires little strength or dexterity to deliver the dose of insulin. It is disposable and thus reduces the additional steps of placing the insulin cartridge into the device. People with impaired cognition have been successfully taught to use this device.

If the person with diabetes is unable to administer their own insulin, insulin pens and other devices such as the Innolet™ may help them accept insulin treatment more readily. Anxiety about syringes and misunderstanding about what might be contained in a syringe can cause resistance to using these devices. Family members, with support, can successfully administer insulin; however, commonly the person with diabetes may be reluctant to have their insulin administered in their abdomen, as is normal practice. Therefore, it may need to be administered into the upper arms or legs; however, the absorption rate may be affected. For example, if insulin is administered into the leg, absorption is reduced and the duration of insulin action is prolonged. In addition, by administering insulin into the leg or arm, the sensation of the injection is increased, possibly even producing pain or discomfort, because muscle tissue contains more nerve fibres compared to fatty subcutaneous tissue.

Newer insulin formulations are becoming more readily available, for example insulin glargine, which is a preparation that releases small amounts of insulin every few minutes for up to 24 hours. Glargine has enormous benefits for people with dementia. For example, it may replace twice-a-day premixed insulins, which may prove very useful if insulin administration contributes towards anxiety and aggressive behaviour from the person with dementia. Another example is if visiting home nursing services are required to administer insulin, doses can be given at any time of the day, as long as the time is consistently the same. Therefore, instead of adding to the strain on such services to meet insulin requirements every morning and evening, glargine could be administered during the middle of the day and be just as effective, thus rationalising home nursing resources.

However, if the person with dementia is quite co-operative and accepting of another person administering their insulin, there is no reason to reduce an insulin regimen to a daily dose. People with Type 1 diabetes usually require three fast-acting insulin doses with meals (bolus) and one longer acting insulin injection at bedtime, the basal dose. However, when glargine is used it is often administered in the morning. In this case it still remains the basal dose.

If the person with dementia is currently prescribed a basal bolus regimen and their food intake varies, rapid-acting insulins such as Novorapid™ and Humalog™ can be administered after meals. This is one situation where a 'sliding scale' might be appropriate. 'Sliding scale' in this context means that the number of serves of carbo-hydrate eaten by the client determines the amount of rapid-acting insulin they receive after completing their meal. Adopting such an approach involves 'working forward' rather than reacting to blood glucose levels, which is common practice in acute settings and often leads to poor glycaemic control (Dunning 2003). This is a very different way of managing insulin dose requirements and administration; however, the complexities involved in caring for a person with diabetes and dementia require health professionals to be innovative and produce workable strategies that are pro-active in nature and therefore respond better to individual needs.

Practice points

(1) Reviewing diabetes medicines and using fewer drugs at the most effective doses and dose intervals may achieve greater compliance and acceptance of medication regimens by the person with dementia and their family.

(2) Recent research suggests that ethno-specific residential aged care facilities benefit people with dementia. Where there is more than one person of the same nationality, they communicate more and often require fewer psychiatric medicines (Australian Nursing Federation Report 2004).

Home blood glucose monitoring

If the person with diabetes is testing their own blood glucose levels without assistance and doing it successfully, there is little reason to make any changes in the early stages of dementia. The person may need prompting to perform blood glucose testing but may still be able to perform the test correctly, which maintains their participation and ownership of their diabetes management.

Family members may need to record results in the client's blood glucose diary, if writing has become difficult. Blood glucose meters have memories that assist family members to know when tests are performed and what levels are being obtained. Blood glucose results in the meter memory can be downloaded onto computers, which helps diabetes health professionals to plan care.

If the person is familiar with an older meter and uses it correctly, it may not be appropriate to 'upgrade' to a newer, 'simpler' blood glucose meter. The person with cognitive impairment may not be able to learn how to use a new meter, yet continue to accurately test using their familiar meter.

If family members perform blood glucose monitoring, they need to be aware of safe practices when handling blood and sharps. Hospital-type lancets can be useful devices for family members to use if they are performing blood glucose monitoring for the client. It is imperative that such devices are available for home visiting nurses performing blood glucose tests to minimise their risk of needlestick injury.

Providing a positive environment during blood glucose testing will assist the resident to co-operate with blood glucose tests. Placing the lancet device on the sides of fingers, rather than directly on the middle of fingertips, reduces the pain associated with capillary blood glucose testing. When the person with diabetes and dementia refuses to have regular blood glucose tests, performing three-monthly HbA_{1c} levels is essential to evaluate glycaemic control.

Hypoglycaemia

Preventing hypoglycaemia is one of the key aims in managing older people with diabetes, regardless of their mental health status. It is evident that people with dementia who experience a hypoglycaemic episode may not present with signs and symptoms in the same way as an older person who is not cognitively impaired (see Chapter 4).

Hypoglycaemia may present with aggressive verbal and/or physical behaviour and dementia. Treatment can therefore be challenging in terms of safety for family or staff when approaching a client experiencing hypoglycaemia. Staff may need to allow time to ascertain if the aggressive behaviour reduces in intensity. Oral treatment is more likely to be achieved without incident to the carer or staff member. However, each person is different so the strategies needed to treat and prevent hypoglycaemia need to be individualised.

Practice point

It is useful to accurately record the signs and symptoms the person with dementia exhibits so that carers and staff can check for hypoglycaemia as the cause of aggressive or negative behaviour, rather than assuming it is only due to dementia.

Behaviour modification

Behaviour management and modification are vital to the treatment of dementia and health professionals providing diabetes services need to be aware of the complexities associated with managing complex behavioural issues. Interventions need to be individualised and existing strategies may require frequent modification. Carers find having specific strategies to manage difficult behaviour useful and supportive of their needs. The more cognitively impaired a person is, the greater the influence their environment will have (Miller 1999). Many researchers have found that excessive stimulation often correlates with deterioration in the behaviour of the person with dementia. Music has been shown to reduce aggressive behaviour during bathing times (Clark *et al.* 1998) and, anecdotally, to assist with other procedures necessary for diabetes management.

Wandering is a common behaviour observed in people with dementia which can be turned into a positive attribute in terms of diabetes management. Diabetes medicines may need to be reduced to alleviate the risk of hypoglycaemia occurring. If clients can wander within a safe and secure environment, such activity can have physical health benefits and often reduce anxiety levels as well as the need for sedation. Holmberg (1997) identified that, by providing a volunteer-facilitated walking programme, such behaviour could be more usefully directed and engendered a greater sense of wellbeing for the person with dementia.

Promoting cognition

Several strategies can help maintain cognitive function (Miller 1999).

- Maintain stable blood glucose levels, if possible between 4 and 10 mmol/L. If hypoglycaemia unawareness is an issue, readings should be maintained between 5 and 15 mmol/L.
- Ensure adequate hydration but ensure the person does not overdrink and become hyponatremic, especially if they have renal impairment.
- Consider dietary supplements such as zinc, choline, lecithin, selenium, magnesium, beta-carotene, folic acid, Vitamin C and Vitamin E.
- Complementary therapies such as *Ginkgo biloba* and aromatherapy (see Chapter 11).
- Exercise.
- Aspirin if the dementia is VaD.

References

Anderson, R., Freedland, K., Clouse, R. & Lustman, P. (2001) The prevalence of comorbid depression in adults with diabetes. *Diabetes Care*, **24**, 1069–78.

Arvanitakis, Z., Wilson, R., Bienias, J., Evans, D.A. & Bennett, D.A. (2004) Diabetes mellitus and risk of Alzheimer disease and decline in cognitive function. *Archives of Neurology*, **61**, 661–6.

Australian Nursing Federation Report (2004) Ethno-specific homes help dementia patients. *Australian Nursing Journal*, **12**(91), 33.

Beeney, L., Bakry, A. & Dunn, S. (1996) Patient psycholgocial information needs when the diagnosis is diabetes. *Patient Education and Counselling*, **29**, 109–16.

Bent, N., Rabbitt, P. & Metcalfe, D. (2000) Diabetes mellitus and the rate of cognitive ageing. *British Journal of Clinical Psychology*, **39**, 349–62.

Biessels, G., van der Heide, L., Kamal, A., Bleys, R. & Gispen, W. (2002) Ageing and diabetes: implications for brain function. *European Journal of Pharmacology*, **441**(1–2), 1–14.

Bird, M. & Parslow, R. (2002) Potential for community programs to prevent depression in older people. *Medical Journal of Australia*, **177**, s107–s110.

Bishop, B. (2000) *The National Strategy for an Ageing Australia*. Commonwealth of Australia, Canberra.

Black, S., Markides, K. & Ray, L. (2003) Depression predicts increased incidence of adverse health outcomes in older Mexican Americans with type 2 diabetes. *Diabetes Care*, **26**(10), 2822–8.

Ciechanowski, P., Katon, W. & Russo, J. (2000) Depression and diabetes: impact of depressive symptoms on adherence, function and costs. *Archives of Internal Medicine*, **160**(21), 3278–85.

Clark, M., Lipe, A. & Bilbrey, M. (1998) Use of music to decrease aggressive behaviours in people with dementia. *Journal of Gerontological Nursing*, **24**(7), 10–17.

Cluning, T. (ed.) (2001) *Ageing at Home: Practical Approaches to Community Care*. Ausmed Publications, Melbourne.

Croxson, S. & Jagger, C. (1995) Diabetes and cognitive impairment: a community-based study of elderly subjects. *Age and Ageing*, **24**, 421–4.

Dunning, T. (2003) *Care of People with Diabetes: A Manual of Nursing Practice*. Blackwell Publishing, Oxford.

Gasparini, L., Netzer, W., Greengard, P. & Xu, H. (2002) Does insulin dysfunction play a role in Alzheimer's disease? *Trends in Pharmacological Sciences*, **23**(6), 288–93.

Goldney, R., Phillips, P. & Fisher, L. (2004) Diabetes, depression and quality of life. *Diabetes Care*, **27**, 1066–70.

Gray, L., Woodward, M., Scholes, R., Busby, W. & Fonda, D. (2002) *Geriatric Medicine*, 2nd edn. Ausmed Publications, Melbourne.

Grodstein, F., Wilson, R., Chen, J. & Manson, J. (2001) Type 2 diabetes and cognitive function in community dwelling elderly women. *Diabetes Care*, **24**(6), 1060–5.

Holmberg, S. (1997) A walking program for wanderers: volunteer training and development of an evening walker's group. *Gerontological Nursing*, **18**, 160–5.

Jeffreys, D. (2004) Update: anxiety disorders in later life. *Medical Observer*, **1**, 20–1.

Kalmijn, S., Feskens, E., Launer, L., Stijnen, T. & Kromhour, D. (1995) Glucose tolerance, hyperinsulinaemia and cognitive function in a general population of elderly men. *Diabetologia*, **38**(9), 1096–102.

Katona, C. (1994) *Depression in Old Age*. John Wiley, New York.

Lo, R. & MacLean, D. (2001) The dynamics of coping and adapting to the impact when diagnosed with diabetes. *Australian Journal of Advanced Nursing*, **19**(2), 26–32.

Logroscino, G., Kang, J. & Grodstein, F. (2004) Prospective study of type 2 diabetes and cognitive decline in women aged 70–81 years. *British Medical Journal*, **328**, 548–51.

Maaravi, Y., Berry, E., Ginsberg, G., Cohen, A. & Stessman, J. (2000) Nutrition and quality of life in the aged; the Jerusalem 70-year olds longitudinal study. *Aging Clinical Experience Research*, **12**(3), 173–9.

McCloskey, R. (2004) Care of patients with dementia in the acute care environment. *Geriatric Nurse*, **25**(3), 139–44.

Medical Research Council (1993) *Health of the UK's Elderly People*. Medical Research Council, London.

Meneilly, G., Cheung, E., Tessier, D., Yakura, C. & Tuokko, H. (1993) The effect of improved glycaemic control on cognitive function in the elderly patient with diabetes. *Journal of Gerontology*, **48**(4), 117–21.

Miller, C. (1999) *Nursing Care of Older Adults*, 3rd edn. Lippincott, Williams and Wilkins, Philadelphia.

Morley, J. & Flood, J. (1990) Psychological aspects of diabetes mellitus in older persons. *Journal of the American Geriatrics Society*, **38**, 605–6.

Moss, S., Polignano, E., White, C., Minichiello, M. & Sunderland, T. (2002) Interaction in Alzheimer's disease. *Jounal of Gerontological Nursing*, **28**(8), 36–44.

Nay, R. & Garratt, S. (1999) *Nursing Older People: Issues and Innovations*. Maclennan and Petty, Sydney.

Ott, A., Stolk, R., Hofman, A., van Harskamp, F., Grobbee, D. & Breteler, M. (1996) Association of diabetes mellitus and dementia: the Rotterdam Study. *Diabetologia*, **39**(11), 392–7.

Petterson, T., Young, B., Lee, P., Newton, P., Hollis, S. & Dornan, T. (1998) Well-being and treatment satisfaction in older people with diabetes. *Diabetes Care*, **21**(6), 930–5.

Phillips, P. & Popplewell, P. (2002) Diabetes and dementia. *Medicine Today*, **3**(11), 30–40.

Posner, H., Tang, M., Luchsinger, J., Lantigua, R., Stern, Y. & Mayeux, R. (2002) The relationship of hypertension in the elderly to AD, vascular dementia, and cognitive function. *Neurology*, **58**(8), 1175–81.

Reaven, G., Thompson, L., Nahum, D. & Haskins, E. (1990) Relationship between hyperglycaemia and cognitive function in older NIDDM patients. *Diabetes Care*, **13**, 16–21.

Reynolds, C. (1999) Depression and aging: a look to the future. *Psychiatry Service*, **50**, 1167–72.

Reza, M., Taylor, C., Towse, K., Ward, J. & Hendra, T. (2002) Insulin improves well being for selected elderly type 2 diabetic subjects. *Diabetes Research and Clinical Practice*, **55**(3), 201–7.

Rouse, R. (2004) Antidiabetic drugs may reduce dementia risk in type 2 patients. Report of the American Diabetes Society Meeting held in Orlando, Florida. *Medical Observer*, **June**, 19.

Sinclair, A., Allard, I. & Bayer, A. (1997) Observations of diabetes care in long-term institutional settings with measures of cognitive function and dependency. *Diabetes Care*, **20**(5), 778–82.

Stewart, R. & Liolitsa, D. (1999) Type 2 diabetes mellitus, cognitive impairment and dementia. *Diabetic Medicine*, **16**(2), 93–112.

Testa, M., Simonson, D. & Turner, R. (1998) Valuing quality of life and improvements in glycaemic control in people with type 2 diabetes. *Diabetes Care*, **21**(suppl 3), c44–c52.

Ushida, C., Umegaki, H., Hattori, A., Mogi, N., Aoki, S. & Iguchi, A. (2001) Assessment of brain atrophy in elderly subjects with diabetes mellitus by computed tomography. *Geriatrics and Gerontology International*, **1**(1–2), 33.

Williams, J., Katon, W. & Lin, E. (2004) The effectiveness of depression care management on diabetes-related outcomes in older patients. *Annals of Internal Medicine*, **140**, 1015–24.

Yaffe, K., Blackwell, T., Kanaya, A., Davidowitz, N. & Barrett-Connor, E. (2004) Diabetes, impaired fasting glucose, and development of cognitive impairment in older women. *Neurology*, **63**, 658–63.

Chapter 9
Effective Medication Management in Older People

Susan Hunt

Key points

- Effective medicine management requires a collaborative and co-operative approach among all health care professionals.
- Older people with diabetes and their carers need to be included as active partners in planning their care.
- Older people are more at risk of experiencing a medicine-related incident.
- Regular medicines review plays an important role in preventing adverse drug events.
- Consumer medicine information is an important and useful component of medication education.

9.1 Introduction

Managing medicines with older people is difficult due to the associated comorbidities, limited evidence for prescribing in frail older people, the risk of adverse events and altered pharmacodynamics. Only 3% of randomised control trials and 1% of meta-analysis include people over 65 and even in specific trials in older people, the inclusion criteria often result in atypical healthy older people being included rather than the frail older group (Le Couteur *et al.* 2004). People with diabetes, particularly older people, are at risk of experiencing a number of medication-related risks, which is not surprising when care systems are examined.

People with diabetes usually interact with a number of different service providers on repeated occasions, which can be confusing and lead to unco-ordinated care. Ideally medication management will be undertaken from a 'quality use of medicines' (QUM) perspective, where the individual is firmly at the centre of any medication-related activity. QUM gives medication management a broad focus by including all the systems related to medicines use and engages a range of health-care services to achieve integrated medicine management and promote positive health outcomes.

9.2   Identifying the complexities

Worldwide, the proportion of people aged 60 years and over is growing faster than any other age group. As the population ages, the demand for medicines to delay and treat chronic diseases, alleviate pain and improve quality of life increases and the medication regimen becomes more complex. Major changes have occurred in the last 30 years in the role of medicines in the treatment of common chronic conditions such as cardiovascular disease, cancer, diabetes, osteoarthritis, pulmonary disease, Alzheimer's disease and psychiatric disorders, most commonly depression and dementia (International Council of Nurses 2004).

The term 'medicine' includes 'prescription, non-prescription and complementary medicines', the latter including 'vitamin, mineral, herbal, aromatherapy and homoeopathic products, which might also be known as alternative or traditional medicines' (Lynne 2003).

As well as increased medicines use, the types, forms and sources of medicines have increased and there have been changes in the degree of supervision/regulation and information provided. For example:

- Medicines may be prescribed by a health professional and dispensed by a pharmacist who provides consumer medicines information (CMI).
- Purchased over the counter from a pharmacy with support and advice from a pharmacist.
- Purchased from a supermarket with minimal information about the medicine or its use.
- Purchased directly from a manufacturer, which is particularly common when using complementary medicines or medicines sourced from the Internet.

The last two options may not supply information to help the consumer understand how to use the medicine safely. In addition, where information is provided the print size is often too small and the colour inappropriate for older people with impaired vision. When medicine information is provided, it is often in the written form and in English, which may not be helpful for people with low literacy or where English is not their preferred language.

Frequently, several health professionals are involved with medicine management. They all have differing levels of knowledge and competence about medicine use, understanding of how medicines are viewed and used by older people and skill at explaining medicines (Consumers' Health Forum of Australia 1997).

Medicines have increased the overall wellbeing of older people but they also increase the risk of medicine-related incidents, especially adverse drug events (ADE). A medication incident includes:

- Adverse drug reactions (ADR).
- Drug–drug or drug–food interactions.
- Problems related to polypharmacy.
- Errors in prescribing, supply or administration (see Chapter 2).

An ADE occurs when a medication incident results in harm to the individual (Australian Council for Safety and Quality in Health Care 2002). ADEs include hospitalisation and, in some cases, death. Hospitalisation as a result of medicine-related

ADRs is predicted to increase because of the numbers of medicines now used to manage chronic diseases (Eaton 2002).

Practice points

(1) All medicines have the potential to cause side effects.
(2) Older people are vulnerable, therefore any symptom they develop should be treated as drug related until proved otherwise (Gurwitz *et al.* 1990).

There is a large body of research concerning medication errors (Meurier *et al.* 1998; Baker 1999; Buerhaus 1999; O'Shea 1999; Thornton *et al.* 1999; Martin *et al.* 2000; Anderson & Webster 2001; Cohen 2001). Most researchers agree that most ADEs are due to system failure, rather than the actions of individuals. In Australia there is a move away from the traditional 'blame and shame' response to a medication error where individuals, usually a nurse, are punished, to an approach that reviews the systems and processes that gave rise to the error (Australian Council for Safety and Quality in Health Care 2002). The UK and the USA are moving in the same direction (Department of Health 2000; Mayor 2000).

9.3   Older people – not a homogeneous group

Young people often think all older people are the same. Yet there is great variety in the social situations, aspirations and health needs of 60-year-old people compared with someone over 90. One of the problems encountered in caring for older people is the limited understanding of many health professionals and policy developers about older people and their lives (Bevan & Jeeawody 1998). In particular, many clinicians hold ageist attitudes that affect their interactions with older people and their expectations of the outcomes of care (Lothian 2001). Many health professionals view older people as being, by virtue of their age, sick, incapable and useless. The reality is very different. The majority of older people live happy, healthy and productive lives in their communities (AIHW 2002).

Over the last 20 years there has been increasing emphasis on 'healthy ageing' as a joint responsibility of the government and the individual. A number of lifestyle initiatives have been encouraged, particularly concerning the role of diet and exercise in maintaining and promoting health (Bevan & Jeeawody 1998) and in preventing chronic diseases such as Type 2 diabetes (Andrews 2001). The notion that older people are passive recipients of care is increasingly being challenged by the ageing 'baby boomers', who are relatively well educated, want to have some control over their health and are very inquiring regarding information and alternative opinions.

Over the last ten years, countries such as New Zealand, the UK and Australia have initiated a number of government programmes that support increasing numbers of frail older people in the community. However, as people age, particularly after 85 years, their level of disability increases and so does the incidence of institutionalised care (AIHW 2002).

The way residential aged care is provided has altered in many countries so that only people in need of care are admitted to residential facilities. Therefore, residents in residential aged care are older, in poorer health and less able to function independently than was the case in the past. In addition, the level of dependency is increasing (AIHW 2003a).

As a result residential aged care accommodates individuals who need intensive levels of care, many of whom would otherwise require hospitalisation (Jenkins 1996). Residents of low-level care facilities generally require assistance with personal care rather than intensive treatment. The concept of 'ageing in place' was introduced in Australia in 1997. Essentially this means that as a person's care needs change, the resident should not have to move to another facility. As a consequence, residents with complex health needs requiring complex medication regimens live in low-level care facilities.

Cognitive impairment is common in residents in both high- and low-level care (AIHW 2002). In addition, over half of the people with a diagnosis of dementia live in the community (AIHW 2004). The incidence of dementia makes it difficult to involve the individual in their medication management (see Chapter 8). Effective medication management needs to be responsive to the different circumstances of older people and their varying levels of ability to be involved in their own care. Therefore, medication management may include:

- The consumer.
- Paid carers such as nurses and personal care workers or attendants.
- Unpaid or informal carers, for example family members and care advocates.
- General practitioners.
- Pharmacists.

9.4   Medicines issues and older people

As already indicated, the level of medicine use increases with age. Approximately 86% of people over 65 years use medicines, compared to 59% of the general population (Australian Bureau of Statistics 1999). Every year about 190 million prescriptions are dispensed in Australia (Department of Health and Ageing 2003). An unknown and unquantifiable number of over-the-counter and complementary medicines are purchased each year, which increases the risk of ADEs. It is difficult to determine the actual rate of ADEs because many ADRs are not recognised or reported. However, an estimated 140 000 hospital admissions each year are medicine related (Australian Council for Safety and Quality in Health Care 2002). The most commonly involved medicines are:

- Cancer chemotherapy.
- Analgesics and anti-inflammatory agents.
- Cardiovascular and antihypertensive agents.
- Anticoagulants.
- Antibiotics.
- Anxiolytics, sedatives and antidepressives.
- Corticosteroids.

The rate of medication incidents is higher in people over 65, partly because they are more likely to be taking one or multiple medicines, particularly those on the above list (Australian Council for Safety and Quality in Health Care 2002). One in twelve community-based older people is prescribed inappropriate or incorrect medicine by their general practitioner (GP) or hospital staff (Tanne 2004). Inappropriate prescribing is prevalent in community-dwelling older people as well as in residential aged care settings (Gurwitz *et al.* 2000).

In addition older people have altered ability to absorb, metabolise and excrete medicines and impaired compensatory mechanisms (National Health and Medical Research Council 1994; McGavock 2003) (see Chapter 2). As a result, a large number of negative health outcomes directly related to medicines occur in older people. These include:

- Falls (Leipzig *et al.* 1999).
- Urinary incontinence (Fonda *et al.* 2002).
- Intellectual impairment including delirium and confusion (Flacker & Marcanonio 1998; Moore & O'Keeffe 1999).

Each of these clinical issues has implications for the individual's quality of life and the cost of providing care, regardless of where the care is provided. There are specific medicine management issues in residential aged care and a growing body of research demonstrates that older people in residential aged care facilities are particularly at risk of ADEs (Field *et al.* 2001). By definition, people living in both high- and low-level facilities are frailer and may have difficulty expressing and ascribing symptoms to their medicines. They frequently suffer from multiple physical problems.

Residents who have multiple comorbidities are often prescribed enough medicines to fulfil the criteria for polypharmacy (Roberts & Bonner 1995; Roberts 1998; Field *et al.* 2001). Polypharmacy increases the risk of ADEs, many of which result in hospitalisation. Although there is no accepted definition of polypharmacy, the two most common definitions are the prescription and administration of more medicines than are clinically indicated to a given patient (Ehms 2000) and the concomitant use of more than five medicines (Le Couteur 2004).

Any contact with health professionals represents an opportunity for the medication regimen to be reviewed and unnecessary medicines ceased (Dhalla *et al.* 2002). However, polypharmacy may be best practice in people with diabetes (see Chapter 2). There is increasing recognition that the issue may not be how to reduce polypharmacy but how to reduce *unnecessary* polypharmacy and emphasising good prescribing (Shakib 2002) and medication management from a quality use of medicines perspective (Australian Pharmaceutical Advisory Council 1999; Department of Health and Ageing 2002).

Conversely, underuse of medicines also occurs. These factors indicate that medicine management is not a simple concept. Some medicines use could be categorised as 'physical abuse' (House of Commons Select Committee 2004). Both over- and underprescribing occur in this context. In particular, there is evidence that analgesia is underprescribed and antipsychotic medication is overused to control the behaviour of people with dementia in community and residential care settings (House of Commons Select Committee 2004).

Assessing older people with cognitive impairment presents special challenges and the problems related to pain management have been well recognised (Parmelee *et al.* 1993; Ebner 1999; Galloway & Turner 1999). Current indications are that care staff may find pain assessment very difficult and therefore do not offer pain relief, particularly in residential aged care facilities. Likewise, medicines are prescribed as chemical restraints to deal with behaviours such as wandering, agitation and unco-operativeness that could be managed using other methods if staff are well trained in dealing with people with dementia (House of Commons Select Committee 2004) (see Chapter 8).

Quality use of medicines encompasses more than merely prescribing appropriately. It involves:

- Appropriate attitudes to older people and medicines.
- Skills in handling difficult situations.
- Skills assessing the need for medicines.
- Not using medicines where possible.
- Monitoring the effects of medicines.

In some cases 'doctors, nurses and nursing assistants need to rethink their approach to the problem of "challenging behaviours"' (Mant & Donnelly 1996). The issues are complex but it appears that adequately trained staff and appropriate staffing levels reduce the risk of inappropriate medicines use and ADEs (House of Commons Select Committee 2004).

Practice point

People monitoring medicine effects, including medicine-related ADEs or ADRs in older people in any setting, may not be registered nurses.

The reduction in the numbers of registered nurses employed in the aged care industry has resulted in greater numbers of unlicensed and inadequately prepared caregivers providing care to this vulnerable population (AIHW 2003b). In the community, the main caregivers are often family members, most often a spouse with their own health problems (see Chapter 2) (AIHW 2002).

9.5   Quality use of medicines

During the 1980s there were increasing calls from a number of sectors to review the role of medicines in health maintenance. The number of medicines available world-wide was increasing and the treatment and prevention of many diseases were trans-formed as a result. However, there was increasing recognition that medicines were costly, did not always lead to positive outcomes and often caused harm. In 1985 the World Health Organisation (WHO) held an international meeting, entitled Rational Use of Drugs, to examine the role of medicines in promoting health and subsequently called on all governments to implement a National Medicinal Drug Policy (WHO 1988). By the beginning of the 1990s, 80 countries, including Australia, had developed national quality or rational medicine usage policies and were implementing various QUM strat-egies (WHO 2001).

Australia's policy on the Quality Use of Medicines (QUM) was launched in August 1992 and was unique in that it emphasised a partnership approach to medicine usage by all those involved:

- Consumers and their carers.
- Health professionals including doctors, pharmacists and nurses.
- Government.
- The pharmaceutical industry (Department of Health and Ageing 2002; Murray et al. 1999).

QUM became an integral component of the National Medicines Policy in 2000. It encompasses the whole spectrum of medicines, including prescription, non-prescription and complementary health-care products. It covers service aspects such as timely access to medicines, safety and quality standards and the need for a viable local pharmaceutical manufacturing industry (Australian Pharmaceutical Advisory Council 1999).

9.5.1   What does QUM involve?

QUM involves selecting management options wisely by:

- Considering the place of medicines in treating illness and maintaining health.
- Recognising there may be better ways than medicines to manage many disorders.
- Choosing suitable medicines, if a medicine is necessary, so that the best available option is selected by taking into account:
  (1)   the individual
  (2)   risks and benefits
  (3)   dosage and duration of treatment
  (4)   coexisting conditions
  (5)   other therapies being used
  (6)   monitoring considerations
  (7)   costs for the individual, the community and the health system as a whole.
- Using medicines safely and effectively to get the best possible results by:
  (1)   monitoring outcomes
  (2)   minimising misuse, overuse and underuse
  (3)   improving people's ability to solve problems related to medicine, such as unwanted effects or managing multiple medication (Department of Health and Ageing 2002).

Five principles underpin QUM and provide a basis for the activities undertaken within medication management. These principles are:

(1)   The primacy of consumers.
(2)   Partnership.
(3)   Consultative, collaborative, multidisciplinary activity.
(4)   Support for existing activity.
(5)   Systems-based approaches (Department of Health and Ageing 2002).

9.5.2   QUM and medication management

To apply QUM to managing medicines with older people, it will be necessary to:

- Develop active partnerships between consumers, carers and health professionals.
- Ensure respect for individuals and their decision to take or not to take medicines.

- Undertake regular medicine review, which is fundamental to ongoing management.
- Make clinical decisions based on systematic and well-documented assessment reviews. The benefits of the medicine should outweigh the potential side effects and the possibility that the medicine could worsen a medical condition or interact with other medicines, herbs or foods the person is taking should be remembered. For example, olanzapine increases blood glucose, worsens hyperglycaemia and puts an older person at risk of hyperosmolar states and falls (see Chapters 2, 4 and 8).
- Refer to the responsible prescriber if medicines are indicated.
- Carry out changes to medicine doses, dose intervals or the medication regimen slowly, ideally over months rather than days or weeks.
- Stop medicines and seek an alternative course of action if there are not obvious benefits; for example, an older person with persistent hyperglycaemia on oral hypo-glycaemic agents may require insulin. However, all the factors related to insulin treatment need to be considered (see Chapters 2, 4 and 8).
- Titrate the dose forms for each person; for example, liquid or patch preparations may be more appropriate for a person on enteral feeds than crushing medicines, which can change their action.
- Start at the lower end of recommended dose ranges. Dosage increments should be gradual and reviewed regularly, especially in a person with renal disease.
- Identify side effects and stop the medicine responsible whenever possible.
- If new symptoms or diseases develop after a new medicine is introduced, assume that the symptoms/disease are due to that medicine until demonstrated otherwise (Ehms 2000).

Figure 9.1 depicts how QUM can be applied to managing medicines for older people with diabetes.

9.5.3 Working in partnership with older people with diabetes

The presence of a chronic disease such as diabetes can result in 'physical and psy-chological difficulties, socio-economic problems, reduced quality of life and sometimes social exclusion' (Department of Health 2001) and an altered life expectancy. However, people with diabetes are often the 'experts', in the sense that they know more about their particular health issues and responses than anyone else.

The concept of the 'expert patient' is gaining increasing attention in the literature and is influencing policy development.

> 'An observation often made by doctors, nurses and other health professionals who undertake long-term follow-up and care of people with particular chronic diseases like diabetes mellitus, arthritis or epilepsy is "my patient understands their disease better than I do".'
>
> (Department of Health 2001)

The term 'expert patient' refers to the concept that the person with the disease has an investment in understanding their health issues and as a knowledgeable person, their expertise is central to managing diseases such as diabetes. Research indicates that many consumers are anxious to use their medicines and other treatment effect-ively to reduce the severity of symptoms and increase the personal control they have over their lives (Consumers' Health Forum 1999).

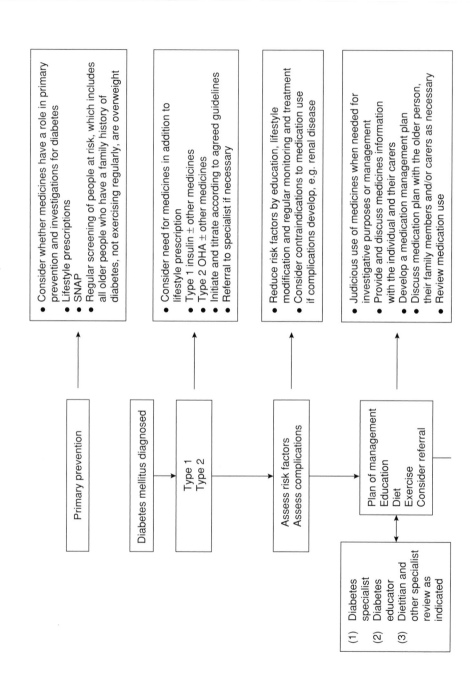

Primary prevention

- Consider whether medicines have a role in primary prevention and investigations for diabetes
- Lifestyle prescriptions
- SNAP
- Regular screening of people at risk, which includes all older people who have a family history of diabetes, not exercising regularly, are overweight

Diabetes mellitus diagnosed

Type 1
Type 2

- Consider need for medicines in addition to lifestyle prescription
- Type 1 insulin ± other medicines
- Type 2 OHA ± other medicines
- Initiate and titrate according to agreed guidelines
- Referral to specialist if necessary

Assess risk factors
Assess complications

- Reduce risk factors by education, lifestyle modification and regular monitoring and treatment
- Consider contraindications to medication use if complications develop, e.g. renal disease

Plan of management
Education
Diet
Exercise
Consider referral

- Judicious use of medicines when needed for investigative purposes or management
- Provide and discuss medicines information with the individual and their carers
- Develop a medication management plan
- Discuss medication plan with the older person, their family members and/or carers as necessary
- Review medication use

(1) Diabetes specialist
(2) Diabetes educator
(3) Dietitian and other specialist review as indicated

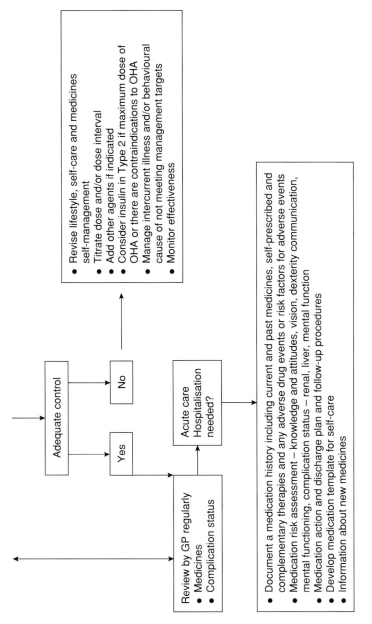

Figure 9.1 How QUM can be applied to managing medicines for older people with diabetes.

Older people are no exception. From a QUM perspective, an older person with diabetes becomes a partner in planning and providing care (Murray *et al.* 1999). Therefore, care is not done *to*, but *with*, the individual, except where the person is extremely frail, acutely ill or cognitively impaired, when other people, such as family members and carers, will be involved in care decisions. Sometimes the older person prepares advance directives to indicate their wishes. Mailed reminders can increase the proportion of people with chronic diseases who continue to take their medicines and improve medicine compliance (Hoffman *et al.* 2003). Table 9.1 outlines the type of information that can be given to people to help them learn about their medicines.

Practice point

As much as is possible, the older person should be involved in planning their care or receive care that complies with their preferences.

9.5.4   Documenting a medication history

A medication history should be taken whenever an older person is admitted to a health service, in order to effectively plan and manage their medication needs. Therefore, it is helpful if the medication history is obtained as early as possible in the episode of care. It should contain information about:

- Known allergies and sensitivities.
- Previous ADEs.
- Over-the-counter (OTC) medicine usage.
- Usage of herbal medicines, vitamins and other complementary products.
- Previous medication-related difficulties such as in obtaining medicines, opening packaging, affording medicines, obtaining or understanding CMI.
- Personal preferences, for instance managing pain.
- Any advance directives concerning medicine use.
- Adherence to their medication regimen and the reason for non-adherence. This may involve observing the person's usual medicine self-care practices such as administering insulin.

9.5.5   Developing a medication action plan

The aim of a medication action plan is to provide an overall framework for the medication activities that will occur as the person moves through an episode of care (Lynne 2003). When devising a medication action plan, it is necessary to work with the person or their carers to identify potential medication management problems and suggest strategies to address them. In some organisations such documentation forms part of risk assessment. Activities might include deciding whether:

- A medication review is needed.
- The individual, their carers or staff require information or education related to the medication/s; for example, when a new drug is first marketed, all of these people will require education about its safe use.

Table 9.1   Consumer education and medicines.

Research has shown that, with good education, many ADEs can be avoided. When educating a person about their medication regimen:

- Ensure a quiet place with minimal interruptions or distractions.
- Take time to build a rapport and encourage questions.
- Use an interpreter if appropriate – do not assume that the technical English regarding medicines will be understood.
- Provide written directions to reinforce your spoken instructions.
- Use consumer medicines information for all medicines, particularly new additions to the regimen.
- With the consumer's consent, include carers or family members who will be involved with medication management.
- Include in your education:
  (1)   what each medicine was prescribed for
  (2)   expected effect
  (3)   most likely side effects. Use discretion; include only the most likely or those that warrant seeking medical advice. For example, when working with an older person it is unlikely that they will experience the same side effects as for a pregnant woman
  (4)   time of day the medicine is to be taken
  (5)   how the medicine is to be used, e.g. taken on an empty stomach, before or after meals, applied to the skin, with milk, etc.
- Check whether the formulation can be managed by the consumer, e.g. tablets versus liquid, crushing to facilitate swallowing or patch formulation.
- Check the compatibility of medicines with any over-the-counter, herbal or complementary medicines also used by the consumer.
- If equipment is needed, demonstrate and then observe use; for example, drawing up appropriate units of insulin, using an administration device.
- Ensure that all bottles and packaging can be opened.
- If there is any difficulty, investigate alternative packaging or a dose administration aid – a compartmental box or blister packaging, which is packed by a pharmacist.
- Ensure the consumer knows how, where and when to obtain repeat prescriptions or supplies.
- If a medication review is indicated, discuss it with the consumer and assist with referral.
- If discharging a person from your service, ensure information is passed on, with the consumer's consent, to local prescriber or general practitioner and other services involved with ongoing care.
- Include telephone number of support organisations and local health services in case of accidental poisoning or an adverse drug event.

Special considerations
- Any precautions needed when driving.
- The need to carry glucose to manage hypoglycaemia.
- The need to wear identification indicating they have diabetes, especially if they are on oral hypoglycaemic agents or insulin.
- Safe disposal of used sharps such as needles and lancets.

- There is a need for education about techniques such as administering insulin or performing blood glucose testing.
- Carers need to be involved.
- Any investigations are needed before commencing a medicine, for example HbA_{1c} and lipids.
- The person is using any complementary therapies that could interact with the medicines.

9.5.6   The medicine review – identifying older people at risk of an ADE

The value of medicine review is well accepted. In a two-month period, Straand & Rokstaal (1999) found that 13.5% of older people were given excessive doses, potentially harmful medicine combinations and medicines that are contraindicated in older people. Ideally, a medication review should involve the individual and their carers, general practitioner and/or other prescribers, a pharmacist accredited to perform medicine reviews, nursing staff delivering care, for example visiting or home nurses, or staff of a residential aged care facility. It may be necessary to include other health-care professionals such as a dietitian on a case-by-case basis. The wishes of the person with diabetes should be taken into consideration when deciding who should be involved in the review.

A medication review can help to identify potential problems with drug–drug, drug–herb and drug–food interactions, medicines that could be ceased and self-management deficits such as inappropriate administration techniques or the need for medication education. A person may be at risk of medication-related problems due to:

- Comorbidities that require multiple drugs to be used. These include diabetes complications that affect drug metabolism and excretion, such as renal disease, and visual and manual dexterity deficits that affect self-care.
- Their age; increasing age is associated with an increased number of medicine-related incidents.
- Social circumstances and available support.
- Characteristics of their medicines.
- Complexity of their medication treatment regimen, for example managing complex regimens and/or delivering enteral feeds.
- Confusion or lack of knowledge about how to use medicines or the skills to use them appropriately, for example inability to see to draw or dial up the correct dose of insulin.
- Unpleasant side effects of medicines.

Compliance, which is also referred to as 'adherence' and 'concordance' (Wade 1999), is said to be one of the greatest challenges to older people attaining positive outcomes from medicines (Shepherd 1998). Compliance is a complex concept and there are many causes of non-compliance, which include:

- Polypharmacy.
- Difficulty opening bottles, packets or blister packs.
- Unpleasant side effects of medicines.
- Not understanding the medication regimen, what their medicines do and why they need to be taken at specific intervals or for a set time, which is often a result of inadequate or inappropriate medicines education.

- Depression and cognitive impairment, which might be due to the side effects of drugs, for example sedatives and diabetogenic drugs that cause hyperglycaemia, lethargy and/or confusion.
- Presence of diabetes complications such as vision deficits and reduced manual dexterity.
- Acute illness or medical or surgical emergencies.
- Beliefs and attitudes towards medicines.
- Financial constraints.
- Loss of independence, for example losing their driver's licence for a period of time if they have a serious hypoglycaemic event (see Chapter 3).

Criteria for undertaking a medication review for people living in the community

Risk factors known to predispose people to medication-related problems include:

- Currently taking five or more regular medicines.
- Taking more than 12 doses of medication per day.
- Significant changes in the medication treatment regimen during the last three months.
- Taking medicines with a narrow therapeutic index and/or requiring therapeutic monitoring, such as warfarin and digoxin.
- The presence of symptoms suggestive of an adverse drug reaction.
- Suboptimal response to treatment with medicines.
- Suspected non-compliance or inability to manage medication-related therapeutic devices.
- Literacy or language difficulties, dexterity problems, impaired sight, confusion or dementia or other cognitive difficulties.
- Attending a number of different general practitioners and specialists for a number of disease entities.
- Discharge from a facility or hospital in the previous four weeks (Department of Health and Aged Care 2001).

Practice points

(1) In addition to regular medication reviews, the registered nurse should exercise clinical judgement to determine whether reviews are required more frequently and take steps to ensure that a referral is made if indicated.
(2) A medication review may be required when a carer becomes frail, depressed, ill or unable to cope. Carers may request a medication review.

Criteria for undertaking a medication review for people in residential aged care

All older people living in residential aged care are, by definition, at risk of an ADE. Those at most risk:

- Are a new resident.
- Have multiple medical conditions.
- Take seven or more medicines.

- Are prescribed:
    (1) opioid medicines
    (2) antipsychotics
    (3) anti-infective agents
    (4) antiepileptic agents
    (5) antidepressant agents (Atkin *et al.* 1994; Gurwitz *et al.* 2000; Field *et al.* 2001).

It is important to note that the criteria listed are not exclusive. They reflect issues that current research has identified as being significant. However, a clinician needs to be mindful that their clinical expertise should also guide practice. As in all areas of nursing practice, the role of the registered nurse in relation to QUM is to exercise sound decision-making skills and professional judgement.

Practice point

People with diabetes may be prescribed antipsychotic and antiepileptic agents to control the pain of diabetic peripheral neuropathy. Therefore, it is important to clarify why medicines were prescribed before ceasing them. The effectiveness of the medicines should be measured according to the reason they were prescribed.

9.5.7 Providing medicine-related information

There is evidence that when consumers feel well informed, they manage their medication regimen with confidence (Consumers' Health Forum 1999) and the incidence of medicines-related ADEs reduces (Krska *et al.* 2001). There are two components to ensuring consumers have sufficient information. The first is a medication record. Consumer organisations and, more recently, governments promote the idea that all consumers should have a record of their current medication regimen that any health professionals involved with their medication regimen can access (Adamson *et al.* 1988). Medicine records play a significant role in minimising the risk of duplicate prescribing or potential interactions between medications. A medication record should also include details of any over-the-counter and complementary items being used, including minerals and vitamins, which can interact with medicines or prevent or delay their absorption.

The second component concerns providing medicine information and education. The specific situation will dictate how education and medicine information will be given; for example, a discharge folio that contains clear, user-friendly information to assist the person to use their medicines appropriately (Lynne 2003). Consumer medicines information (CMI) is required to accompany all medicines listed on the Pharmaceutical Benefits Scheme (PBS) in Australia. CMI information must be kept up to date, be easy for consumers to use and be consistent with the technical product information (PI) that medicine manufacturers are required to submit to the government when they seek approval for a medicine to be used in Australia. Copies of the relevant CMI can be included in the folio.

CMI can be provided by the prescriber at the time of the consultation or, more commonly, by a pharmacist when the medicines are dispensed. Registered nurses also find CMI helpful to explain medicines to the people in their care and their family members. CMI provides information about the medicine, its expected effects and what side effects to be aware of. Answers to some of the more common questions about the medicine and how to use it wisely are included. Nurses should also have access to non-biased information about medicines such as *The Australian Medicines Handbook, The Endocrinology Guidelines* and the *British National Formulary*.

Practice point

CMI is only available for prescription and pharmacist-only medicines in Australia. Therefore, many over-the-counter medicines and medicines sold in the supermarket do not have CMI inside the packaging.

It is much harder to ensure that residents in aged care facilities have access to CMI, because many residents do not manage their own medication regimen. However, using relevant CMI can be very helpful when discussing medicines with family members and resident advocates. In this way family members become part of the care plan, which is a fundamental principle underpinning the Aged Care Act 1997 (Department of Health and Family Services 1997).

Practice point

Medication management, assessment and activities, particularly medication education, should be given in the person's preferred language and might require interpreters. Given the nature of medication education, it is generally inappropriate for family members to interpret technical information.

9.5.8 Liaison about medicines

One of the continuing problems is the difficulty of ensuring that accurate and timely information is communicated between health professionals or health services, especially on discharge from an acute care service to a community-based service such as general practitioner or visiting nursing service. Liaison between hospital and community health-care providers is central to discharge planning (Australian Pharmaceutical Advisory Council 1998). However, information might also need to be passed between community-based health professionals, for example a general practitioner, pharmacist, community nursing services or the staff of a residential aged care facility. In the past, discharge information was generally sent by mail but most organisations now accept electronic transfer including fax or email.

It is important to communicate:

● Details of the admission, including the reason for the admission and the duration of the episode.
● Changes to the medication regimen.
● Any reported/identified adverse drug reactions.
● Specific needs such as ongoing education or supervision with blood glucose monitoring or insulin administration.
● Arrangements for follow-up care.

QUM requires registered nurses to foster a co-operative, collaborative approach between health-care professionals. Any questions or concerns regarding a person's medicines must be directed to either the prescriber or the pharmacist.

9.6 Nursing responsibilities

(1) Registered nurses play an important role in medication management, not only in administering medicines. The role encompasses a duty of care to practise quality use of medicines; that is, to ensure medicines are used judiciously, appropriately, safely and effectively.

(2) Medication administration is largely governed by practices sanctioned within law, for example by relevant legislation and regulations, and professional associations and regulatory bodies such as the Australian Nursing Federation and the UK Nursing and Midwifery Council.

(3) Nursing regulatory authorities require each registered nurse to check, to their own satisfaction and on the written order of a medical practitioner, the following:
- that it is the right medicine
- that it is the right dose
- that it is the right time
- that it is the right route
- that it is the right person (Australian Nursing Federation 2002).

(4) Appropriately document any medicines administered.

(5) Ensure the individual and/or their family or carers are involved in all aspects of medicine-related decision making.

(6) Exercise clinical decision-making skills and professional judgement to identify medication-related problems and refer to other health professionals as indicated.

(7) Maintain up-to-date knowledge of pharmacokinetics, pharmacodynamics and pharmacogenetics in older people.

(8) Use CMI in all client and family medicine-related education.

(9) Actively monitor and document and where relevant report/discuss the effects of medicines.

(10) Report all concerns related to medication regimens to the prescriber and/or pharmacist.

Practice points

(1) Many medicines cannot be crushed for administration. Check with a reliable, independent source, for example the *Australian Medicines Handbook, British National Formulary* or a pharmacist, about whether a particular medicine can be crushed before it is administered and the availability of alternative formulations, particularly if the medicine is to be administered via a PEG tube (see Chapter 2).

(2) It is important to ensure the medicine order is clear and not ambiguous; for example, insulin doses should be written as 'units' not 'u/s' or 'u'. These abbreviations have led to dose errors and litigation.

References

Adamson, L., Kwok, Y. & Smith, S. (1988) *Too Much of a Good Thing: Older Consumers and Their Medications.* Australian Consumers' Association and Combined Pensioners' Association, Melbourne.

Anderson, D. & Webster, C. (2001) A systems approach to the reduction of medication error on the hospital ward. *Journal of Advanced Nursing,* **35**(1), 34–41.

Andrews, G.R. (2001) Promoting health and function in an ageing population. *British Medical Journal,* **322**, 728–9.

Atkin, P.A., Finnegan, T., Ogle, S., Talmont, D. & Shenfield, M. (1994) Prevalence of drug related admissions to a hospital geriatric service. *Australian Journal on Ageing,* **13**(1), 17–21.

Australian Bureau of Statistics (1999) *National Health Survey Use of Medications Australia.* Australian Bureau of Statistics, Canberra.

Australian Council for Safety and Quality in Health Care (2002) *Second National Report on Patient Safety: Improving Medication Safety.* AusInfo, Canberra.

Australian Institute of Health and Welfare (AIHW) (2002) *Older Australia at a Glance,* 3rd edn. AusInfo, Canberra.

Australian Institute of Health and Welfare (AIHW) (2003a) *Residential Aged Care in Australia 2001–02. A Statistical Overview.* AusInfo, Canberra.

Australian Institute of Health and Welfare (AIHW) (2003b) *Nursing Labour Force 2001.* AusInfo, Canberra.

Australian Institute of Health and Welfare (AIHW) (2004) *Extended Aged Care at Home (EACH) Census: A Report on the Results of the Census Conducted in May 2002.* AIHW, Canberra.

Australian Nursing Federation (Victoria) (2002) *Policy Statement. Double Checking In Medication Administration.* ANF, Victoria.

Australian Pharmaceutical Advisory Council (1998) *National Guidelines to Achieve the Continuum of Quality Use of Medicines Between Hospital and Community.* Australian Government Publishing Service, Canberra.

Australian Pharmaceutical Advisory Council (1999) *National Medicines Policy 2000.* Commonwealth Department of Health and Aged Care, Canberra.

Baker, H. (1999) Medication errors: where does the fault lie? In: *Nursing and the Quality Use of Medicines* (eds S. Hunt & R. Parkes). Allen & Unwin, Sydney.

Bevan, C. & Jeeawody, B. (1998) *Successful Ageing. Perspectives on Health and Social Construction.* Mosby, Sydney.

Buerhaus, P.I. (1999) Lucian Leape on the causes and prevention of errors and adverse events in health care. *Image: Journal of Nursing Scholarship,* **31**(3), 281–6.

Cohen, M. (2001) 'High-alert' medications and patient safety. *International Journal for Quality in Health Care,* **13**(4), 339–40.

Consumers' Health Forum (1999) *Understanding Consumer Behaviour and Experiences in Relation to the Use of Medicines. Literature Review.* Consumers' Health Forum, Canberra.

Consumers' Health Forum of Australia (1997) *Cost of Chronic Illness and Quality Use of Medicines.* Consumers' Health Forum of Australia, Canberra.

Department of Health (2000) *An Organisation with a Memory. Report of an Expert Group on Learning from Adverse Events in the NHS.* Department of Health, London.

Department of Health (2001) *The Expert Patient: A New Approach to Chronic Disease Management for the 21st Century.* Department of Health, London.

Department of Health and Aged Care (2001) *Domiciliary Medication Management – Home Medicines Review.* AusInfo, Canberra.

Department of Health and Ageing (2002) *The National Strategy for Quality Use of Medicines. Executive Summary.* Department of Health and Ageing, Canberra.

248   *Chapter 9*

Department of Health and Ageing (2003) *Australian Statistics on Medicines 1999–2000.* AusInfo, Canberra.

Department of Health and Family Services (1997) *The Residential Care Manual.* Department of Health and Family Services, Canberra.

Dhalla, I.A., Anderson, G., Mamdani, M., Bronskill, S., Sykora, K. & Rochon, P. (2002) Inappropriate prescribing before and after nursing home admission. *Journal of the American Geriatrics Society,* **50**, 995–1000.

Eaton, L. (2002) Adverse reaction to drugs increase. *British Medical Journal,* **324**, 8.

Ebner, M.K. (1999) Older adults living with chronic pain: an opportunity for improvement. *Journal of Nursing Care Quality,* **13**(4), 1–7.

Ehms, S.-A. (2000) *Quality Use of Medicines. Reference Guide.* Veterans' Medication Management Consortium of NSW and ACT, Sydney.

Field, T.S., Gurwitz, J., Avorn, J. et al. (2001) Risk factors for adverse drug events among nursing home residents. *Archives of Internal Medicine,* **161**(13), 1629–34.

Flacker, J. & Marcanonio, E. (1998) Delirium in the elderly. *Drugs and Aging,* **13**(2), 119–30.

Fonda, D., Benvenuti, F., Cottenden, A. et al. (2002) *Urinary Incontinence and Bladder Dysfunction in Older Persons. 2nd International Consultation on Incontinence.* Health Publications, Paris.

Galloway, S. & Turner, L. (1999) Pain assessment in older adults who are cognitively impaired. *Journal of Gerontological Nursing,* **July**, 34–9.

Gurwitz, J.H., Soumerai, S. & Avorn, J. (1990) Improving medication prescribing and utilization in the nursing home. *Journal of the American Geriatrics Society,* **38**(5), 542–52.

Gurwitz, J.H., Field, T. & Avorn, J. (2000) Incidence and preventability of adverse drug events in nursing homes. *American Journal of Medicine,* **109**, 87–94.

Hoffman, L., Enders, J., Luo, J., Segal, R., Pippins, J. & Kimberlin, C. (2003) Impact of an antidepressant management program on medication adherence. *American Journal of Managed Care,* **9**(1), 70–80.

House of Commons Select Committee on Health (2004) *Second Report.* Stationery Office, London.

International Council of Nurses (2004) *Nursing Matters. ICN on Healthy Ageing: A Public Health and Nursing Challenge.* ICN, Geneva.

Jenkins, A. (1996) *Client Profiles for Aged Care Services in Australia.* Australian Institute of Health and Welfare, Canberra.

Krska, J., Cromarty, J., Arris, F. et al. (2001) Pharmacist-led medication review in patients over 65: a randomized controlled trial in primary care. *Age and Ageing,* **30**, 205–11.

Le Couteur, D. (2004) Prescribing in older people. *Australian Family Physician,* **33**(10), 777–81.

Leipzig, R.M., Cumming, R. & Tinetti, M. (1999) Drugs and falls in older people: a systematic review and meta-analysis: I. Psychotropic drugs. *Journal of the American Geriatrics Society,* **47**(1), 30–9.

Lothian, K. (2001) Maintaining the dignity and autonomy of older people in the healthcare setting. *British Medical Journal,* **322**, 668–70.

Lynne, T. (ed.) (2003) *Medication Management Manual.* Queensland Health, Brisbane.

Mant, A. & Donnelly, N. (1996) Drug use in nursing homes: some new evidence. *Medical Journal of Australia,* **165**, 295.

Martin, E.D., Burgess, N. & Doecke, C. (2000) Evaluation of an automated drug distribution system in an Australian teaching hospital. *Australian Journal of Hospital Pharmacy,* **30**(4), 141–5.

Mayor, S. (2000) English NHS to set up new reporting system for errors. *British Medical Journal,* **320**, 1689.

McGavock, H. (2003) *How Drugs Work. Basic Pharmacology for Healthcare Professionals.* Ausmed, Melbourne.

Meurier, C.E., Vincent, C. & Parmar, D. (1998) Nurses' responses to severity dependent errors: a study of the causal attributions made by nurses following an error. *Journal of Advanced Nursing*, **27**, 349–54.

Moore, A.R. & O'Keeffe, S. (1999) Drug-induced cognitive impairment in the elderly. *Drugs and Aging*, **15**(1), 15–28.

Murray, M., Hunt, S. & Parkes, R. (1999) Nurse involvement in QUM. In: *Nursing and the Quality Use of Medicines* (eds S. Hunt & R. Parkes). Allen & Unwin, Sydney.

National Health and Medical Research Council (1994) *Medication for the Older Person.* Australian Government Publishing Service, Canberra.

O'Shea, E. (1999) Factors contributing to medication errors: a literature review. *Journal of Clinical Nursing*, **8**, 496–504.

Parmelee, P.A., Smith, B. & Katz, I. (1993) Pain complaints and cognitive status among elderly institution residents. *Journal of the American Geriatrics Society*, **41**(5), 517–22.

Roberts, M.S. (1998) *Medication Use in Aged Care Hostels. A Team Approach Applied to Defining and Optimising Quality Use in Residents of Aged Care Hostels.* The Quality Use of Medication Care Group, Departments of Medicine, Pharmacy and Social and Preventative Medicine, University of Queensland.

Roberts, M.S. & Bonner, C. (1995) *Project to Optimise the Quality of Drug Use in the Elderly in Long Term Care Facilities in Australia.* Departments of Medicine, Pharmacy and Social and Preventative Medicine, University of Queensland.

Shakib, S. (2002) Problems of polypharmacy. *Australian Family Physician Online*, **31**(2), 125–7.

Shepherd, M. (1998) The risks of polypharmacy. *Nursing Times*, **94**(32), 60–2.

Straand, J. & Rokstaal, K. (1999) Elderly patients in general practice: diagnosis, drugs and inappropriate prescriptions. A prescription study. *Family Practitioner*, **16**(94), 380–8.

Tanne, J.H. (2004) One in 12 people are prescribed the wrong drug. *British Medical Journal*, **328**, 424.

Thornton, P.D., Simon, S. & Mathew, T. (1999) Towards safer drug prescribing, dispensing and administration in hospitals. *Journal of Quality Clinical Practice*, **19**, 41–5.

Wade, T. (1999) Consumers or patients – partnerships or compliance? In: *Nursing and the Quality Use of Medicines* (eds S. Hunt & R. Parkes). Allen & Unwin, Sydney.

World Health Organization (WHO) (1988) *The World Drug Situation.* WHO, Geneva.

World Health Organization (WHO) (2001) *National Drug Policies.* WHO, Geneva.

Chapter 10
Sexuality and Older People with Diabetes

Trisha Dunning

Key points

- Health professionals need to be comfortable with their own sexuality to counsel effectively.
- Sexual problems are common in people with diabetes, especially men.
- The presence of a sexual problem and diabetes does not mean one led to the other.
- Physical, psychological and social factors should be considered.
- Sex education is part of preventive diabetes care.
- The focus should be on what is normal and achievable for the individual rather than focusing on dysfunction and abnormality.
- The relationship between sex, intimacy and dementia is not well understood.
- People with dementia may display a need for sexual intimacy in inappropriate ways that put other people and staff at risk.

10.1   Introduction

The majority of books and papers concerning diabetes in older people do not adequately address sexuality. People with diabetes expect nurses to have some knowledge about the impact of diabetes on their sexual health. Nurses are ideally placed to be able to emphasise the need for primary prevention and early identification of sexual difficulties and to dispel sexual mythology.

10.2   Sexual health

Sexual health is a core aspect of the general wellbeing of an individual. Sexual identity, sexual desire and the need for intimacy continue throughout life, including in older people. Unfortunately, society often appears to perceive sexual activity as inappropriate for older people and portrays sexually inaccurate stereotypes, which affect older people's sexual self-image. Self-image, of which sexuality is only one aspect, is linked to perceptions of usefulness to society (Littler 1997).

Sexual functioning is contingent on the integration of many components into a unified complex system, which involves endocrine hormonal regulators and the vascular, nervous and psychological systems. Diabetes can profoundly affect an individual's sexual identity and the physical ability to engage in sexual activity. These things are further affected by increasing age. The sexual aspects of an individual's life should be an integral part of a holistic management plan for all people with diabetes and must be considered when placement in a care facility is necessary, especially when people are in a relationship. Sexual issues are highly sensitive and must be approached with tact and consideration of the person's culture, privacy and confidentiality.

Many factors concerned with increasing age, presence of diabetes, gender, resilience, self-efficacy, the environment and societal attitudes affect sexual relationships (see Table 10.1). The World Health Organization (WHO 1975) defined the ideal for sexual health and stressed the importance of considering sexuality as an integral component of health. The WHO defined sexual health as:

> 'The capacity to control and enjoy sexual and reproductive behaviour, freedom from shame, guilt and false beliefs which inhibit sexual responsiveness and relationships. Freedom from medical disorders that interfere with sexual responsiveness and reproduction.'

(WHO 1975)

The reality is far more complex and difficult to measure than the WHO ideal definition implies. In fact, there is no single universally recognised measurement scale for sexual dysfunction (Najman *et al.* 2003). Therefore, actually defining 'sexual dysfunction' is difficult. It may be even more difficult to define in older people with cognitive impairment or dementia.

Masters and Johnson first described the human sexual response in 1970. They described four phases: arousal, plateau, orgasm and resolution (Masters & Johnson 1970). These phases blend into each other and sexual difficulties can occur in one or all of these stages. Later, Kaplan (1979) described the parasympathetic nerve activity causing vasocongestion, vaginal lubrication and erection, and sympathetic nerve activity that results in reflex muscle contraction, orgasm and ejaculation, as a biphasic response. Kaplan's description makes it easier to see how diabetes can affect physical sex in men, given that autonomic neuropathy causes nerve damage. Masters & Johnson and Kaplan found that sexual responsiveness is more varied in women than men.

Sexual difficulties do not occur in isolation from other aspects of an individual's life and relationships and the society in which they live. Therefore, a thorough assessment and history is necessary to identify what is normal for the individual.

10.3   Sexual development

Sexual development and sexual identity develops throughout the lifespan. In broad terms, the following stages occur (Dunning 2003).

- Chromosomal sex is determined at fertilisation.
- 3–5 years: diffuse sexual pleasure, fantasies and sex play. The child often forms a close relationship with the parent of the opposite sex.

Table 10.1 Possible causes of sexual difficulties. Sexual difficulties may be present as a result of normal ageing, the effects of diabetes and other illnesses, relationship difficulties and environmental factors. Often the causes of sexual difficulties are multifactorial.

Normal ageing	Effects of diabetes and other illness	Psychological and relationship factors	Environmental factors
Men Less rigid erections. Erections do not last as long. Erection subsides during intercourse. Penis becomes less sensitive. Orgasms less intense. Fewer erections on waking. *Women* Increased vaginal dryness. Reduced vaginal size and tone. Orgasms less intense. Rapid resolution. More frequent postcoital urethral irritation. *Both* Take longer to become aroused. Reduced frequency of intercourse. Require more direct, intense and prolonged genital stimulation. Interpersonal relationship becomes important.	*General* Body image changes. Body changes due to normal ageing (see Chapter 1). Physical pain. Reduced mobility and ability to used/favourite sex positions. Anxiety and depression. Fatigue and lack of energy. Fear of failure and of dying during intercourse. Need for intimacy in dementia can be misinterpreted and put others at risk. Effect of drugs, e.g. vaginal dryness, reduced libido, erectile dysfunction, polyuria. Odours due to incontinence or other factors. *Diabetes* Hypoglycaemia. Hyperglycaemia. Complications such as neuropathy that alters sensation or causes erectile dysfunction. Infections such as thrush. Pain. Constipation due to reduced gut mobility. Anxiety, stress and depression.	Ignorance. Guilt and shame. Poor communication generally and/or due to cognitive deficits and dementia. Myths and stereotypes. Fear of 'dropping dead while doing "it"'. Loss of a partner. Stress, anxiety and depression. Focus may be on giving and receiving pleasure rather than penetration. Frottage can often be very fulfilling.	Comfort and ambience. Privacy, fear of 'being caught'. Attitudes of others. Opportunity. Ample time. Safety.

- 5–8 years: interested in sexual differences between boys and girls. Sex play is common.
- 8–9 years: begin to evaluate personal attractiveness and are curious about sex.
- 10–12 years: preoccupation with changes in their body and puberty.
- 13–20 years: puberty, development of self-image and sexual identity.
- Late 30s–early 40s: peak sexual responsiveness.
- Menopause: variable onset and highly individual effect on sexuality. Debate about whether male menopause occurs is still continuing.
- Old age: physical difficulties may be present and opportunities for sexual expression is often limited.

Many factors influence a person's sexual attitudes and needs, including age-related changes, and disease processes that can affect their body image, sexual responsiveness and self-esteem (Riley 1999). Sex is often not as satisfying for older people and may cause embarrassment and guilt. Interpersonal relationships, monotony, unresolved grief and seeking new partners in later life when there are fewer opportunities for relationships, with and without sex, make this aspect of life difficult for many older people.

However, these generalisations have little predictive value for a 'normal' sexual identity and functioning for older individuals (Heath 2002). Societal attitudes, experience and prevailing norms are among the factors that affect sexuality. The fact that a person is growing older does not mean they do not have sexual needs, although the type of sexual activity may change with increasing age. Some people with Alzheimer's disease exhibit increased sexual activity (Gibson 1992; Depuesne *et al.* 1996). Recognising these sexual needs and helping the individual, family and staff to deal with them appropriately is an ongoing challenge for nurses working in aged care settings. Sexual issues in people with Alzheimer's disease include:

- Sexual modesty, which can make providing intimate nursing care procedures very intrusive and can result in verbal and physical abuse.
- Specific sexual behaviours, including disinhibition, which may put staff and other residents at risk.
- Changed sexual activities in relationships, relationship breakdown, stress in partners and trauma.
- The effects of sexual behaviours on family members and staff.
- Illicit sexual relationships, putting the individual at risk of sexually transmitted diseases.

The causes of sexual changes in older people are multifactorial and occur as a result of change in the cerebral cortex, effects of medicines and the inability to continue to enjoy other aspects of life. In addition, many residential aged care facilities are not adequately set up to facilitate sexual activity and there is an emphasis on single rooms and single beds. In addition, a great deal of intimate care of older people is given by younger women, which can be stressful for some older people. A book published by the UK Relatives and Residents Association highlighted the fact that aged care facilities do not meet the sexual needs of older residents (O'Dowd 2001). Likewise, the document *Improving Care for Older People* (Department of Human Services Victoria 2003) makes no mention of sexual needs.

Elderly people experience a range of health problems that affect their sexuality. In addition to erectile dysfunction in men as a consequence of diabetes, these include breast and genital atrophy in women as a result of changed hormone status. The vaginal mucosa becomes thin, which increases the risk of trauma, inflammation and infection as a result of sexual activity or nursing procedures such as catheterisation or taking vaginal swabs. Women over 65 are interested in discussing sexual issues with their doctors but rarely do so because the doctors do not seem to understand or be concerned (Nusbaum 2004).

Women report reduced interest in sex, unmet intimacy needs and the desire for sex education, despite being over 65. In addition, older women are less likely to be concerned about adopting safe sex practices or contracting sexually transmitted disease, although the risk remains, even late in life (Nusbaum 2004).

Men are able to reproduce to a much later age than women because testicular atrophy occurs late. Prostatic hypertrophy, which leads to difficulty voiding and incomplete emptying of the bladder, is relatively common and increases the risk of urinary infection in older men with diabetes. Premature ejaculation appears to be the most common sexual dysfunction in men of all age groups (Najman *et al.* 2003), followed by performance anxiety. However, the main issue discussed with respect to men with diabetes is erectile dysfunction, which occurs in ~50% of men with diabetes and may reduce sexual activity, since management recommendations rarely suggest other ways of giving and receiving sexual pleasure besides intercourse.

Arousal needs to be more direct, intense and prolonged and involve genital stimulation for both older men and women, and orgasm usually takes longer. Therefore, ensuring uninterrupted time and privacy is essential. In addition, helping people communicate their sexual needs to their partner is important, especially given that inadequate communication leads to many sexual difficulties. Effective sexual communication can be complicated by cognitive deficits and resultant inappropriate sexual behaviours.

The cumulative effects of intercurrent illness apply to both men and women with diabetes and include:

- Fear of:
  (1) hypoglycaemia, especially older people with Type 1 diabetes
  (2) myocardial infarction
  (3) stroke.
- Pain, due to sexual activity or fear of causing pain in a partner, or existing pain due to other reasons such as arthritis and vaginal dryness.
- Osteoporosis that can lead to stress fractures and pain during sexual activity.
- Arthritis, which may limit the sexual positions and the type of touch the couple can use without causing discomfort.
- Medicines that affect erectile function, cognition or strength and energy.
- Psychological and psychiatric factors such as job loss, death of a spouse, loss of home and moving to a care facility or to live with family, loss of usual activities.
- Dementia.

Despite these limitations many older couples enjoy an enhanced relationship where they can be a couple and develop a different type of closeness, sexual intimacy, and companionship in their relationship. Developing a new relationship can be daunting in the face of family opposition and societal stereotyping, especially when there is an age disparity, for example 'dirty old man' and 'mutton dressed as lamb'.

Effective sex education and diabetes education should be part of the diabetes management plan so intimacy and sexual health issues can be identified early. Health professionals and people with diabetes often have limited information about the impact diabetes can have on intimacy and sexuality. Sex education, good metabolic control, early identification and management of sexual problems are important, often neglected aspects of the diabetes care plan.

When sex issues are considered, the focus is often on dysfunction and performance, rather than what is normal for the individual or couple, which can have a negative psychological impact on sexuality. The focus can be altered to concentrate on what the individual can achieve and how to promote intimacy, love and warmth in a relationship and improve sexual wellbeing, remembering that sexual satisfaction is a combination of physical and emotional factors. Sexual activity has other health benefits. It is a good cardiovascular exercise, increases blood flow, improves muscle tone in women and makes people feel valued and needed (Gibson 1992).

10.4   Sexual problems

Defining the nature of the 'sexual problem' is central to effective management. Sexual problems can be:

- Primary – usually defined as never having an orgasm.
- Secondary – difficulties occur after a period of normal functioning. Most sexual difficulties fit into this category.
- Situational – where the situation itself inhibits sexual activity. Other primary or secondary sexual problems may also be present. Situational problems are often an issue for older people.

10.4.1   Overview of the causes of sexual difficulties

Sexual difficulties usually involve two people. The specific difficulty may be a shared problem or each person may have individual issues that need to be considered. Interpersonal factors, the relationship and environmental and disease factors need to be explored with the couple involved.

Individual factors

- Ignorance and misinformation are common despite the sexually permissive society of today. A great deal of readily available literature in magazines and on television overemphasises performance and sets up unreal expectations.
- Guilt, shame and fear, which may be fear of not pleasing the partner, being rejected by them or of having a hypoglycaemic or heart attack.
- Non-sexual concerns such as worry about finances or children or moving out of the family home.
- Past sexual abuse.
- Current physical health such as the status of diabetes, complications or other illnesses such as osteoporosis or arthritis that can inhibit giving and receiving pleasure.

- Inadequate information or misinformation about sex. Most sex education is developed for young people.

Interpersonal factors

A sexual relationship is one of the most complex relationships two people ever make, yet most people prepare for sexual relationships casually as young people and are often ignorant of the effects of increasing age, mechanics and psychological issues on their sexuality.

- Changes in lifestyle such as moving into an aged care facility or in with a family member.
- Communication problems are the most common sexual difficulty.
- Lack of trust.
- Different sexual preferences and desires, for example a desire for intimacy rather than intercourse.
- Relationship difficulties that can include problems associated with alcohol and violence or be related to disease processes, including diabetes, or environmental constraints on the relationship.

Chronic disease sequelae

Psychological
Depression, anger, guilt, anxiety, fear, feelings of helplessness, changed body image and self-identification as a victim, lowered self-image and self-esteem may or may not accompany the disease. Loss of libido is one of the classic signs of depression.

Physical changes such as arthritis and diabetic neuropathy
- Pain and debilitation associated with changed mobility such as arthritis, bad odour associated with infections, cardiac or respiratory problems, sleep apnoea and snoring can all inhibit sexual activity.
- Disease processes and hormonal imbalance, including diabetes, as well as other endocrine and reproductive conditions.
- Medicines such as antihypertensive and antidepressive agents can lead to erectile dysfunction and altered sexual activity.
- Alcohol consumption.

Diabetes related
- Hypoglycaemia during intercourse can be frightening and offputting, especially for the partner, and reduce spontaneity and enjoyment in future encounters.
- Tiredness and decreased arousal and libido are associated with hyperglycaemia.
- Mood disorders such as depression and other psychological problems may be present but mood can change with hypo- and hyperglycaemia and can cause temporary sexual problems.
- Autonomic neuropathy leading to erectile dysfunction in men and possibly decreased vaginal lubrication in older women. Vaginal dryness is also associated with normal ageing, not being aroused and painful intercourse and has not been definitively linked to diabetes as a cause.
- Infections such as vaginal or penile thrush or urinary tract infections.

Environmental factors

- Lack of privacy.
- Limited opportunity, especially in aged care facilities or when a partner dies or leaves.
- Uncomfortable, noisy surroundings.

10.5   Effects of diabetes on sexual functioning

10.5.1   Women

The biological effect of diabetes on male sexual functioning has been well documented. The effects of diabetes on sexual function in women are poorly understood and the evidence for any effect is less conclusive than the evidence for the effects on male sexual functioning (Leedom *et al.* 1991). There is no real evidence that physical function is impaired by diabetes in the same way as it is in men, except that older women with Type 2 diabetes report decreased vaginal lubrication, which could be due to reduced oestrogen and normal ageing, related to diabetic neuropathy or other causes such as inadequate arousal.

Women who have difficulty accepting that they have diabetes report higher levels of sexual dysfunction than those who accept their diabetes and integrate it into their lifestyles, but Type 2 diabetes has a pervasively negative effect on women's sexuality (Schriener-Engel *et al.* 1991). Fear of hypoglycaemia during sexual activity is well described in younger people and may occur in older people but the incidence is not known. There is a positive correlation between the degree of sexual dysfunction and the severity of depression which illustrates the connection between physical and psychological factors and the need for a holistic approach, especially in older people in whom the incidence of depression is high and often unrecognised.

Fluctuating blood glucose levels can have a negative transient effect on sexual desire and responsiveness in both men and women. Women often report slow arousal, decreased libido and inadequate lubrication during hyperglycaemia. However, these factors are also an aspect of normal ageing. There appears to be no correlation between the presence of diabetes complications and sexual difficulties in women with diabetes (Campbell *et al.* 1989; Dunning 1993).

10.5.2   Men

Longer time to achieve erections and difficulty sustaining an erection are part of normal ageing and can lead to fear of failure. Age-associated erectile dysfunction (ED) is common in men with diabetes, especially if other diabetic complications are present; 50% of men develop ED 10 years after diagnosis. Normal erections are defined as the ability to achieve or maintain an erection sufficient for satisfactory sexual performance – penetration and ejaculation. Smoking may be a predictor of cardiovascular risk and there is a higher incidence of undiagnosed coronary disease in men with ED. Lowered sperm counts are associated with obesity, smoking and poor diet and these factors can all reduce sexual activity in older men with diabetes.

Elevated blood fats and hypertension and antihypertensive agents may also play a part in the development of ED. ED is not confined to men with diabetes. Other causes include:

- Vascular damage, due to systemic atherosclerosis and microvascular disease.
- Neurological diseases such as diabetic neuropathy, spinal cord damage and multiple sclerosis.
- Psychological causes such as performance anxiety, depression and mood changes associated with hypo- or hyperglycaemia.
- Endocrine disease causing androgen deficiencies (SHBG, prolactin, FSH, LH, testosterone).
- Surgery and trauma to the genitalia or the nerves and vascular supply.
- Anatomical abnormalities such as Peyronie's contracture, which is often associated with other glycosylation diseases such as Dupuytren's contracture.
- Medicines such as thiazides, beta blockers, lipid-lowering agents, antidepressants.
- Smoking, alcohol and illicit drug use.
- Hypogonadism can occur in chronic disease.

ED causes a significant reduction in the man's quality of life, especially in the emotional domain, and has a negative effect on their self-esteem. When sexual functioning improves, improvement in mental and social status follows.

Management of erectile dysfunction

A thorough history and physical examination are required. This includes identifying the causative factors, determining blood glucose control and the extent of the dysfunction using devices such as the Rigiscan and snap gauges to discover if nocturnal erections occur. Sleep apnoea studies may be useful as there is an association between poor sleep, sleep apnoea and ED. Doppler studies are carried out to measure penile blood flow. Blood tests for testosterone, FSH, LH, SHBG and prolactin are necessary to determine hormone status.

- Good metabolic control.
- Early recognition and management by modifying risk factors where possible.
- Assess fitness for sexual activity and modify and give appropriate advice and education.
- Appropriate diet and exercise programme.
- Stop smoking and limit alcohol intake if applicable.
- Diabetes education.
- Counselling should include partners and inform them about treatment options and help them find fulfilling sexual alternatives, if the ED cannot be alleviated.

Medicines such as Viagra, Levitra and Cialis are vasodilators that enhance the natural sexual response. Viagra can cause transient hypotension and unmask cardiac ischaemia. These medicines should not be taken at the same time as GTN patches are applied and when some forms of cardiovascular disease are present. Cimetidine and ketoconazole increase Viagra levels.

10.6   Sex education

Sex education is important and needs to include:

- Revision of diabetes knowledge and self-care and the importance of blood and lipid control.

- Knowledge about sex and sexuality and what 'normal' functioning is.
- Sexual health and the need for protected intercourse. Regular monitoring of sexual health, pap smears, mammogram and prostate checks are advisable.

Hormonal changes and associated fatigue and depression may also inhibit sexual enjoyment. Often long-term partners have different sexual needs, which affects their sexual relationship. There are fewer partners and opportunities for sexual activity for older people, especially those in care facilities.

10.7   Complementary therapies

Men use a range of complementary therapies to enhance their sexual attractiveness and ability to achieve and maintain erections. Many preparations are unsafe and ineffective. In addition, hunting some animal species reputed to be aphrodisiacs, such as rhinoceros horn, has put many species on the endangered list. It is important to ascertain if any such products are being used before commencing conventional therapies.

10.8   Sexual counselling

Establishing good communication and trust with older people is essential. Knowledge of the human sexual response, the effects of normal ageing and the potential effects of diabetes on sexual functioning is needed to counsel effectively. Sexual questions can be included when taking a nursing history. Taking a sexual history can be simple and identify sexual problems and determine whether a more detailed history or referral is required. Respect and regard for the person, empathetic understanding and privacy are essential (Ross & Channon-Little 1991). Table 10.2 gives an outline of the main areas to be covered when taking a sexual history.

Practice points

(1)   There is a fine line between taking a sexual history and voyeurism.
(2)   Nurses need to clarify their own feelings and attitudes towards the sexual activity of older people and be aware of the possibility of transference, e.g. 'it's like my grandparents having sex'.

The main areas to ask about are:

- Social – number of children, whether the individual is sexually active, sex orientation.
- Sex – knowledge, problem (as described by the person).
- Psychological – acceptance of diabetes, body image, perceived effects of sex, depression, mental status.
- Physical – normal, diabetes complications, concomitant disease processes, ADLs.
- Diabetes – knowledge and self-care skills.

Table 10.2 An outline of important aspects to be enquired about when taking a sexual history.

---

(1) Social aspects
  - Childhood experiences.
  - Marital status.
  - Family relationships.
  - Number and sex of any children.
  - Interests, activities.
  - Job demands/retirement activities.
  - Religious and cultural beliefs.

(2) Sexual aspects
  - Sexual knowledge, education, fears, fantasies.
  - Previous sexual experiences.
  - If there is a current problem:
      - whose problem does the person believe it to be?
      - description of the problem in the person's own words.
      - is the partner aware of the problem?
      - does the problem follow a period of poor diabetic control or illness?
      - have there been any previous sexual problems?
      - what were those problems?
      - how were they resolved?

(3) Psychological aspects
  - Acceptance of diabetes by self and partner.
  - Body image concepts.
  - Presence of depression or other psychological problem.

(4) Diabetes knowledge
  Self-care skills and knowledge of effects of poor diabetic control.

- Counselling – the PLISSIT model (Annon 1975; Table 10.3) is a useful framework to use in sexual counselling. It also helps the nurse identify their level of knowledge and competence in the area. A general sexual history should be part of any health history and specific questions can be included where a sexual problem is identified.

10.9   Role of the nurse

The nurse has an important role in the early identification of sexual problems and helping the individual or couple develop a health plan that includes sexual health. Some sexually transmitted diseases must be notified to government health authorities in some countries.

Some specific nursing actions include:

- Considering and clarifying own beliefs and attitudes about older people engaging in sexual activity.

Table 10.3 Overview of the PLISSIT Model, which was first described by JS Annon in 1975. Although it is old it is still a very effective framework for nurses to use to ascertain their level of knowledge and competence to deal with sexual issues and to develop assessment and management strategies.

PLISSIT is an acronym for: Permission giving, providing Limited Information, offering Specific Suggestions, and Intensive Therapy. The model uses four phases to address sexual problems and moves from simple to complex issues. It can be used in a variety of settings and adapted to the individual's needs (Annon 1975).

(1) Permission giving

Being open and non-judgemental allows the person to discuss their problem by offering:

- Brochures and information in waiting areas.
- Reassurance.
- Acceptance of the person's concerns.
- A non-judgemental attitude.
- Acceptable terminology.

Questions about the person's sexuality can be asked or the nurse can respond to questions the person asks. These actions establish that it is appropriate and acceptable to discuss sexual issues.

(2) Providing limited information

This involves giving limited information and general suggestions that might include:

- Practising safe sex.
- Diabetes and sex education.
- Some references and information for home reading.

(3) Making specific suggestions

These are usually made by a qualified sex therapist and can include sensate focus exercises and the squeeze technique for premature ejaculation (Clarke & Clarke 1985).

- Specific ways about how to have sexual intercourse or give pleasure.
- Involve the partner.
- Provide sex education.

(4) Intensive therapy

Therapy at this stage may include:

- Referral to a sex psychologist/psychiatrist.
- Psychotherapy.
- Marital therapy.

- Providing opportunities for people to discuss sexual issues that include considerations of privacy and confidentiality. Often men with sexual difficulties feel more comfortable speaking about the issue with a nurse.
- Taking a sexual history and watching for important body language cues and using appropriate language, considering the person's culture, gender and general health.
- Relevant care during investigative procedures and surgery.
- Medication advice and management.
- Advice about safe sex and how to give and receive pleasure.
- Advice about monitoring quality sexual health.
- Providing a variety of relevant education material on sexual health in waiting areas.
- Knowing the availability of local services and referral mechanisms for people who wish to receive counselling or other therapies.

There are a growing number of sexual health clinics but not all offer expert, knowledgeable services. Investigation and management of the issues may be inadequate and costly. Useful resources in Australia include the impotence telephone helpline (1800 800 614, www.impotenceaustralia.com.au), and Relationships Australia (1300 364 277, www.relationships.com.au). In the UK, contact the Sexual Dysfunction Association (0870 774 3571, www.sda.uk.net).

Table 10.4 provides some example questions that can be used when taking a sexual history.

Table 10.4   **Some example questions to use when taking a sexual history.**

- Many people in your age group experience sexual difficulties. Do you have any issues you would like to discuss?
- Many people who take this medicine notice an alteration in their sexual function. Have you noticed any changes?
- It is normal to have some vaginal dryness after menopause. Have you experienced dryness?

References

Annon, J. (1975) *The Behavioural Treatment of Sexual Problems*. Enabling Systems, Honolulu.

Campbell, L., Redelman, M., Borkman, M., McLay, S. & Chisholm, D. (1989) Factors in sexual dysfunction in diabetic female volunteer subjects. *Medical Journal of Australia*, **151**(10), 550–2.

Clarke, M. & Clarke, D. (1985) *Sexual Joy in Marriage. An Illustrated Guide to Sexual Communication*. Adis Health Science, Sydney.

Department of Human Services Victoria (2003) www.dhs.vic.gov.au

Depuesne, C., Guigot, J., Chermat, V., Winchester, N. & Lacomblez, L. (1996) Sexual behavioural changes in Alzheimer's disease. *Alzheimer's Disease and Associated Disorders*, **10**, 2.

Dunning, P. (1993) Sexuality and women with diabetes. *Patient Education and Counselling*, **21**, 5–14.

Dunning, T. (2003) *Care of People with Diabetes. A Manual of Nursing Practice*. Blackwell Publishing, Oxford.

Gibson, C. (1992) *The Emotional and Sexual Lives of Older People. A Manual for Professionals.* Chapman and Hall, London.

Heath, H. (2002) *The Challenge of Sexuality in Health Care.* Blackwell Publishing, Oxford pp. 133–52.

Kaplan, H. (1979) *Making Sense of Sex.* Simon and Schuster, New York.

Leedom, L., Feldman, M., Procci, W. & Zeidler, A. (1991) Severity of sexual dysfunction and depression in diabetic women. *Journal of Diabetic Complications,* **5**(1), 38–41.

Littler, G. (1997) Social age cohort control: a theory. *Generations Review,* **7**, 11–12.

Masters, W. & Johnson, V. (1970) *Human Sexual Inadequacy.* Little, Brown, Boston.

Najman, J., Dunne, M., Boyle, F., Cook, M. & Purdie, D. (2003) Sexual dysfunction in the Australian population. *Australian Family Physician,* **32**(11), 951–4.

Nusbaum, M. (2004) Older women no less likely to have sexual health care needs. *Journal of the American Geriatrics Society,* **52**, 117–22.

O'Dowd, A. (2001) It's that devil I called love. *Nursing Times,* **97**(17), 13.

Riley, A. (1999) Sex in old age. Continuing pleasure or inevitable decline? *Geriatric Medicine,* **29**, 325–8.

Ross, M. & Channon-Little, L. (1991) *Discussing Sexuality. A Guide for Health Practitioners.* MacLennan and Pretty, Sydney.

Schriener-Engel, P., Schiavi, P., Vietorisz, D. & Smith, H. (1991) The differential impact of diabetes type on female sexuality. *Diabetes Spectrum,* **4**(1), 16–20.

World Health Organization (WHO) (1975) *Education and Treatment of Human Sexuality – the Training of Health Professionals.* WHO, Geneva.

Chapter 11

Using Complementary Therapies Wisely in Older People

Trisha Dunning

Key points

- Over 30% of older people use complementary therapies.
- Nurses need to be able to use complementary therapies safely if indicated and provide objective, accurate information about them.
- Complementary therapies can be used with conventional medical treatment to improve diabetes balance and quality of life.
- Herb–drug and herb–herb interactions and other adverse events can occur when conventional and complementary therapies are combined inappropriately.
- Complementary therapy use and the reasons for their use should be ascertained when taking a routine history and assessment.

11.1   Introduction

The term 'complementary therapies' refers to healing practices that are not usually part of conventional nursing and medical practice. Holistic nursing uses complementary therapies (CT) to enhance nursing care as part of the evolution of a new health paradigm. Complementary therapies include a range of practices, which are outlined in Table 11.1.

Although complementary therapies are primarily used therapeutically in aged care, some are incorporated into recreational activities (Quirk 2003) and to enhance the environment. Most complementary therapies require specific training and expertise to be used safely and effectively. Nurses are advised to ensure they are appropriately qualified to use these therapies or to refer to qualified practitioners if the therapy is outside their level of education and competence.

Practice point

The International Diabetes Federation used the yin yang symbol as its logo on World Diabetes Day in 2003.

Table 11.1 Complementary therapies commonly used in aged care facilities.
Many therapies are used in combination, for example aromatherapy and massage.
Complementary therapies are used therapeutically, in recreational activities and to
enhance the environment. Adapted with permission from Dunning (2003).

Acupuncture and acupressure	Kinesiology
Aromatherapy	Massage (many forms and traditions)
Art therapy	Meditation and guided imagery
Ayurveda (traditional Indian medicine system)	Music therapy
	Naturopathy
Chiropractic	Nutritional therapies
Counselling (a range of techniques)	Pet therapy
Dance therapy	Reflexology
Flower essences	Reiki
Herbal medicine (from several traditions – Indian, Chinese, European, North American, Australian Aboriginal)	Therapeutic touch
	Traditional Chinese medicine: a complex medicine system that uses several techniques, e.g. herbs, cupping, moxibustion and exercise.
Homeopathy	Spiritual therapies
Hydrotherapy	
Hypnosis	

Over 50% of the general population of most Western countries use complementary
therapies, particularly people with chronic diseases and especially women who
choose to be actively involved in their own care (Eisenberg *et al.* 1993; Lloyd *et al.*
1993; MacLennan *et al.* 1996). For example, 48% of older community-dwelling women
who reported disability in ADLs, had poor health, frequent visits to the doctor
and chronic diseases, including diabetes, used herbal therapies in the preceding
12 months (Gozum & Unsal 2004). Likewise a US study found that 30% of people
65 and over used a complementary therapy in the previous year compared to 26%
of people younger than 65. The most common therapies used were chiropractic,
herbs, relaxation techniques, high-dose megavitamins and spiritual healing (Foster
et al. 2000). Interestingly, people with a primary care provider used complementary
therapies more frequently than those without (34% versus 7%) but 57% did not tell
their doctor they were using complementary therapies.

In the community, people use complementary therapies to maintain their health
and manage the unpleasant symptoms of conditions such as arthritis, as well as
to cope with stress. A BBC Radio 5 survey in 2000 (Ernst & White 2000) found
that 20% of people surveyed used complementary therapies, especially aromatherapy,
massage, reflexology, herbs, acupuncture and homeopathy. The majority of respond-
ents were aged between 35 and 64 years.

The prevalence of use by people with diabetes is largely unknown but three studies (Leese *et al.* 1997; Ryan *et al.* 1999; Dunning 2003) found that between 17%
and 25% of people with diabetes in diabetic outpatient settings were using a range
of complementary therapies, particularly herbs, massage and vitamin and mineral
supplements such as zinc. The pattern of use is similar to that in the general population. However, up to 80% of people in developing countries use complementary therapists as their primary source of care. The World Health Organization

(WHO 2002) supports the use of complementary therapies provided there is evidence of their efficacy and safety.

Older people with diabetes usually do not abandon conventional treatments that have been rigorously tested for complementary therapies. They choose therapeutic options that are congruent with their life philosophy, knowledge, experience and culture. Therefore, conventional practitioners need to ask about complementary therapies and learn to discuss their use in an objective non-judgemental manner with patients to encourage them to disclose complementary therapy use and prevent adverse events. Older people with diabetes are particularly at risk of adverse events, inter-actions and renal and liver damage from complementary therapies, especially if they combine them with conventional medicines.

Many health professionals, especially nurses and GPs, incorporate complementary therapies into their practice to provide holistic care (Stone 1999). However, many health professionals who use complementary therapies do not have formal qualifications and often do not adequately or objectively document or monitor the goals of complementary therapy use or the effects. For example, Dunning (2003) found that 47% of 37 diabetes educators reported using complementary therapies in their practice and none had any complementary therapy qualifications.

The Cochrane Collaboration (2000) defined complementary therapies as:

'All health systems, modalities and practices and their accompanying theories and beliefs, other than those intrinsic to the politically dominant health system of a particular society or culture in a given historical period. They include all such practices and ideas self-defined by their users as preventing or treating illness or pro-moting health and wellbeing. The boundaries within and between complementary therapies are not always sharp or fixed.'

This definition highlights the changing nature of health care. Integration is happen-ing informally and there are increasing calls for formal integration strategies (WHO 2002). The slowly increasing amount of research into complementary therapies by conventional researchers is a step forward.

11.2   Complementary therapy philosophy

Despite the diversity of complementary therapies and the differences between them, they have a common underlying philosophy that is consistent with current diabetes empowerment strategies and the focus on developing effective professional–patient partnerships, good communication and preventive health care. This philosophy is based on a salutogenic (health) model rather than pathogenesis and encompasses the following key concepts.

- The individual is a unique person with their own beliefs, attitudes, life experi-ences and goals.
- Achieving balance is important. Balance usually refers to the physical, emotional, spiritual and social aspects of a person's life.
- The body has the capacity to heal itself. Complementary therapists seek to enhance that capacity and manage 'the whole person', not just the symptoms of 'disease'.

- A positive attitude is important to health and wellbeing and can be enhanced by appropriate actions and self-care.
- The patient–therapist relationship is integral to the healing process.
- Mind, body and environment cannot be separated – what affects one affects the others (mind–body medicine).
- Illness is an opportunity for positive change.

Most of this philosophy is consistent with the current focus on empowerment and patient-centred care and the emerging concept of 'the expert patient' evident in diabetes management. In the context of complementary therapies, 'healing' does not mean curing. It refers to a process of bringing the physical, mental, emotional, spiritual and relationship aspects of an individual's self together to achieve an integrated balanced whole where each part is of equal importance and value (Dossey *et al.* 1995).

Understanding complementary philosophy is important to understanding why people use complementary therapies. People seek answers to their health problems that are congruent with their existing beliefs. Their health choices are part of their overall attitude to life and their general and specific health beliefs and are not made in isolation from their beliefs and attitudes. People frequently mix and match complementary and conventional therapies to suit their needs at any given time.

Adverse events can arise when due consideration is not given to the potential effects of such combinations, which includes drug–herb interactions. Alternatively, complementary therapies, if used appropriately, can enhance the effects of conventional medicines, allow lower doses of conventional drugs to be used, reduce unwanted side effects and improve healing rates (Braun 2001), which is consistent with the quality use of medicines (see Chapter 9).

11.3 Goals of complementary therapy use for older people with diabetes

Complementary therapies have the potential to contribute to the holistic care of older people (Brett 2002). They are used in aged care to:

- Promote healing.
- Prevent physical, psychological and social problems by:
    (1) respecting personal choice
    (2) boosting immunity, e.g. aromatherapy massage
    (3) managing stress and depression
    (4) reducing the need for or dose of conventional drugs
    (5) reducing airborne infections.
- Enhance quality of life and wellbeing.
- Improve sleep.
- Enhance appetite and enjoyment of food.
- Improve wound care.
- Enhance relationships and reduce isolation, e.g. healing touch.
- Manage pain.
- Improve mobility.
- Enhance the environment.
- Manage specific problems.

It is necessary to determine individual needs, based on a thorough assessment. Once goals are established, the effectiveness of the therapy needs to be monitored and reviewed appropriately.

11.4   Integrating complementary and conventional care

Many health institutions are concerned about regulatory, manufacturing and supply issues relating to complementary therapies and products, as well as the benefits and risks for individuals. These factors influence the safe use of complementary therapies. The degree of statutory and professional regulation varies from country to country and from therapy to therapy. Frequently, there are no legislated regulatory processes in place; however, many complementary therapy professional associations have stringent self-regulation, education and ongoing professional development processes in place. Some also require current competence in first aid, for example the International Federation of Aromatherapists.

In many countries, complementary products are subject to regulation under existing medicines and/or manufacturing regulations, acts, standards and codes, for example the Therapeutic Goods Association (TGA) in Australia, Food and Drug Administration (FDA) in the USA and COSHH and CHIPS in the UK. There may be differences between the ingredients listed on the label and the actual contents of the product.

The safe, effective combination of complementary and complementary or complementary and conventional therapies involves considering the following issues.

- The safety of the individual, based on a thorough history and assessment, allowing for their personal choices unless contraindicated, for example an allergy to an essential oil or herb.
- Facilitating people to make informed choices based on an understanding of the risks and benefits involved in using any therapies, especially combining complementary and conventional therapies. When the person is not competent to give informed consent, guardianship issues may arise. Consent may be formal and in writing or implied by the person accepting the therapy.
- The knowledge and competence of health professionals to give advice about complementary therapies and the knowledge of how to refer to a suitable practitioner if necessary. Therapies need to be appropriate to the individual's physical, mental and spiritual status and only used after a thorough assessment considering potential interactions with conventional therapies or other complementary therapies. The suitability of the therapy should be reviewed regularly, because diabetes is a progressive disease and changes in health status can occur suddenly, especially in older people, which could make continued use dangerous, for example when renal function declines. In addition, conventional medicine doses should be monitored and may need to be reduced if hypoglycaemic complementary therapies are used. When complementary and conventional therapies are combined, they need to be considered together and as part of the overall management plan.
- Guidelines for using complementary therapies should be followed where they exist. Consent from the person receiving a complementary treatment is required in some

settings. Policies and guidelines need to include processes for communication between complementary and conventional practitioners, as well as defining collaboration and referral mechanisms to prevent fragmented care (Dunning *et al.* 2001). Where possible, guidelines should be evidence based to support best practice. They need not be prescriptive or inflexible.

- Processes for monitoring outcomes and accurately documenting the effects, both beneficial and harmful, of the therapy should be in place and structured in such a way as to enable objective data to be collected.
- Ensuring that safe, quality products are used is important. Dose variations, contamination and/or adulteration with potentially toxic substances, such as heavy metals, and unsubstantiated claims made about products can lead to serious adverse events, including irreversible kidney failure (Ko 1998). Evidence for using the particular therapy for the specific application should be available, where possible, and could be included with research papers in a portfolio on the ward.
- It is important that an accurate diagnosis is made, and thorough health history and assessment carried out, prior to using *any* therapy. These considerations are often overlooked, especially when the person with diabetes self-diagnoses and self-treats. Such practices can delay appropriate management and lead to a deterioration in general health and/or diabetic status.

11.5 Complementary therapy guidelines

Many general and aged care facilities have documented guidelines for using complementary therapies and nurses need to practise within these guidelines. In addition, a number of professional and regulatory bodies such as the Royal College of Nursing, Australia, and the Nursing and Midwifery Council in the UK have addressed complementary therapy use in nursing practice. Any new policies developed should be based on evidence where possible and be consistent with these regulatory bodies' policies. The prime aims of such policies are to safeguard the individual, assist nurses to identify competent practice and define their scope of practice.

11.6 Do complementary therapies benefit older people with diabetes?

In order to manage diabetes effectively, an individual must achieve balance. Frequently, a range of therapies, used holistically, is needed to achieve metabolic and quality-of-life balance. Complementary therapies can contribute to balance by assisting people to:

- Accept the diagnosis of diabetes and incorporate diabetes into their lives.
- Manage their diabetes by reducing stress, which helps reduce stress hormone levels and insulin resistance, making it easier to control blood glucose and achieve balance.
- Develop strategies to recognise issues that cause stress and implement methods to prevent or reduce stress in specific circumstances.
- Take an active part in decision making and increase their self-esteem, self-efficacy and sense of being in control, by improving their quality of life and allowing

personal growth. Personal growth is always possible, even in older people, even when they are terminally ill.

- Increase insulin production and/or reduce insulin resistance, either by the direct effects of therapies, such as some herbs, by reducing stress or by enhancing the effects of conventional medications.
- Manage the unpleasant symptoms of diabetic complications such as pain and nausea.
- Reduce the risk of long-term complications and prevent adverse events such as foot pathology, maintaining skin integrity and preventing problems such as cracks that increase the potential for infection and its consequences.
- Engage in education programmes and facilitate knowledge acquisition, retention and recall.

11.7   Some complementary therapies commonly used by people with diabetes

11.7.1   Ayurveda and traditional Chinese medicine

Ayurveda and traditional Chinese medicine (TCM) are complete medical systems that use a range of therapies including herbs, massage, surgery, exercise and diet.

11.7.2   Herbal medicines

There are several herbal traditions including American Indian, Chinese, Indian, European and Australian Aboriginal. There is a growing body of research into many complementary therapies, including herbs; the Cochrane database lists some 700 trials. Some herbs have been shown to reduce blood glucose, HbA_{1c} and lipids. These include:

- Many species of ginseng but American ginseng (*Panex quinquefolius*) is the most promising species (Vuksan *et al.* 2000).
- Gymnema/gurmar (*Gymnema sylvestre*) (Baskaran *et al.* 1990).
- Fenugreek (*Trigonella foenumgraecum*) (Sharma *et al.* 1996).
- Oolong tea in combination with oral hypoglycaemic agents (Hosoda *et al.* 2003).
- Cinnamon, which lowers glucose and lipids in Type 2 diabetes (Khan *et al.* 2003).
- Bitter melon (*Momordia charantia*), which is both a food and a medicine and has similar effects to chlorpropamide.

Herbal teas are commonly used and usually represent a very low dose of the herb.

Hypoglycaemic herbs have primarily been used in people with Type 2 diabetes but some, such as fenugreek, have also been shown to lower blood glucose in people with Type 1 diabetes (Anderson 1996). Hypoglycaemic herbs might be the prime diabetes treatment in some countries when conventional medicines are not available or are not affordable by sections of the community. They might be useful for people with IGT as part of a diet and exercise plan; however, the QUM principle of using non-drug options where possible must also be considered (see Chapter 9).

Most herb trials to test the hypoglycaemic properties of herbs have not included older people, so there may be unknown effects due to altered absorption, metabolism and excretion. In addition, the active ingredients in many herbs have not been identified so the herbal product can have unknown effects and interactions. However, people may not be using herbal therapies to control their blood glucose, they may be using them as sedatives, antidepressants and laxatives and to prevent prostate disease.

11.7.3　Minerals and supplements

Chromium

Chromium deficiency is associated with impaired glucose tolerance. However, most people with diabetes are not chromium deficient. Many people with diabetes use chromium to manage blood glucose levels and there is some evidence to support its hypoglycaemic effects and improvements in fasting and postprandial blood glucose, but more clinical trials are needed (Finney & Gonzalez-Campoy 1997). Chromium appears to work with insulin to facilitate glucose uptake. Postulated effects include increased insulin binding to receptors. The most common preparation used is chromium picolinate.

Magnesium

Magnesium is a cofactor in glucose oxidation and transcellular glucose transport. It is said to reduce insulin resistance. Hypomagnesaemia is common in people with diabetes but its clinical significance is unclear.

Supplements can act in the same way as many drugs and may interfere with drug absorption and cause adverse events in large doses; for example, Vitamin B toxicity can cause numb fingers (Carter 2002) that could be mistaken for diabetic neuropathy. Supplements have a preventive role, for example reducing the incidence and effects of infections by enhancing immunity (see Chapter 2).

Antioxidants

Antioxidant therapies have received significant press coverage in the last few years. It is speculated that diabetes and its complications are associated with increased levels of free radicals, which produce a range of effects. There is accumulating evidence that oxidation plays a role in the development of vascular disease. Antioxidants may delay the progression of retinopathy (O'Brien & Timmins 1999; Verdejo *et al.* 1999) and possibly other complications.

Antioxidants such as Vitamin E increase blood flow to eyes and kidneys, Vitamin C replenishes Vitamin E, and the B group vitamins are necessary for normal nerve function. However, consensus has not been reached about the benefits of using antioxidants, the dose needed and when in the course of diabetes or complication development they should be used. The potential interactions between antioxidant preparations and conventional medicine need to be considered. For example, some antioxidant vitamins, such as niacin, may blunt the lipid-lowering effects of simvastatin (Brown 2001).

11.7.4   Acupuncture

Acupuncture has been shown to reduce the pain in diabetic peripheral neuropathy (Abuaisha *et al.* 1998). Acupuncture and electrical stimulation into spastic limbs daily for 5–6 weeks, when the person's condition stabilises, improves nerve function and stimulates endogenous opioids and neurotransmitters, which reduce pain and improve disability but may not change motor recovery (Kron 2002). Specific acupuncture points are used depending on the limbs and neural pathways affected.

11.7.5   Hot baths

It has been reported that baths could help reduce blood glucose levels (Hooper 1999). The claims have not been substantiated and there are real risks such as postural hypotension, falls and burns to neuropathic feet if the water is too hot. Faster uptake of injected insulin or reduced stress levels could be methods whereby blood glucose was reduced in the cases reported. Hot baths are not recommended for older people with diabetes.

11.7.6   Aromatherapy

Aromatherapy is probably one of the most popular complementary therapies used in aged care settings. It consists of using essential oils applied using a variety of methods, especially applied to clothing or bedding, in massage and carrier oils, baths and a range of vaporisers.

Aromatherapy can be used to enhance wellbeing, aid relaxation and reduce stress, which benefits metabolic control, and for physical conditions such as alleviating pain, reducing hypertension, improving sleep and in skin and foot care. It can also alleviate stress during procedures such as CAT scans and after cardiac surgery (Buckle 1997) and in turn improves the individual's quality of life and psychological wellbeing.

However, people's odour associations are highly individual and certain essential oils may trigger adverse psychological reactions and behavioural problems. Taking a careful 'smell history' is important if essential oils are used. In addition, topical application can initiate allergic reactions or sensitivity, especially in susceptible people, for example those with fragile skin, skin allergies or asthma. Ambient odours can enhance the environment for patients and staff.

11.7.7   Pet therapy

Pets are very important to many people and often become constant companions to older people in the community. In some cases they replace human companionship. Some health facilities also incorporate visiting or house pets into their daily regimens, often on a formal basis. In such cases the wellbeing and health of the pets are as important as that of the residents and a health management programme for the pet, including regular vetinerary checks, is essential. Some residential facilities develop specific care plans for their pets.

Guide dogs are familiar sights assisting visually impaired people to lead independent lives. There were several media reports in late 2001 of dogs being able to recognise when their owners with diabetes were hypoglycaemic and alert them early enough to enable the person to manage the episode themselves or to alert another person.

11.8 Complementary therapies used for specific diabetes comorbidities

11.8.1 Cardiovascular system

Complementary therapists prescribe a range of diets focused on achieving optimal nutrition which are low in fat, high in fibre and organic foods. A herbal product, Vascupan, is currently in phase two clinical drug trials and appears to reduce cardiovascular risk by normalising cholesterol levels, reducing oxidative cell damage and the effects of homocystine. Homocystine is implicated in many diabetes complications. Vascupan contains globe artichoke, Vitamins B_6 and B_{12}, coenzyme Q10 (CQ 10) and folate. CQ 10 reduces blood pressure and improves exercise capacity (Rosenfeldt *et al.* 2003).

Biofeedback, acupuncture and exercise are associated with improved function and reduced oedema in people after stroke. A range of biofeedback, relaxation, meditation and counselling therapies can improve attitudes and 'fighting spirit' after vascular events but do not increase survival. They reduce stress by attenuating the effects of increased autonomic activity and catecholamine production and have also been shown to improve mood and reduce blood glucose levels (McGrady *et al.* 1991).

Ginkgo biloba is often used to improve memory, peripheral circulation and neurological sequelae after a stroke. Care needs to be taken if the person is also using anticoagulants and aspirin because of the risk of bleeding. Bilberry stabilises capillary membranes and can reduce the likelihood of further haemorrhage after stroke. Brahmi (*Bacopa monniera*) improves cognition, memory and concentration and aids in the recovery of function. Several phytochemicals reduce cholesterol, for example policosanol which is equivalent to the statins and has fewer side effects. It can be used alone or in combination with lipid-lowering agents (Sasser & Barringer 2004). It can be purchased over the counter, in which case appropriate monitoring may not take place.

11.8.2 Urinary tract infections

Plants in the berry family such as cranberry (*Vaccinium macrocarpon*) and blueberry contain two compounds, fructose and non-dialysable polymeric compound, that inhibit certain strains of *E. coli* by reducing their ability to adhere to mucosal surfaces (Avorn *et al.* 1994; Howell & Foxman 2002). Tablet forms are preferable to juice, which can predispose the person to Candida due to the high sugar content. Prophylactic doses are often given and the dose may be increased temporarily to 10 000 mg to combat acute urinary tract infections. A microculture and sensitivity should also be performed to ensure appropriate treatment is administered.

Other important preventive measures include:

- Frequent bladder emptying, including after sexual activity.
- Appropriate cleansing of the perineal region after toileting.
- Drinking water to help flush the bladder and urinary tract unless fluid intake is restricted.
- Wearing cotton underclothes.
- Managing pain if voiding is uncomfortable.
- Medication review to ascertain the need for antibiotics, steroids and oestrogen preparations.
- Managing hyperglycaemia, which might mean a change of medicines.

11.8.3 Wound care

Honey is becoming increasing popular in wound care, especially in aged care settings for burns, diabetic ulcers and pressure ulcers. Aristotle defined the power of honey according to its colour and constituents. Modern research has identified the healing properties of honey from particular plant species, *Leptospermum scoparium* and *Leptospermum polygalifolium*, which have antibacterial, anti-inflammatory, antioxidant and deodorising effects to improve healing. Honey produced from these plants is marketed as 'MediHoney'.

The active ingredients in honey from these plants consist of glucose, caffeine, benzoic acid, flavonoids, peroxide and inhibin. It stops the growth of a number of organisms including *E. coli*, *Salmonella typhimurium*, *Shigella sonnei*, *Listeria monocytogenes*, *Staph. aureus*, *Bacillus cereus* and *Strep. mutans*. Honey is warmed and evenly applied to clean wounds, extending beyond the wound margins. The dressing usually needs to be changed every 1–2 days but can be changed less frequently.

11.8.4 Pain management

A range of complementary therapies can help relieve pain. The psychological and hidden aspects of pain should be considered in older people who have difficulty communicating. Aromatherapy massage with or without the addition of analgesic essential oils relieves joint stiffness and improves mobility. A recently introduced complementary product, Body EZE patches, appears to relieve muscle and joint pain. The patches are placed over the painful area and act by increasing blood flow to the area. Acupuncture and exercise can also be beneficial depending on the cause and site of the pain.

Glucosamine sulphate is frequently used in arthritis. Glucosamine is a normal component of joint cartilage and synovial fluid. A dose of 1.5 g/day significantly reduces osteoarthritic knee pain and cartilage loss in people with normal body mass index. It does not appear to lead to hyperglycaemia. The Arthritis Foundation in Australia recommends it as one management strategy.

11.8.5 Mental health and depression

Many older people want to handle stress and depression without involving a doctor. Complementary and self-help treatments for anxiety with the best evidence for effectiveness in a systematic review were kava, exercise and relaxation therapies for generalised anxiety and bibliotherapy for specific phobias. There was limited evidence for acupuncture, music, meditation and autogenic training (Jorm *et al.* 2004). People use a range of other complementary therapies including:

- Meditation, prayer and counselling, using a range of techniques.
- Massage, with or without antidepressant essential oils such as bergamot, orange, geranium, sandalwood and frankincense.
- St John's wort, which is effective for mild to moderate depression. It has similar effects to antidepressants and concomitant use is contraindicated. However, it interacts with a range of conventional medicines, including anticoagulants, and should be used under the direction of qualified practitioners.
- SAMe, which is a natural amino acid, phenylalanine, that is a precursor of neurotransmitters. There is little evidence to support its efficacy.
- Folate to increase the efficacy of antidepressant medications.
- Acupuncture. Specific points stimulate serotonin production and reduce the risk of relapse.
- Fish oils and selenium to improve mood.
- Light exposure, especially in the winter and for people who suffer from seasonal affective disorder or SAD syndrome.

11.8.6 Intercurrent illness

Complementary therapies are also used to manage intercurrent illnesses such as colds and flu. These include echinacea, zinc, garlic and Vitamin C. Therapies are also used to boost the immune system to increase immunity to infections.

11.9 Adverse events associated with complementary therapies

A number of adverse events in people with diabetes using complementary therapy have been reported. They include:

- Stopping insulin in a person with Type 1 diabetes, which precipitated ketoacidosis (Gill *et al.* 1994).
- Trauma and burns to neuropathic feet and legs from cupping and moxibustion (Edwins *et al.* 1993).
- Allergies, drug–herb interactions and hospital admissions, largely from using adulterated traditional Chinese medicine (Beigel & Schoenfeld 1998; Ko 1998).
- Hypoglycaemia following prolonged massage, and using hypoglycaemic herbs (Goudie & Kaye 2001).
- Bleeding from herb–anticoagulant interaction, including during surgical procedures and investigative procedures.
- Kidney damage.

In addition, a range of herb–drug interactions have been reported and these are shown in Table 11.2. Five main potential mechanisms for herb–drug interactions have been suggested.

Table 11.2 Commonly used herbs and supplements, their potential interactions, reported adverse events and some suggested management strategies should an adverse event occur. Adapted with permission from Dunning 2003.

Botanical name, herb and uses	Potential interactions	Reported adverse events	Management strategies
Echinacea	• Hepatoxic drugs, e.g. anabolic steroids, amiodarone, methotrexate, ketoconazole • Immunosuppressants, e.g. corticosteroids, cyclosporin	Allergic reactions, especially in atopic people. Impairs the action of immunosuppressive drugs. Can cause immunosuppression if taken for long periods. In acute surgery impairs wound healing.	Do not use continuously for more than 8 weeks at a time.
Garlic	Aspirin Warfarin Cholesterol-lowering agents	Risk of bleeding, especially when taken with anticoagulants. Increased GIT activity. Decreased effectiveness of antacids. Inhibits platelet aggregation. Has additive effects.	Discontinue 7 days before surgery. Do not use concomitantly with antacids.
Ginkgo biloba	Aspirin Warfarin SSRI MAO inhibitors	Bleeding risk if used with anticoagulants.	Stop 36 hours before surgery. Do not use concurrently with these drugs.
Fenugreek	Anticoagulants. Oral hypoglycaemic agents (OHA)	Bleeding. Hypoglycaemia.	Do not use concurrently with these drugs. Monitor. Adjust dose of OHA or the herb.
Ginseng. Note: there are several species in common use	Corticosteroids Oral contraceptives Warfarin Digoxin Oral hypoglycaemic agents MAO inhibitors Tricyclic antidepressants	Increased risk of bleeding with anticoagulants. Suppresses immune system, which increases the risk of infections. Hypoglycaemia. Headache. Additive effects.	Stop 7 days before surgery. Do not use concomitantly with these drugs.
Ginger	Antacids Warfarin	Decreased effectiveness of antacids.	Do not use at the same time.

Substance	Drug/Interaction	Effect	Precautions
Guar and bulking agents	Antibiotics	Decreased food absorption, which increases the risk of hypoglycaemia.	Do not administer at the same time.
Glucosamine		GIT complaints. Allergy if allergic to sea foods. Nausea, vomiting, abdominal pain. Sleepiness. Hyperglycaemia.	Avoid with sea foods.
Zinc	Increased HbA$_{1c}$ in Type 1 diabetes		
Valerian and hops	Anaesthetic agents / Barbiturates / Hypnotics / Antidepressive drugs	Enhance/potentiate the effects of sedatives. If used long term the amount of anaesthetic needed is increased.	Withdrawal symptoms resemble valium addiction. Taper dose preoperatively.
St John's wort contains hyperfourin Affects metabolism by inducing liver cytochrome P450 3A4. Said to affect 50% of conventional drugs	MAO inhibitors / SSRI / Decreases effect of HIV medications / Warfarin / Anticonvulsants / Activates liver enzyme, hastening drug metabolism and reducing their effectiveness	Alters metabolism of some drugs, e.g. cyclosporin, warfarin, steroids. Interacts with psychotrophic drugs and can increase their effect. Skin allergies.	Stop 5 days before surgery. Do not use concomitantly with other drugs.
Slippery elm		Decreases GIT absorption. Hypoglycaemia.	
Vitamin C and E, B group; often used as antioxidants	Vitamin toxicity / Niacin	Decreases the beneficial effects of statins on HDL levels.	
Feverfew	NSAIDS and warfarin offset the herb's effect for migraine and might alter bleeding time	Changed bleeding time.	
Hawthorn	Antihypertensive agents	Additive effects – hypotension.	Monitor drugs and herbs.
Coenzyme Q10	OHA / Statins	Hypoglycaemia.	Lower dose of statin.

(1) Induction of liver enzymes, especially cytochrome P450, which leads to reduced drug availability.
(2) Induction of intestinal D-glycoprotein, which leads to reduced drug absorption and metabolism, which can be clinically significant.
(3) Stimulation of neurotransmitter production, especially serotonin, which enhances the effects of some drugs; that is, both the drug and the herb do the same thing.
(4) Reduction of the effects of serotonin-inhibiting drugs (Braun 2001).
(5) Herbs compete with drugs for serum protein binding sites, which increases the amount of free drug available. People with low serum albumin, such as the elderly and those with malnutrition, are especially at risk.

Herb–drug interactions are complex. Alone, neither the drug nor the herb might be a problem but when they are used together, the *combination* can be potentially dangerous. It should also be noted that between 20% and 30% of cases of liver failure and 30% of kidney damage are recognised side effects of readily available conventional medicines. In most of these drugs, the benefits are considered to outweigh the risks.

Practice point

When using complementary therapies in the elderly, kidney and liver and hydration status need to be considered and carefully monitored.

Elderly people most at risk of herb–drug interactions are those who:

● Take drugs with a narrow therapeutic window such as lithium, phenytoin, barbiturates, warfarin and digoxin.
● Are at risk of, or have, renal and/or liver disease and therefore, altered ability to metabolise and excrete herbs and drugs.
● Have atopic conditions such as allergies, asthma or dermatitis.
● Take several drugs (polypharmacy) and herbs at the same time.
● Take alcohol or drugs of addiction.
● Lack knowledge or do not consult knowledgeable practitioners about complementary therapy use.
● Self-diagnose, delay seeking medical advice, do not tell their conventional or complementary practitioners about the therapies/drugs they are using.
● Import products or use products when travelling that are not subject to standards, regulations or good manufacturing practices. The danger of contaminated and adulterated products from some countries is significant.

Practice point

Touch is an aspect of many complementary therapies and nursing procedures required in the care of older people. Touch can be comforting and reassuring. It can also be confronting, threatening and culturally inappropriate. Touch may be mistaken for a sexual invitation.

11.10   How can complementary therapies be used safely for older people?

Safety is a complex issue and consists of four main interrelated factors.

(1)   The therapy and how it is administered. Some methods are more likely to cause harm than others.
(2)   The practitioner's knowledge and competence, including their knowledge of the person seeking care and ability to conduct a thorough holistic assessment.
(3)   The person seeking care.
(4)   The environment in which the therapy is delivered.

Giving people appropriate advice so they can make informed decisions is an important aspect of nursing care. The following information could help nurses assist people with diabetes to use complementary therapies safely and choose therapies appropriate for the problem they want to treat. Patients need to know that there could be risks if they do not follow conventional evidence-based diabetes management practices. People should not be made to feel guilty or lacking in judgement if they choose to use a complementary therapy. People can be advised to:

● Develop a holistic health plan and decide what they hope to achieve by using a complementary therapy and then use a therapy best suited to achieve their goals; for example, to reduce stress, use massage, counselling or time line therapy.
● Find out as much about the therapy as possible before using it. Seek information from unbiased sources and be wary of information they find in chat rooms on the Internet and in advertising material. If in doubt, clarify with a suitably qualified reputable practitioner.
● Consult a reputable practitioner, such as a member of a relevant professional association, and buy products from reputable sources that follow good manufacturing and labelling processes and are prepared to guarantee their products and have relevant safety data available.
● Store and maintain products appropriately.
● Read labels carefully.
● Ensure the condition for which they want to use a complementary therapy is correctly diagnosed before commencing treatment, otherwise appropriate treatment could be delayed and the condition deteriorate.
● Recognise there are risks if conventional evidence-based diabetes management recommendations are not followed.
● Not stop or change recommended conventional treatments without the advice of a doctor.
● Inform all practitioners, conventional and complementary, about the therapies being used so the health plan can be co-ordinated.
● Be aware that some complementary therapies should not be used continuously for long periods.
● Take great care if they have kidney or liver damage or are taking a lot of other treatments because of the increased risk of adverse events.
● Seek advice about how to manage the therapy if surgery or investigative procedures are required or conventional treatment is changed or new treatments initiated.

- Seek advice quickly if any of the following occur:
  (1) hypoglycaemia
  (2) hyperglycaemia
  (3) mental or behavioural changes
  (4) abdominal pain
  (5) skin rashes
  (6) nausea, vomiting, diarrhoea.
- Monitor the effects of the complementary therapies on their diabetes status. Regularly check their blood glucose, lipids and HbA_{1c} as well as the way they respond to the therapy; for example, if they choose massage to manage pain, did it actually reduce the pain?

11.11   Nursing responsibilities

Nurses have a responsibility to respect people's choices and not to be judgemental. They are also responsible to their employer, other patients, visitors and staff. Nurses can use complementary therapies as part of holistic nursing care but they have a duty of care to practise at the level of their education and competence, obtain consent and use safe therapies. The following general advice applies. Specific information about individual complementary therapies should be sought before using or giving advice.

- Be sensitive to the philosophical and cultural views of older people with diabetes and be aware that they may perceive risks and benefits differently from health professionals.
- Follow guidelines for using complementary therapies where they exist, for example guidelines produced by the NMC in the UK. In Australia, the state nurse registering authorities, the Australian Nursing Federation and Royal College of Nursing, Australia, have all produced guidelines for nurses using complementary therapies (McCabe 2001).
- Ensure you are appropriately qualified and competent if you decide to use, recommend or offer advice about complementary therapies to a person with diabetes or their carers.
- Look for evidence of safety and efficiency but do not be too quick to accept or reject 'evidence'.
- Communicate the risks and benefits to people with diabetes and their families/carers. If the person chooses not to follow advice, you should document the information that you gave in the medical record.
- Develop a portfolio of evidence for any therapies in regular use as a reference on the ward.
- Use herbs and essential oils within the framework of the quality use of medicines and prescribe, administer, document and monitor within that philosophy (see Chapter 9). Nurses should ask about complementary therapy use as part of any holistic nursing assessment. People are not always willing to disclose such information and skilful questioning is required. Questions should be asked in a framework of acceptance. The patient has a responsibility to disclose.
- Value the nurse–client relationship as an essential aspect of the healing process.
- Consider the reaction of and effects on other staff of environmental therapies such as vaporising essential oils and playing music.

- Know how to contact the Poisons Advisory Service.
- Have mechanisms in place to check, clean and maintain any equipment needed, for example aromatherapy vaporisers and disposable acupuncture needles. Processes should be in place to deal with any complementary products the patient brings with them.
- Appropriate disposal of used and unused products; for example, spilled massage oil on wood or linoleum surfaces represents a falls risk for staff and older people.
- Document therapy use appropriately in the same way that conventional treatment is documented. Document the type, dose, dose interval and duration of the therapy, condition it is used for, advice given, expected outcome and actual outcome and report any adverse events as appropriate to the specific therapy.

References

Abuaisha, B., Boulton, A. & Costanz, J. (1998) Acupuncture for the treatment of chronic painful diabetic peripheral neuropathy: a long-term study. *Diabetes Research and Clinical Practice*, **39**(2), 115–21.

Anderson, R. (1996) Beneficial effect of chromium for people with Type 2 diabetes. *Diabetes*, **45**, 124–5.

Avorn, J., Monane, M., Gurwitz, J.H., Glynn, R.J., Choodnovskiy, I. & Lipsitz, L.A. (1994) Reduction of bacteriuria and pyuria after ingestion of cranberry juice. *Journal of the American Medical Association*, **271**(10), 751–4.

Baskaran, K., Kizar, A., Radha, K. & Shanmugasundaram, E. (1990) Antidiabetic effect of leaf extract from *Gymnema sylvestre* in non-insulin dependent diabetes mellitus patients. *Journal of Ethnopharmacology*, **30**(3), 295–3000.

Beigel, Y. & Schoenfeld, N. (1998) A leading question. *New England Journal of Medicine*, **339**, 827–30.

Braun, L. (2001) Herb drug interactions: a danger or advantage? *Diversity*, **2**(6), 31–4.

Brett, H. (2002) *Complementary Therapies in the Care of Older People*. Whurr Publishers, London.

Brown, B. (2001) Simvastatin and niacin, antioxidant vitamins or the combination for prevention of coronary disease. *New England Journal of Medicine*, **345**, 1583–92.

Buckle, J. (1997) *Clinical Aromatherapy in Nursing*. Arnold, London.

Carter, H. (2002) Numb fingertips could be a sign of vitamin B toxicity. *Medical Observer*, 17 May, 9.

Cochrane Collaboration (2000) *The Cochrane Library Complementary Medicine Field*. Cochrane Review, Oxford.

Dossey, B., Keegan, L., Guzzetta, C. & Kolkmeier, L. (1995) *Holistic Nursing: A Handbook for Practice*. Aspen Publications, Gaithersburg.

Dunning, T. (2003) Complementary therapies and diabetes. *Complementary Therapies in Nursing and Midwifery*, **9**(2), 74–8.

Dunning, T., Chan, S.P., Hew, F.L., Pendek, R., Mohd, M. & Ward, G. (2001) A cautionary tale on the use of complementary therapies. *Diabetes in Primary Care*, **3**(2), 58–63.

Edwins, D., Bakker, K., Youn, M. & Boulton, A. (1993) Alternative medicine: potential dangers for the diabetic foot. *Diabetic Medicine*, **10**, 980–2.

Eisenberg, D., Kessler, R. & Foster, C. (1993) Unconventional medicines in the United States. *New England Journal of Medicine*, **328**, 246–53.

Ernst, E. & White, A. (2000) Survey of complementary medicine use in the UK. *Complementary Therapies in Medicine*, **8**, 32–6.

Finney, L. & Gonzalez-Campoy, J. (1997) Dietary chromium and diabetes: is there a relationship? *Clinical Diabetes*, **Jan./Feb.**, 6–8.

Foster, D., Phillios, R., Hamel, M. & Eisenberg, D. (2000) Alternative medicine use in older Americans. *Journal of the American Geriatrics Society*, **48**, 1560–5.

Gill, G., Redmond, S., Garratt, F. & Paisley, R. (1994) Diabetes and alternative medicine: cause for concern. *Diabetic Medicine*, **11**, 210–13.

Goudie, A. & Kaye, C. (2001) Contaminated medicine precipitating hypoglycaemia. *Medical Journal of Australia*, **11**, 210–13.

Gozum, S. & Unsal, A. (2004) Use of herbal therapies by older community dwelling women. *Journal of Advanced Nursing*, **46**(2), 171–8.

Hooper, P. (1999) Hot tub therapy for Type 2 diabetes. *New England Journal of Medicine*, **341**, 924–5.

Hosoda, K., Wang, W., Chuang, C., Iha, M., Clevidence, B. & Yamamoto, S. (2003) Antihypertensive effect of Oolong tea in Type 2 diabetes. *Diabetes Care*, **26**(6), 1714–18.

Howell, A.B. & Foxman, B. (2002) Cranberry juice and adhesion of antibiotic-resistant uropathogens. *Journal of the American Medical Association*, **287**(23), 3082–3.

Jorm, A., Christensen, H., Griffiths, K., Parslow, R., Rodgers, B. & Blewitt, K. (2004) Effectiveness of complementary and self-help treatments for anxiety disorders. *Medical Journal of Australia*, **7**, s29–s41.

Khan, A., Safdar, M., Khan, M., Khattak, K. & Anderson, R. (2003) Cinnamon improves glucose and lipids of people with type 2 diabetes. *Diabetes Care*, **26**(12), 3215–18.

Ko, R. (1998) Adulterants in Asian patent medicines. *New England Journal of Medicine*, **339**, 847.

Kron, J. (2002) Modality in focus: acupuncture. *Journal of Complementary Medicine*, **1**(3), 32–7.

Leese, G., Gill, G. & Houghton, G. (1997) Prevalence of complementary medicine usage within a diabetic clinic. *Practical Diabetes International*, **14**(7), 207–8.

Lloyd, P., Lupton, D. & Wiesner, D. (1993) Choosing an alternative therapy: an Australian study of sociodemographic characteristics and motives of patients resident in Sydney. *Australasian Journal of Public Health*, **7**(2), 135–44.

MacLennan, A., Wilson, D.M. & Taylor, A. (1996) Prevalence and cost of diabetes in Australia. *Lancet*, **347**, 569–73.

McCabe, P. (ed.) (2001) *Complementary Therapies in Nursing and Midwifery*. Ausmed Publications, Melbourne.

McGrady, A., Bailey, B. & Good, M. (1991) Controlled study of biofeedback assisted relaxation in Type 1 diabetes. *Diabetes Care*, **14**(5), 360–5.

O'Brien, R. & Timmins, K. (1999) Trends. *Endocrinology and Metabolism*, **5**, 329–34.

Quirk, L. (2003) Complementary therapies. In: *Aged Care Nursing. A Guide to Practice* (eds S. Carmody & S. Forster). Ausmed Publications, Melbourne.

Rosenfeldt, F., Hilton, D., Pepe, S. & Krum, H. (2003) Systematic review of effect of Coenzyme Q10 in physical exercise hypertension and heart failure. *Biofactors*, **18**(1–4), 91–100.

Ryan, E., Pick, M. & Marceau, C. (1999) Use of alternative therapies in diabetes mellitus. Paper presented at the American Diabetes Association Conference, San Diego, USA.

Sasser, H. & Barringer, T. (2004) Policosanol: a natural alternative for lipid management? *Alternative Medicine Alert*, **7**(4), 37–41.

Sharma, R., Sarkar, A. & Hazra, D. (1996) Use of fenugreek seed powder in the management of non-insulin dependent diabetes mellitus. *Nutritional Research*, **16**, 1331–9.

Stone, J. (1999) Using complementary therapies within nursing: some ethical and legal considerations. *Complementary Therapies in Nursing and Midwifery*, **5**, 46–50.

Verdejo, C., Marco, P., Renau-Piqueras, J. & Pinazo-Duran, M. (1999) Lipid peroxidation in proliferative vitreorentinopathies. *Eye*, **13** (part 2), 183–8.

Vuksan, V., Stavro, M., Seivenpiper, J. *et al.* (2000) Similar postprandial glycaemic reductions with escalation of dose and administration time of American ginseng in Type 2 diabetes. *Diabetes Care*, **23**, 1221–6.

World Health Organization (WHO) (2002) *Traditional Medicine Strategy 2002–2005*. WHO, Geneva.

Chapter 12
Resources

Trisha Dunning and Michelle Robins

A number of resources are available to help nurses understand and care for older people with diabetes and assist family and carers to manage in the community. Diabetes is a rapidly changing specialty and new information, medications and products appear frequently. Local diabetes associations are important sources of up-to-date information.

12.1   Diabetic associations

Diabetic associations have been established in most countries, including the UK (Diabetes UK) and Australia (Diabetes Australia). Membership of these associations consists of lay people and health professionals who work together to develop management policies and educational material/programmes for the care of people with diabetes and to promote and support research into diabetes.

Diabetes Australia

Diabetes Australia (DA) is the national diabetes organisation in Australia. It has branches in all states. A magazine, *Diabetes Conquest*, is produced quarterly. Diabetes education material in several languages can be downloaded from the website. A National Diabetes Services Scheme (NDSS) is organised through Diabetes Australia and allows diabetic equipment (blood and urine test strips, syringes, meters) to be purchased at subsidised prices. People must enrol in the scheme and a doctor's signature is required on the enrolment form. There is no cost to enrol. Supplies can be ordered and received by mail under this scheme. Medications are not available through the NDSS scheme.

Diabetes Australia
GPO Box 3156
Canberra, ACT 2601
Australia
Tel: +02 6232 3800
www.da.com.au

Diabetes UK

Diabetes UK is the national diabetes organisation in the UK, with 400 branches and groups. It provides education, develops education material and trains volunteers. A magazine, *Balance*, is produced six times each year.

Diabetes UK
10 Parkway
London NWI 7AA
Tel: 020 7424 1000
Email: info@diabetes.org.uk

American Diabetes Association

This provides similar services in the USA. Enquiries can be directed to:

American Diabetes Association
1701 North Beauregard Street
Alexandria, VA 22311
USA
Tel: +1 800 342 2383
Email: membership@diabetes.org

Health professional diabetes associations

Health professional groups with a particular interest in diabetes also work to ensure uniformity of diabetic information, a high standard of care and the professional development of their members. Such associations include:

- American Association of Diabetes Educators: www.aadenet.org
- Australian Diabetes Educators' Association: www.adea.com.au
- Australian Diabetes Society: www.racp.edu.au/ads
- European Association for the Study of Diabetes: www.easd.org
- Federation of European Nurses in Diabetes: www.fend.org
- Juvenile Diabetes Research Foundation International: www.jdrf.org.uk

International Diabetes Federation

The IDF is an international federation of most of the national diabetes associations in the world. An International Diabetes Federation Congress is held every three years in a different part of the world.

The IDF has specific sections devoted to diabetes education, the IDF Consultative Section on Diabetes Education (DECS) and the IDF Consultative Section on Paediatric and Adolescent Diabetes. It regularly produces publications, guidelines and a journal for people with diabetes, *Diabetes Voice*.

International Diabetes Federation
1 rue Defacqz
B1000 Brussels, Belgium
Tel: +32 2 538 5511
Email: idf@idf.org

12.2   Other associations providing services relevant to older people with diabetes

Other associations often have diabetes interest groups within their membership. They include:

- National heart foundations
- Kidney foundations
- Dietetics associations
- Podiatry associations.

Alzheimer's Australia
Helpline: 1800 639 331
www.alzheimers.org.au/

12.3   Pharmaceutical companies

Many of the pharmaceutical companies produce diabetic products and supply patient and health professional information and products, although very little is specifically related to older people. The major companies producing diabetic products are:

- Synofi Aventis
- Bayer Diagnostics
- Becton Dickinson
- GlaxoSmithKline
- Hoechst Pharmaceuticals
- Novo Nordisk
- Roche
- Servier Laboratories
- Terumo Corporation
- Medisense Abbott
- Johnson & Johnson.

Addresses and telephone numbers can be found in the telephone directory or from the diabetic association in your country.

12.4   Government departments concerned with health and ageing

Guardianship and protective authorities
Complaints and advocacy services
Consumer organisations such as:
   Continence Foundations of Australia and UK
   Carers' organisations
   Dementia services
   Hearing and vision services.

12.5   Recommended reading

For people with diabetes

Court, J. (1998) *Modern Living with Diabetes for All Ages*. Diabetes Australia, Canberra.
Hammond, C. & Jilek, R. (2003) *Caring for the Aged*. ACP Publishing, Sydney.
Krall, L. & Beaser, R.J. (1999) *Joslin Diabetes Manual*. Lea and Febiger, Philadelphia.
Parker, J. & Parker, P. (2002) *The 2002 Official Patient's Source Book on Diabetes – Directory of Internet Use*. Icon Health Publishing, San Diego.
Phillips, P., Dunning, T., Brown, L. & Ayers, B. (eds) (1999) *Diabetes and You: The Essential Guide*. Diabetes Australia, Canberra.
Sonksen, P., Fox, C. & Judd, S. (1998) *Diabetes at your Fingertips: The Comprehensive Diabetes Reference Book for the 1990s*. Class Publishing, London.

Diabetes Conquest, *Diabetes Forecast* and *Balance* are magazines for people with diabetes produced by the diabetic associations of Australia, the USA and the UK, respectively. They are available to people who become members of the relevant association.

For health professionals

Health professionals should be familiar with material recommended for people with diabetes.

Applegate, W., Blass, J. & Williams, T. (1990) Instruments for the functional assessment of older patients. *New England Journal of Medicine*, **322**, 1376–8.
Brett, H. (2002) *Complementary Therapies in the Care of Older People*. Whurr Publishers, London.
Dunning, T. (2003) *Care of People with Diabetes: A Manual of Nursing Practice*. Blackwell Publishing, Oxford.
Nazarko, L. (2002) *Nursing in Care Homes*, 2nd edn. Blackwell Publishing, Oxford.
Sinclair, A. & Finucane, P. (1995) *Diabetes in Old Age*. John Wiley, Chichester.

Index